POWER TO THE PATIENT

Live Now, Age Later

Dr. Rosenfeld's Guide to Alternative Medicine

Doctor, What Should I Eat?

The Best Treatment

Symptoms

Modern Prevention

Second Opinion

The Complete Medical Exam

The Electrocardiogram and
Chest X-ray in Diseases
of the Heart

ISADORE ROSENFELD, M.D.

POWER TO THE PATIENT

THE TREATMENTS TO INSIST ON WHEN YOU'RE SICK

WARNER BOOKS

An AOL Time Warner Company

Warner Books, Inc., 1271 Avenue of the Americas, New York, NY 10020
Visit our Web site at www.twbookmark.com.

 An AOL Time Warner Company

Printed in the United States of America
First Printing: February 2002
10 9 8 7 6 5 4 3

Library of Congress Cataloging-in-Publication Data

Rosenfeld, Isadore.
        Power to the patient : the treatments to insist on when you're sick / Isadore Rosenfeld.
            p. cm.
        Includes index.
        ISBN 0-446-52694-0
            1. Medicine, Popular. I. Title.

RC81 .R829 2002
616—dc21   2001046645

Book design by Giorgetta B. McRee

For Camilla

My guiding light and the love of my life

Acknowledgments

Joni Evans has stayed the course with me through all nine of my books. She started as my editor for *The Complete Medical Exam* more than twenty years ago and then became my agent. Despite the change in title, she has continued to be a de facto editor for every single book I've written. As soon as I finish a chapter, it goes to Joni first for her input. Thanks, Joni, for helping me with this and the other eight books.

My thanks too for their help, patience, and understanding to Diana Baroni, her editorial staff, and the entire team at Time Warner headed by my friend Larry Kirshbaum. It's not easy for any editor or publisher to cope with a medical book that must stay up to date. There's no such thing as a finished manuscript, what with all the advances happening virtually every day. *Power to the Patient* is no exception. I have frantically presented to Diana a new version literally to the final galley in an attempt to keep the information up to date—and she has always accepted the revisions with grace and only minimal irritation.

Finally, I wanted to make sure that the information I presented to my readers was entirely accurate. To do so, I asked the following specialists with whom I work and whose opinions I value to review the manuscript for any errors or omissions. Whenever they dared disagree with me, I must confess that I deferred to them! I thank them again for their help and friendship. Here is the roster of medical stars upon whom I called:

Phyllis August, M.D.
   Chief, Division of Hypertension and Professor of Medicine, Cornell University–Weill Medical College, NY; Attending Physician, New York-Presbyterian Hospital, NY
Myron I. Buchman, M.D.
   Attending Obstetrician and Gynecologist, Clinical Associate Professor of Obstetrics and Gynecology, Cornell University–Weill Medical College, NY
Harry L. Bush, Jr., M.D.
   Associate Professor of Surgery, Cornell University–Weill Medical College, NY; Clinical Director, Vascular Diagnostic Center, New York-Presbyterian Hospital, NY
Thomas Caputo, M.D.
   Director of Gynecologic Oncology, Professor and Vice Chairman, Department of Obstetrics and Gynecology, Cornell University–Weill Medical College, NY
Richard B. Devereux, M.D.
   Professor of Medicine, Director of Echocardiography Laboratory, Division of Cardiology, Cornell University–Weill Medical College, NY
Philip Felig, M.D.
   Attending Physician, Senior Staff, Lenox Hill Hospital, NY
Christine L. Frissora, M.D.
   Assistant Professor of Medicine, Division of Gastroenterology and Hepatology, Cornell University–Weill Medical College, NY

Antonio M. Gotto, Jr., M.D.
    The Stephen and Suzanne Weiss Dean and Provost, and Professor of Medicine, The Joan and Sanford I. Weill Medical College and Graduate School of Medical Sciences, NY
Richard Granstein, M.D.
    George W. Hambrick, Jr. Professor, Chairman Department of Dermatology, Dermatologist in Chief, Cornell University–Weill Medical College, NY
Ira M. Jacobson, M.D.
    Chief of the Division of Gastroenterology and Hepatology, Vincent Astor Distinguished Professor of Clinical Medicine, Attending Physician, and Medical Director, Center for the Study of Hepatitis C, Cornell University–Weill Medical College, NY
Warren D. Johnson, M.D.
    Professor of Clinical Public Health, B.H. Kean Professor of Tropical Medicine, Attending Physician, Cornell University–Weill Medical College, NY
Lawrence J. Kagen, M.D.
    Professor of Medicine, Cornell University–Weill Medical College, NY; Attending Physician, Hospital for Special Surgery and New York-Presbyterian Hospital, NY
Marilyn G. Karmason, M.D.
    Associate Clinical Professor of Psychiatry, Cornell University–Weill Medical College, NY
Barney J. Kenet, M.D.
    Assistant Attending Physician, Cornell University–Weill Medical College, NY
Bruce B. Lerman, M.D.
    Professor of Medicine, Chief of Cardiology, Attending Physician, Hilda Altschul Master Professor of Medicine, Cornell University–Weill Medical College, NY
Daniel Libby, MD, FCCP
    Clinical Professor of Medicine, Pulmonary and Critical Care Medicine, Cornell University–Weill Medical College: Attending Physician, New York Presbyterian Hospital
Michael D. Lockshin, M.D.
    Professor of Medicine, Joan and Sanford Weill School of Medicine of Cornell University, NY; Director, the Barbara Volcker Center for Women & Rheumatic Disease at Hospital for Special Surgery, and Director, Mary Kirkland Center for Lupus Research at Hospital for Special Surgery, NY
Steven K. Magid, M.D.
    Associate Professor of Clinical Medicine, Associate Attending Physician, Cornell University–Weill Medical College, NY; Associate Attending Rheumatologist, Hospital for Special Surgery, NY
James P. McCarron, Jr., M.D.
    Diplomat American Board of Urology, and Surgeon, Cornell University–Weill Medical College, NY
Kevin P. Morrissey, M.D.
    Associate Attending Surgeon, Clinical Associate Professor of Surgery, Cornell University–Weill Medical College, NY
Martin Nydick, M.D.
    Associate Attending Physician, Clinical Associate Professor of Medicine, Cornell University–Weill Medical College, NY
Frank A. Petito, M.D.
    Attending Neurologist, Professor of Clinical Neurology, Cornell University–Weill Medical College, NY
Samuel Rapoport, M.D.
    Assistant Clinical Professor of Neurology, Cornell University–Weill Medical College, NY

Contents

Introduction

Times have changed—and so has medical-care delivery in this country. Remember the days when you phoned your doctor because you were sick and his nurse told you to come right over? If you weren't up to leaving home, chances were the doctor would come to see you. That was referred to as "making a house call," a relic of the past that's probably unfamiliar to anyone under the age of forty. Remember, too, when it was your doctor who decided what tests and treatments you should have—and he didn't need anyone's approval to order them? Remember when medication was affordable? Remember when you and your doctor—and no one else—decided whether or not you required hospitalization and for how long? Remember when your doctor had the time actually to sit, talk with you, and listen to your complaints?

All that is history for most of us. Many physicians are no longer free agents; the companies or health carriers for whom they work have the last word on the critical decisions that affect you. You can no longer be sure that you're getting the definitive test to diagnose what ails you—or the best treatment for it. That's because insurance companies, despite their pious pronouncements, are in business to make money—for themselves, their CEOs, and their stockholders. The only way they can earn a profit is to pocket the premiums you pay them. If there is a cheaper way to treat you, your carrier will probably choose it, even if it's not quite the most effective treatment.

The other harsh reality is that doctors today are spending less time with you and are busy filling out endless numbers of insurance forms instead. Important questions about family history and lifestyle that should be asked and answered face-to-face are filled out on printed questionnaires. The friendly nurse has been replaced by the efficient gatekeeper whose main function is to keep the number of your office visits to a minimum. It is she who triages calls and decides whom the doctor will see, how soon, and for how long. You can no longer count on getting an immediate appointment when you're sick unless you're virtually at death's door. Instead of sharing with you his unlisted home phone number as he once did, the doctor uses an answering machine that replies with, "Office hours are nine to five. If this call is urgent, go to the nearest emergency room. If not, try again in the morning." For millions, the hospital emergency room has replaced the family doctor's office.

All this means that today, more than ever, you're essentially on your own when it comes to your health. Yes, you can still get treatment for a really obvious emergency, like when you're hemorrhaging, but most symptoms and health concerns are not as dramatic as that. We often want and need to know what to do about such mundane symptoms as a nagging ache; a low-grade fever; heart palpitations; transient diarrhea or constipation; more fatigue than usual. Ordinarily, these complaints do not warrant a visit to the emergency room, but they can be worrisome and potentially serious. You should know what they mean and what to do about them and whether it's important that your doctor sees you quickly. You should understand what caused your illness and how you can prevent it from happening again; you should be aware of the most reliable way to confirm its diagnosis and the most effective way to treat it. That kind of information from a reliable source is not easy to come by, which is why I wrote this book and called it *Power to the Patient*. For knowledge is power, and when it concerns your health, it can save your life.

The current state of our health-care system is such that frustrated patients often wonder, How do I know if my doctor and my insurer are treating me correctly? Are they providing me with the best therapy regardless of how much it costs them? How can I be sure that I'm getting the right tests and whether I need a second opinion, or should be admitted to the hospital? You'll find the answers to these questions—and more—in this book.

Even if your carrier is a nonprofit organization and your doctor an independent practitioner, free to recommend what he or she believes is best for you regardless of cost, it's still important for you to understand all your options. You should be able to discuss them intelligently and be confident that what you are being offered is optimal. This book will arm you with those facts. It describes in detail virtually every aspect of some forty major illnesses one or more of which you may well develop sometime during your life—everything from acne to cancer, and including such diverse disorders as Parkinson's disease, infertility, gallstones, and diabetes. You will learn how to recognize and interpret their telltale symptoms; how they're most accurately diagnosed; the latest and best ways to treat them; under what circumstances to insist on a second opinion or consultation; and when to demand hospitalization. That kind of knowledge means "power" to you, the patient—the power to share in the decisions that affect your life.

Your rights are protected by law. If you are not being given or offered the best care, there are impartial appeal mechanisms that you can invoke, independent panels of experts that can assess your case and decide whether you're getting what you need and deserve. And all you need to do is request that your doctor initiate the appeal process. (Don't confuse these independent panels with the politically charged "right to sue" issue. Suing is not relevant to your immediate problem; it takes years. You need a quick decision when you're sick, and the panels to whom you "insist" can act in time to make a difference.)

Keep this book handy. Browsing through it even when you're well will help you stay healthy. And when you're sick, refer to the appropriate chapter to see how best to handle whatever ails you. Throughout these pages, whenever you see the word "insist" you will know that, in my opinion, you're on solid ground and entitled to what you're asking for. That's the meaning of "power to the patient."

POWER TO THE PATIENT

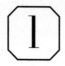

ACNE

When Zits Are the Pits

There are at least ten different forms of acne, two of which are extremely important: acne vulgaris (meaning "common," not "vulgar") and acne rosacea (adult acne). The former is the subject of this chapter.

Acne vulgaris is a skin disorder that plagues most teenagers and young adults. It starts in puberty and can persist into young adult life. Some 80 percent of us develop the pimples and bumps of acne vulgaris some time or another while we're growing up. In most cases, the pimples (often referred to as zits) and their variants—blackheads, whiteheads, pustules, and cysts—as a rule clear up by the mid- to late twenties, but they can last longer. They are not usually severe, but can have a serious impact on physical or emotional health when they recur and persist in large numbers on the face, the shoulders, the neck, and the upper back.

Acne vulgaris runs in families; if any of your close family members have it, chances are you do, or will, too. More young men are affected than women, but the ratio changes when acne continues into adult life.

Despite great progress in its treatment, the most important advance in dealing with acne has been the debunking of the many myths that have for so long surrounded it. The following beliefs were inviolable until fairly recently and are unfortunately still held by many:

- Myth: Acne is due to poor personal hygiene—dirt and skin oil that haven't been washed away often enough.
- Fact: There is no evidence that acne is caused by dirt or an excess of skin surface oils. In fact, you can worsen matters by scrubbing the skin too vigorously. Gentle washing with normal soap is all you need; don't waste your money on expensive "cleansers." Also, keep your fingers away from your pimples. Squeeze your sweetheart, not your zits. Use oil-free "non-comedogenic" cosmetics.
- Myth: The wrong diet causes acne—too many french fries, too much chocolate, pizza, and junk food.
- Fact: No connection has ever been established between diet and acne. Vitamins don't help either. Strangely enough, many patients insist that their skin breaks out after they eat a particular food, usually chocolate. In such cases my advice is to avoid that food even though there is no scientific study linking diet to acne. But whenever a patient does make such an association, I sneakily take the opportunity to promote a balanced diet with lots of grains, fruits, vegetables, and fish. It won't necessarily help the acne, but it will reduce the risk of heart disease and cancer!
- Myth: Acne is the result of unhealthful sexual habits, including masturbation and "tainted" sex partners.
- Fact: "Loose" living, as it used to be called, can give you AIDS and sexually transmitted disease, but not acne. Nor will masturbation!
- Myth: Stress causes acne.
- Fact: Actually, the opposite is true. Acne causes stress; stress per se does not result in acne, although lack of sleep and chronic tension do increase androgen pro-

duction in some people and may lead to a breakout. More important, picking, squeezing, and rubbing your pimples when you're nervous aggravates them. So if you're under stress, keep your hands in your pockets.

- Myth: Acne should be left untreated and allowed to run its course because it's a normal cosmetic problem.
- Fact: This is a good tack for insurers to avoid paying for doctors' visits. The physical and emotional fallout from acne can be devastating. Prompt and continuing treatment can prevent outbreaks and reduce the likelihood of developing permanent scars.
- Myth: Acne vulgaris always clears up after adolescence.
- Fact: One adult in nine, aged twenty-five to forty-five, continues to have acne.

How Acne Develops

Why does acne begin at puberty? Why does it affect younger men more commonly than women? Why does it usually clear up as we get older? The answers lie in our hormones. In adult life each gender has some of the other's hormone. (Thankfully, men have lots of androgens—testosterone—and only nominal amounts of estrogen, and vice versa for females. That's why I shave and my wife doesn't.) But when the body first produces its sex hormones at puberty it makes large amounts of both in boys and girls, in order to ensure adequate bone growth and sexual maturation. The high concentration of male hormones in both causes acne in both genders. Here's why:

Hair follicles in the skin are surrounded by sebaceous glands that make oil that is delivered to the skin surface. The extra amounts of male hormone at puberty increase the production of this oil, and the glut eventually clogs the ducts and their openings on the skin surface. This results in pimples, either blackheads or whiteheads (doctors call them comedones). Since boys produce more male hormones than do girls, they have more pimples—and more acne.

If you're lucky, the process stops right there, leaving you with only a few pimples. No big deal. Complications set in when "normal" bacteria on the skin surface penetrate and inflame the obstructed, bulging ducts. In order to deal with these bacteria, the immune system mobilizes its warrior white blood cells and sends them in droves to prevent the ducts from becoming infected. An excess of these white blood cells and other debris forms pus, which when added to the sebaceous ducts already choked with oil, make the pimples bigger and bigger. When the engorged ducts can enlarge no more, they burst under the skin, forming bumps of various kinds and sizes. These bumps may be papules (slightly raised and red), pustules (filled with pus), or cysts (larger, inflamed, and painful). When a cyst opens onto the skin, it scars and disfigures it. That's why so many untreated acne patients have unsightly defects.

Acne can have a serious emotional and social impact on adolescents when it mars and scars the skin: withdrawal, depression, loneliness, frustration, and in some cases suicide have all been reported among such youngsters.

Too many doctors and patients view acne as a normal and inevitable phenomenon—a rite of passage, so to speak. Youngsters are told they must live with it, despite its social consequences. *The worst thing parents can do is to make light of their youngster's acne. Insist on the proper medical care to treat it.* If the lesions are extensive, see a dermatologist, for, as you will see below, there are measures that can control acne, modify its course, and even cure it! These consist basically of proper skin care, antibiotics to control the bacteria that infect the ducts, hormones in some cases to prevent overproduction of sebum (the fatty substance made by the glands), and dermatological procedures to deal with whatever scarring has occurred. The sooner such therapy is begun, the less emotional trauma there will be in the short run, and the fewer permanent disfiguring scars.

Treating Acne

Don't rush to the doctor just because you've found a pimple or two. Try some home remedies first. Sun helps, but too much is bad for the skin over the long term. Avoid putting anything greasy on your skin, especially cosmetics, cleansers, and moisturizers. Use water-based makeup and oil-free moisturizers; keep away from heat and humidity whenever possible; use non-oily sunscreens; and never pick or squeeze the pimples.

The first treatment step, one you can start yourself, is benzoyl peroxide (for example, Clearasil). You can get it at the pharmacy without a prescription. It comes in gel, cream, or lotion. I suggest starting with the weakest strength of the lotion, especially if you have sensitive skin. You can then switch to the 2.5 percent gel and increase the strength all the way to 10 percent if necessary. Benzoyl peroxide dries the pimples and prevents infection by reducing the number of bacteria on the skin; it often unplugs the black or white comedones. It's a peeling agent as well. Don't wear expensive clothes when you're using it because it can bleach them. Sometimes benzoyl peroxide is all you need for your acne, but it can also be combined with several of the other therapies described below.

There are other popular over-the-counter preparations you can safely try if the benzoyl doesn't help. I have found the most effective to be products containing salicylic acid (2 percent), glycolic acid, resorcinol, and sulfur (whose anti-inflammatory properties keep the pimples from swelling). They come in a variety of brands, whose names you can check at your cosmetic counter. I have also found benzoyl peroxide combined with erythromycin (marketed as Benza-mycin) to be especially effective.

If none of these treatments work, consult your skin doctor, who might recommend topical lotions of antibiotics such as clindamycin, erythromycin, or products that contain sulfa-cetamide for mild acne. Apply them once or twice a day to the affected skin.

If these antibiotics are not successful, the next step is tretinoin (Retin-A). This preparation, which requires a pre-scription, is especially good against blackheads and white-heads because it unclogs the ducts and allows the oil to flow freely to the skin surface. It also lightens dark spots caused by old acne lesions. I prefer the gel or cream; the liquid can be irritating. Start with a tiny amount of the weakest strength (that's 0.01 percent for the gel and 0.025 percent for the cream) every couple of days and work your way up gradually as needed. Too much causes peeling, dryness, and irritation. Keep away from strong sunlight when using it and wear sun-screen in sunny weather. Tretinoin will irritate your skin at first, but you will see some improvement in two to three weeks, although maximum effect may take three or four months. Differin and Tazorac are related products.

Azelaic acid cream is a new, effective, and well-tolerated topical preparation recently approved for the long-term treat-ment of mild to moderately severe acne. Apply it to the af-fected area once or twice a day. It works very much like Retin-A and also prevents thickening, pigmentation, and dis-coloration of the top skin. Try it if the topical antibiotics don't work.

When the acne does not respond as well as you'd like to any of these topical applications, you may need to take oral antibiotics in low doses on an ongoing basis, sometimes for as long as a year or more. Your doctor will recommend any of the following, all of which slow the growth of the offend-ing bacteria: tetracycline (taken with a full glass of water on an empty stomach), erythromycin (harder on the stomach; although it's safe, it makes the skin more sensitive to sun, so cover up in bright sunlight or use sunscreen), minocycline (my preference), and doxycycline (also very popular). Unlike tetracycline, the latter three can be taken with food. However, take them hours apart from iron or antacids, both of which can interfere with their absorption. Pregnant women should not take tetracycline because it can discolor the teeth of their newborns.

For maximum effect, the various topical therapies can be taken together with oral antibiotics.

There is something new and effective for adult women with acne. It's called Diane-35, a low-dose oral contraceptive that combines estrogen and cyproterone; the latter neutralizes the androgens that are responsible for the increased production of sebum. This preparation takes six to twelve months to work, and the acne is apt to return when the drug is discontinued.

When all else fails and acne is severe, you may need isotretinoin (Accutane) orally, *but never if you're pregnant or of childbearing age unless you use appropriate contraception—without fail!—because it can cause birth defects.* Accutane works by preventing the sebaceous glands from producing oil and can permanently shrink them. Even the most severe and resistant cases usually respond within weeks to Accutane. As many as 40 percent of patients can be cured by 1–2 mg per kilo of body weight taken for five to six months. Always take this drug under the close supervision of a dermatologist. And while you're doing so, check your cholesterol and triglyceride levels; they can be increased by Accutane. Be careful with your diet during the treatment period. Never take vitamin A supplements with Accutane. Also, because it makes the skin fragile, never use it to remove hair and don't get a facial peel.

If you have been scarred by acne, several cosmetic and/or dermatological treatments are available. These include dermabrasion, in which the superficial layers of the skin are planed down, the new Cooltouch laser, and chemical facial peeling. Pitting scars, however, do not usually respond to these measures. *If you require such treatment, insist on a second opinion from a dermatologist as to which approach is best for you.*

WHAT TO INSIST ON IF YOU HAVE ACNE

Although acne is extremely common, it can be dramatically alleviated and often cured. *Insist on a consultation with a dermatologist* to avoid the devastating emotional impact that extensive acne can have on vulnerable adolescents. Rupture of untreated cysts can cause permanent scarring that can be improved by a variety of dermatological and cosmetic procedures. *Insist on guidance from a specialist.*

A variety of topical solutions—ranging from over-the-counter preparations to prescription tretinoins and antibiotics that unplug the blocked ducts and reduce the bacteria on the skin surface—are effective. *When topical measures fail, insist on low-dose antibiotics,* either alone or in conjunction with these other measures, to reduce the severity of acne. In some women, hormonal therapy can control the disorder. *If other treatments aren't working, insist on Accutane.* It can dramatically improve acne and cure it in almost half the cases by preventing the production of the oils that obstruct the ducts. However, do not use Accutane if you are of childbearing age unless you scrupulously practice birth control because it can cause severe fetal abnormalities.

2

AIDS

Serious Monkey Business

AIDS, the modern-day plague, currently affects some 4 million Americans and strikes about 40,000 more every year in this country alone. Although everyone is vulnerable to AIDS, regardless of age or gender, most patients in the United States are men between the ages of twenty-five and forty-four. Fully one-quarter of the population in parts of Africa are infected, and since most of them do not have access to therapy, millions are expected to die in the next few years.

The virus that causes AIDS attacks the human immune system, leaving it unable to protect the body against infection and cancer, which is why it is called HIV (human immunodeficiency virus). Stripped of their natural defense mechanisms, AIDS patients eventually die from either overwhelming infection or malignancies.

History of AIDS

In 1981 several investigators at the Centers for Disease Control (CDC, the clearinghouse for information dealing with all diseases, including infections, in the United States), noted that an inordinate number of people in Los Angeles were suddenly developing *Pneumocystis carinii Pneumonia* (PCP), a lung infection that occurs when the immune system is impaired. Pursuing this lead, the CDC discovered that the majority of patients with PCP were gay men. At about the same time, other reports began to surface that a type of skin cancer called Kaposi's sarcoma, which also strikes persons whose immune systems are compromised, was occurring in unusually large numbers of male homosexuals—this time in New York. Scientists began to wonder what was destroying the resistance of these men on both coasts. Some speculated that it might be the amyl nitrite they frequently were known to inhale in order to obtain a "high." Cases of PCP then began to appear across the country in other groups of people: drug addicts, women and their babies, persons who'd received blood transfusions, especially hemophiliacs who required them frequently, and, curiously, Haitian refugees in Miami.

When you feel lousy and your doctor can't pinpoint the cause, chances are he blames it on a virus. The scientific community, true to form, has decided that AIDS has the characteristics of a virally transmitted disease. It's been around for so long now that you may have forgotten that the letters stand for "acquired immunodeficiency syndrome."

This discovery opened a Pandora's box. Where did the virus come from? How did it evolve? Continuing research has revealed that there are two human AIDS viruses (HIV-1 and HIV-2), and both are probably descended from a previously identified monkey virus. Whatever its origin, HIV has probably been around for much longer than we thought, perhaps even a hundred years or more. Once humans began to harbor HIV, the virus spread like wildfire via infected blood—through transfusions, needles shared by drug users, and certain sexual practices, all accelerated by the fact that we do live in one world, thanks to international travel.

How AIDS Is Transmitted

The virus is present in blood but not in urine, feces, vomit, or sweat. It has been found in infectious amounts in semen, vaginal and cervical secretions, and breast milk. It doesn't survive long in the open air, so inhaling it can't infect you. Neither will shaking hands, sitting on a toilet seat, sneezing, coughing, or sharing a swimming pool or eating utensils.

The most common ways the AIDS virus is transmitted in this country are as follows:

- Mainly by contact with contaminated blood. The majority of infections occur among intravenous drug abusers who share contaminated needles. Transfusions in hospitals are no longer an important cause, since we are now able to screen donor blood for the virus. Although it is impervious to freezing, a temperature of sixty degrees centigrade or higher kills HIV. Make sure that your barber uses disposable blades when shaving you so as not to receive infected blood from his last customer.

- Sexual contact, especially during anal intercourse continues to be an important route of infection. (Spread is less common during vaginal sex.) Don't worry about smooching; deep or open-mouth kissing rarely spreads the disease. In fact, there is a protein called lysozyme in the tears, saliva, and urine, which, along with other natural proteins, breaks down the genetic material of the HIV and prevents it from replicating. Oral sex is not an important route of HIV transmission, although a woman giving oral sex to a man can be infected by his semen, if she has any open cuts or sores in her mouth. Still, this risk is less than that of unprotected vaginal or anal sex. Infection from a female's sexual fluids is possible but uncommon, except when menstrual blood is present.

- Children born to HIV-positive mothers can be infected before and during delivery, and also from breast milk.
- Health workers can be infected by contact with amniotic fluid, spinal fluid, and the fluid around bone joints, and must be careful not to stick themselves with contaminated needles.

How to Prevent HIV Infection

Here's how to avoid contracting or spreading AIDS:

- Always use condoms during vaginal, oral, or anal intercourse unless you're in a marriage or a long-term relationship in which neither you nor your partner has strayed.
- Avoid unprotected sexual contact with someone who has AIDS or who you know is an intravenous drug user.
- Don't have sex with anyone whose sexual history is not an "open book."
- Never accept any blood products unless you're absolutely sure they were screened. This is especially important if you find yourself in a developing country.

Symptoms of HIV

HIV infection can damage virtually any body organ or tissue, but most commonly the lungs, the gastrointestinal tract, the nervous system, and the skin. Here's what to look for if you have been exposed. Remember, however, that symptoms may not appear for days, weeks, months, or even years after exposure.

- Flulike symptoms such as low-grade fever, weakness, and feeling lousy generally
- Fatigue and weight loss
- Diarrhea and night sweats
- Recurrent skin and respiratory infections, and a cough that persists for more than a couple of weeks
- Swelling of the lymph glands throughout your body, not just one or two painful ones. (This is an ominous sign, but it can also reflect other diseases, including certain types of cancer.)
- Sores in your mouth. (They may be only herpes or benign cold sores, but check them out.)

If there is even the slightest possibility that you were exposed to HIV infection, let your doctor know if you develop any of these symptoms, but fess up even if you feel perfectly well. You may be infected with the HIV for a long time, sometimes years, before AIDS becomes apparent, and it may take six months or longer after infection for the blood test to become positive.

If You Test Positive for HIV

Insist on being referred to a specialist if you test positive. Progress against AIDS is being made very rapidly, and your best chance of receiving the most effective therapy is from someone who is an expert in this particular infection. In addition to the specific therapy described below, there are some lifestyle steps you should take immediately:

- Avoid close contact with anyone who's sick. You're now susceptible to whatever ails them, and they, of course, are vulnerable to your infection. I give all my HIV patients the usual prophylactic vaccinations such as those against the flu, hepatitis, and pneumococcal pneumonia.

- Late in the course of the disease, consider finding a new home for your pets. Cats, dogs, and birds can transmit a variety of diseases. These are not a great threat to normal persons, but can be dangerous to someone with impaired immunity. Should you decide to keep your pets (as I suspect most owners do), then get someone to clean their boxes or cages.

- Tuberculosis poses a special threat. Many of us are exposed to and develop immunity to this disease early in life. Although we have "positive" skin tests, there is no evidence of the disease. But the tubercle bacillus is nevertheless hibernating in our bodies, held in check by a strong immune system. Such resistance decreases as we grow older, and the TB organisms, which have been dormant for years, are reactivated and can cause overt tuberculosis in the debilitated elderly. This is especially true for persons with HIV, who should be skin-tested for TB. If positive, they should receive prophylactic isoniazid, the drug used to treat tuberculosis.

- Get lots of rest. Fatigue lowers resistance.

- Don't drink alcohol to excess.

- Eliminate tobacco. It aggravates the lung problems (PCP mentioned above) that AIDS commonly causes.

- Eat sensibly. AIDS often interferes with absorption of nutrients from the bowel, so take vitamin supplements, especially if you're losing weight. Avoid raw eggs and unpasteurized milk, both of which may contain organisms that can infect you.

- Contact an AIDS support group in your community. You'll need all the help you can get. Belonging to one is also the best way to learn about any breakthroughs in the field.

How Is AIDS Treated?

Billions of dollars are spent every year on AIDS research. Although a cure has not yet been found, treatment has improved dramatically. For many years after AIDS was discovered, all we could do was treat its complications. That depended on what organ the virus attacked "opportunistically." If it was the lung, drugs were given to eradicate the various organisms that had taken advantage of the lax immune system and infected it. If it was the brain, or the intestinal tract, or the skin, other therapy was available. However, none of these dealt with the virus itself. Although such symptomatic treatment is still an important part of the management of patients with AIDS, other measures that attack the virus have now been developed.

The most common and serious bacterial infection of the sinuses, bronchial tubes, and lungs is caused by the organism *Pneumocystis carinii*. Most experts treat it with co-trimoxazole. Other frequent "opportunistic" infections are herpes zoster (shingles), thrush, yeast infection of the mouth, vagina, or respiratory tract, and fungal infiltration of the skin and brain. All of the latter usually respond to an appropriate antifungal agent such as amphotericin B.

The most common malignancies associated with HIV are Kaposi's sarcoma (it affects the skin and occurs almost exclusively in male homosexuals) and non-Hodgkin's lymphoma. Kaposi's also occurs in non-HIV-infected persons, particularly in Africa, and is treated with several anticancer drugs and recombinant alpha interferon.

The major breakthrough in the management of AIDS is the development of drugs that attack the HIV itself and interfere with its ability to replicate. These agents fall into three main categories and yield the best result when used together. But even the most effective combinations do not cure the infection. Even when they eradicate the virus from the bloodstream, it simply moves to other areas of the body, where it continues to replicate, albeit at a much slower rate. During this latent interval, patients feel better, their symptoms abate, and they can often resume a virtually normal life—although the symptoms eventually recur. These medications do buy valuable time, and in so doing, prolong both the duration and the quality of life.

The new drugs against HIV described below can cost as much as $10,000 a year or more. This means that the poor and/or uninsured usually cannot afford them—a problem that society has not yet solved, but it should be high on our agenda. Patients of limited means try to cut corners and take less of the medication than was prescribed. This can be disastrous because it is crucial that these drugs be taken *exactly* as prescribed and at the precise time. Lower doses lead to viral resistance and an HIV rampage.

The New Antiretroviral Drugs

The new antiretroviral drugs, as they are called, are potentially very toxic. In some studies half the patients abandoned them because of intolerable side effects. Their regimen is also inconvenient, often requiring twenty or more pills a day taken at exact times from which you must not deviate. Finally, although these agents represent a major breakthrough, my enthusiasm for them is tempered by the fact that no one is sure how long they will continue to be effective—one, two, or three years. They've only been around a short time, and HIV is a very resourceful enemy.

As of 2002, there are some sixteen drugs approved for the treatment of HIV infection. They fall into three different groups, all of which inhibit the replication of the HIV by neutralizing one or more of the enzymes that the virus needs in order to multiply and do its dirty work. However, each antiretroviral group acts on a different enzyme. By combining them, we can hit three or four enzymes and paralyze the virus, at least for a while. Every AIDS specialist has his or her own favorite combination of these drugs.

The first group consists of the *nucleoside reverse transcriptase inhibitors* (NRTI), which block a crucial viral enzyme called reverse transcriptase. The NRTIs are never used alone (except in pregnant women, in whom they can successfully prevent transmission of the virus to the infant) because they have been shown to increase mutation of the HIV and actually make it more resistant to therapy unless combined with other agents. The first drug in this category was zidovudine (ZDV, Retrovir), formerly known as AZT. It was introduced in 1987 and remains a key drug today. There are currently five other medications in this category; their trade names are Viramune, Videx, Hivid, Zerit, and Epivir. (A product called Combivir contains both Retrovir and Epivir.) *Every combination of anti-HIV therapy contains at least one drug in the NRTI category.*

The second group of drugs, called *protease inhibitors,* represents a major therapeutic breakthrough. Protease inhibitors inhibit viral protease, another enzyme that the HIV needs in order to replicate. There are currently six protease inhibitors on the market. They are marketed as Crixivan, Norvir, Fortovase, and Viracept. Others are in the works. Taken together with one or more of the NRTIs, the drugs in this group have prolonged the life of AIDS patients and delayed the onset of opportunistic disease.

The third and most recent addition to the anti-AIDS armamentarium are the *nonnucleoside reverse transcriptase inhibitors* (NNRTIs). They inhibit the same enzyme as does the nucleoside group, but do so in a different way. The NNRTIs are never used alone, only in combination with drugs in the other two categories, whose effectiveness they enhance. This group includes Rescriptor, Viramune, and Sustiva, with several others in development.

At the present time, most AIDS specialists start therapy with one protease inhibitor—for example, Crixivan—and two NRTIs, such as Retrovir and Epivir. If the results are not satisfactory, they switch agents in each category and/or add one of the NNRTIs. As new drugs are developed, different combinations will undoubtedly be tried. Treatment protocols change with experience and new knowledge. That's why it's so important to insist on continuing input from an AIDS specialist. The gatekeeper and general internist may not be qualified to provide it.

When to Start Treatment

The next big question is *when* to start therapy. After HIV enters the body, it goes into hiding for months or years. However, during this "silent" interval, it is active, gradually destroying the immune system. If you've been infected for months or years and have never been treated, the toxicity of therapy is so great that most doctors will postpone initiating therapy until either symptoms of AIDS appear or the T cell count (see below) drops to 350. However, if you've been infected *recently* with HIV, it is critically important to start treatment immediately. If the probability of infection is high but hasn't yet been documented, don't wait for a positive test. For example, a health worker stuck with a needle that is contaminated with blood of a known AIDS patient should receive therapy immediately.

The HIV first targets the CD4 cells in the blood (also known as T lymphocytes or helper cells) that fight infection and cancer. The total CD4 cell count is an important indicator of the level of HIV activity. For years it was the sole index of the activity or severity of the HIV infection because we were unable to assess how much of the virus itself had entered the patient. The CD4 cell count in normal persons ranges from 800 to 1,200 cells. Doctors arbitrarily used 500 as the cutoff point in deciding on the timing of therapy in HIV-infected individuals. There has recently been a major breakthrough in this regard.

It is now possible to measure the actual viral concentration in the blood as well as the number of CD4 cells. This test, called the *viral load,* is a sensitive indicator of the effectiveness of any treatment. Whereas the CD4 count reflects the state of the immune system, the viral load indicates the actual level of viral activity. It is very useful in determining how aggressive the disease is and is also a measure of the patient's response to treatment. The viral load can fall as early as two weeks after effective therapy is begun. But remember that even an undetectable viral load in the blood does not mean you've been cured. You are still infected, and what's more, can potentially continue to transmit the disease. Unless you receive the treatment *exactly* as prescribed, you may relapse.

Current official guidelines advise delaying therapy until the CD4 count is less than 350, or when an opportunistic infection or cancer has developed, or when the viral load is between 500 and 10,000. However, no two patients are the same. *Insist on a second opinion concerning when to start your anti-AIDS therapy.*

If you're receiving antiretroviral therapy, you should have a physical exam, CD4 cell count, and viral load determination twice during the first month and once every three months thereafter if your condition is stable. There are several different tests to determine viral loads, and their numbers may not be comparable, so make sure you're getting the same one each time. This is particularly true if you've been moving from place to place and the test was done in different clinics. Your blood should also be checked for evidence of toxicity from the drugs.

Side effects from the antiretroviral agents include depression of the bone marrow, which can cause you to become anemic and more vulnerable to infection, gastrointestinal symptoms, lack of appetite, fever, and just feeling poorly. If you notice any change in your energy level, let your doctor know. *Do not stop the treatment on your own, because that may reactivate your disease.* Many drugs, especially certain antibiotics and painkillers, can affect the potency of the anti-HIV agents, so let your doctor know what you're taking. Also be sure that your doctor spells out for you whether you should be taking these medications with food or on an empty stomach, and whether they should be stored in a refrigerator or kept at room temperature. Every drug is different.

Remain optimistic if you have HIV. Research is moving quickly ahead in this area. What's more, testing positive for HIV doesn't necessarily mean that you are going to develop AIDS. One of my patients received several blood transfusions in the early 1980s, long before we were able to screen for HIV in donor blood. Ten years later the hospital where he had received the blood notified me that a donor of one of the pints of blood he had received subsequently developed AIDS. I checked my patient's blood, not expecting to find it positive because he was so healthy. Alas, the HIV antibodies were there. Three or four years later he developed a type of lymphoma associated with AIDS and was successfully treated for it. Now, almost twenty years after receiving the tainted blood, this man continues to enjoy good health, is married, has a child, and his viral load is zero!

WHAT TO INSIST ON IF YOU HAVE HIV OR AIDS

AIDS is a serious disease for which there is no cure. However, dedicated research over the years has resulted in new knowledge and some important advances in drug therapy. These have improved the quality of life and prolonged its duration for thousands of people. *The management of HIV infection and AIDS is highly complicated and ever changing. If you are so diagnosed, you must insist on care from a specialist in this field. The progress and problems are usually beyond the expertise of a general internist. Specific questions for you to ask are when to start treatment and what the best combination of drugs is. The drugs are expensive. Make sure you get them regardless of the cost.*

There has been an important breakthrough in the development of medications (antiretrovirals) that interfere with the ability of the virus to replicate. They fall into three categories, all of which block different enzymes that the virus requires in order to replicate. These agents are rarely used alone, but combinations can prolong the duration and improve quality of life for AIDS patients.

There has been a major change in the timing of therapy. Formerly, it was deferred until either symptoms appeared or the CD4 count dropped dramatically. Most specialists now believe that treatment of HIV should begin as soon as exposure is certain, and before the onset of symptoms. However, because of the toxicity of the drugs involved, those who have been infected with HIV for several months should wait until their T cell (CD4) count drops to 350 or less, or the viral load ranges between 500 and 10,000, or they develop symptoms of AIDS.

If you do not believe that you are receiving the best combination of drugs or the best treatment options, insist on a second opinion.

3

ALZHEIMER'S DISEASE

Forget About It

Alzheimer's disease (AD) has replaced cancer, stroke, heart attacks, and AIDS as the most feared affliction of mankind. It's insidious, devastating, and incurable, engulfing not only the patient but his or her loved ones as well. Families must witness for years the inexorable, tragic deterioration of a vital, active human being. What begins with subtle memory loss ends in total dementia. To make matters worse, spending time with an AD patient whom you love may leave you identifying with him or her and fearing for your own sanity. Harmless memory lapses such as forgetting where you left your keys or where you parked your car may trigger panic and raise the question "Is this the beginning for me too?"

What Is Alzheimer's?

Although the incidence of Alzheimer's is rising, it's by no means a new disease. Ancient Greeks and Romans described it thousands of years ago. Alzheimer's is named after a German doctor, Alois Alzheimer, who in 1908 discovered twisted strands of fiber in the brains of some persons with "mental illness." These "neurofibrillary tangles" remain the only objective proof of Alzheimer's—and they're found only at autopsy.

Not until seventy-five years later did scientists discover that the characteristic Alzheimer plaques contain beta amyloid, a string of forty or more amino acids whose parent protein is called amyloid precursor protein (APP). This observation may be very important because researchers are now testing a vaccine that prevents this protein from forming. If it works, it may cure or prevent Alzheimer's. The tangles also contain another protein called tau, which too is being studied.

AD starts in an area of the brain called the entorhinal cortex, moves to the hippocampus (important for memory formation), then moves deep inside the brain, and finally to the centers of higher function in the cerebral cortex that are concerned with thought, language, and reason.

In addition to these anatomic changes, the Alzheimer brain loses 90 percent of its acetylcholine, a neurotransmitter used predominantly by neurons (nerve cells in the brain) in the areas most important for memory. Drug therapy of this disease, such as it is, is based on replenishing this missing acetylcholine.

The best guesstimate is that there are 4 million cases of Alzheimer's in this country alone, and the numbers are increasing as our population ages. There are two main types; one accounts for 95 percent of cases and is "sporadic"—that is, it occurs randomly and for no apparent reason; the other 5 percent are genetically determined and develop in families in whom as many as half the members are afflicted.

Alzheimer's is not an immediate threat to life. Some patients survive for twenty years or more. However, many die a few years after the diagnosis is made, usually from pneumonia or some other disease. AD costs Americans $100 billion a year, whether caring for its victims at home or in nursing facilities.

AD is *not* an inevitable consequence of aging. Yes, you are more likely to develop it as you grow older, but there is no such thing as "natural" senility. When you "lose" your mind at any age, it's because some disease or disorder has affected it. Alzheimer's is one of several such conditions, and the most common.

The memory loss and other behavioral abnormalities of AD can usually be accurately assessed by neurological and psychiatric tests. Some are as simple as asking, "What's the date, the day of the week, the year, and who's the president of the United States?" However, since there is presently no objective test to diagnose Alzheimer's *with certainty* during life, everyone suspected of having it should undergo a careful neurological and medical evaluation to rule out the various *other* disorders that can produce similar symptoms. *Do not accept a diagnosis of Alzheimer's until you've had such an evaluation. Insist on it.*

Although several Alzheimer genes have been identified, many people without the genes have the disease, while others who possess them never develop it.

Several drugs and herbs can improve some of the symptoms of Alzheimer's, but there is no cure for it, and no way to stop its inevitable progress.

What Is Dementia and How Can You Recognize It?

"Dementia" refers to deterioration of mental function due to *any* cause. You forget someone's name at a cocktail party but remember it later. Is that dementia? Or you suddenly draw a blank on a telephone number you've dialed every day for months. Or you decide to phone a friend, dial the number, and then can't remember whom you're calling. Should you worry? Not if it only happens *now and then*. But if these lapses occur frequently, they may be early signs of serious trouble. The following should prompt a visit to your doctor:

- Forgetfulness is affecting your job performance. Customers or colleagues ask for your input on important matters, and you promise to get back to them but forget to do so. Even worse, you don't even recall the conversation in the first place.
- You're preparing dinner and forget that you've left the rice on the stove. That's bad enough, but if you then leave the house to go to a movie, you'd better tell your doctor about it.
- Dan Quayle and George W. Bush have trouble using the right word, like saying "hostile" instead of "hostage." That's not too serious, but when your sentences as a whole are gibberish, you're in trouble.
- You don't know the day, the month, or the year.
- While driving your car you suddenly forget where you were going.
- You've lived in the same part of town for years, have gone for the same daily ten-minute walk for as long as you can remember, but now don't know where you are, how you got there, why you went in the first place, and can't find your way home.
- Your color coordination may not qualify you to be a design consultant—neither does mine—but wearing one black shoe and one white one is cause for concern. As is putting on two shirts.
- Most people dislike the task of balancing their checkbooks, but if you stare blankly at the numbers and don't know what they mean, you need help.
- Everyone forgets occasionally where he or she has put something—a book, keys, wallet, glasses, or any one of the countless personal items we carry with us. But when you find one of your shoes in the refrigerator or your pocket comb in the sugar bowl, you've got problems.

- It's normal to feel angry, depressed, or frustrated once in a while, but sudden dramatic mood swings from one moment to the next for no apparent reason may suggest dementia.
- Our tastes change as we grow older. What gave us pleasure and made us smile years ago may bore us today. That's normal. But demented individuals often undergo a fundamental change in their personality: They become aggressive, paranoid with a persecution complex, confused, or withdrawn *for no apparent reason.*
- Everyone needs a vacation from time to time to regain the energy necessary to get on with the job. A demented individual loses interest that cannot be rekindled and needs constant prompting to get on with life.
- When the above behavior patterns become habitual, they may progress to inability to speak intelligibly and communicate effectively; loss of appetite; no control of the bowels and bladder; and finally the need for a round-the-clock caregiver.

Most of us, even doctors who should know better, almost reflexively attribute these signs and symptoms to Alzheimer's, but several other disease processes can also cause them. The distinction should be made as quickly as possible because dementia caused by something other than Alzheimer's can often be cured or arrested if diagnosed and treated promptly. Here are a few of the conditions, some common, others rare, that *must* be ruled out before you accept the Alzheimer diagnosis.

Conditions That Mimic Alzheimer's and What to Do About Them

- Multiple small strokes, often unrecognized, are the most common cause of non-Alzheimer's dementia. When arteriosclerosis affects the brain, plaques form in its arteries, eventually obstructing them. Blood supply to the brain is cut off, often causing dementia. "Thinning" the blood with anticoagulants, lowering cholesterol levels, and normalizing elevated blood pressure in such cases may prevent more strokes and worsening of the dementia. When such vascular disease coexists with AD, preventing small strokes can slow down the progress of the dementia.

- Blood clots that travel to the brain from the carotid arteries in the neck or from the heart (especially in an untreated cardiac rhythm disturbance called atrial fibrillation) can also result in brain damage—and dementia. Anticoagulants can prevent these clots from reaching the brain.

- Seniors take an average of seven different medications every day. These drugs often accumulate and can become toxic because as we age, our bodies do not excrete them as efficiently. Painkillers, antidepressants, tranquilizers, sleeping pills, steroid hormones (cortisone family of drugs), and even some medicines that lower high blood pressure and treat heart disease can obtund, confuse, depress, and result in irrational behavior. So when an older person starts acting strangely for no apparent reason, take a good look in his or her medicine cabinet.

- Excess alcohol consumption over the years can cause *alcoholic dementia,* which should not be confused with AD.

- *Subdural hematoma* is a collection of blood between the skull and the surface of the brain. It develops when fragile blood vessels in the skull burst after even a gentle blow to the head. Blood then forms a pocket on the outside of the brain and presses on it. I have seen several patients become demented after a head injury of which they were often unaware. All it takes to make the diagnosis is an X ray, CT scan, or MRI of the brain. *Insist on these procedures in anyone whose behavior has become bizarre.* Subdural hematomas can be removed by either withdrawing them with a needle, or dissolving them with medication. Once the pressure on the brain is relieved, symptoms usually disappear.
- Nutritional deficiency is an important and fairly common cause of dementia. Older people who live alone may not have the means, the energy, or the teeth to eat nutritiously. Many are depressed and can't be bothered to prepare a meal. Whatever the reason, they are apt to be deficient in several key nutrients, especially vitamin B. So always take a good look in a demented senior's refrigerator. These individuals respond dramatically to a good diet and multivitamins. I prescribe a multivitamin to every older patient—just in case. I even take one myself.
- Severe depression can mimic dementia. I remember one of my patients, a widower in his seventies, whose personality began to change after he lost his wife two years earlier. He no longer smiled, even when his grandchildren did the cutest things; he was preoccupied; previously a gourmand, he lost his appetite; he was totally disinterested in his environment and his family. All he wanted to do was sleep. One of his sons, a radiologist, advised his siblings that their dad had Alzheimer's and would be better off cared for in a nursing home. So without consulting their family doctor (and why would they want to when one of their own was an M.D.?) they

suggested to their father that he might be happier living among people his own age. He offered no resistance; he didn't seem really to care. His children moved him out of his apartment and enrolled him in a very nice retirement home in the suburbs.

For the first few weeks after his arrival, there was no change in his behavior. When his family visited him on weekends, he did not complain about the food—or anything else, for that matter. However, a few months later he was suddenly a changed man. His children were puzzled. Was it better nutrition or a medication prescribed by one of the home's doctors? Not at all. Their father had found romance! After living alone for so long and grieving for his departed spouse, he'd struck up a friendship with another resident in the facility, an attractive widow a few years younger than he. They had many interests in common—American history, politics, antique furniture, and movies. They spent hours walking on the grounds, going to movies, and enjoying each other's company. It wasn't long before "Dad" proposed—and was accepted. The couple was married (the radiologist son who had made the wrong diagnosis was best man), and they moved to a small apartment, where they lived happily ever after.

So depression can and does mimic dementia. But depressed seniors don't necessarily have to find romance to improve their state of mind. There are many antidepressants that can lift their spirits and "cure" their "Alzheimer's."

- Any chronic disease can result in dementia. One of the most common is underfunction of the thyroid gland. Lack of thyroid hormone can produce sluggishness, disinterest, slow thinking, and halting speech, all of which suggest dementia. Replacing the missing thyroid results in a "miracle." Disorders of the kidney, liver, and lung (when the latter is associated with low oxygen levels in the blood) can also affect behavior.

- Infections such as HIV, as well as a host of viral agents, can affect the brain and cause dementia.
- Several neurological diseases other than Alzheimer's are associated with brain damage that causes behavioral changes. These include Parkinson's disease, malignant brain tumors, Creutzfeldt-Jakob disease and Mad Cow disease, one of its variants, and several others.

To confirm the diagnosis of AD beyond the shadow of a doubt, dementia requires that the doctor take enough time to assess the patient's mind as well as the body, to determine how appropriate are the responses to pertinent questions, to size up the dress and grooming, to decide whether depression is playing a role, to determine whether the patient is agitated, repetitious, confused, or irritable. This is critical information that cannot be obtained from a printed questionnaire or an untrained office aide. So here's what to *insist* upon to determine the underlying cause of dementia:

A complete history. One or more family members who can describe the lifestyle that may be contributing to the symptoms should always accompany the patient. In today's "in and out" office visits, such time is not easy to obtain. *Insist on it in advance.*

A careful and thorough physical exam. Although the focus should be on the neurological status, the evaluation should include other body systems as well. For example, kidney and liver disease, severe anemia, and malignancies can have an impact on behavior. As for the neurological exam, a well-trained family doctor can detect an obvious neurological disorder such as a stroke or Parkinson's. Ideally, the patient should also undergo a brief mental function test such as the Mini-Mental State Test or the Short Portable Mental Status Questionnaire. These take only five or ten minutes and provide a good idea of the severity of mental impairment.

You must insist, too, that all of the following be done:

- Complete blood count to uncover evidence of anemia and infection
- Electrolyte panel to measure the level of such minerals as sodium and potassium
- Screening metabolic panel to assess kidney and liver function as well as blood sugar
- Thyroid function tests
- Vitamin B_{12} and folate levels. (They're reduced in pernicious anemia and other vitamin deficiencies.)
- HIV test
- Urinalysis
- Electrocardiogram

If the history, physical exam, and these other tests suggest the presence of dementia but don't establish the cause, you must *insist* on a consultation with a neurologist. He or she may advise a formal psychiatric interview. In any event, MRI (magnetic resonance imaging) of the brain should be done. *Insist on it.* This procedure costs more than a CT scan but is more sensitive and therefore more likely to detect small strokes, tumors, and other structural abnormalities in the brain. It also has the advantage of not exposing the patient to radiation.

Several other procedures are currently being evaluated to help determine the cause of dementia. They include spinal fluid analysis for the presence of certain proteins, PET (positron emission tomography), SPECT (single photon emission computed tomography), and MRSI (magnetic resonance spectroscopy imaging). However, these are still largely experimental.

I recently read of a fascinating experiment done at Columbia Presbyterian Medical Center in New York City in which ninety men and women whose average age was sixty-seven and who had minor memory problems were given a "scratch and sniff" test. They were asked to identify forty different distinctive odors such as menthol, peanuts, and soap over a fifteen- to twenty-minute period. None of thirty subjects who identified all the smells correctly developed Alzheimer's during the next twenty months, but nineteen who had trouble doing so did become demented. If this study is repeated and found to be accurate, the smell test may be a useful screen. But don't take it if your sense of smell is less than perfect because of chronic allergies or nasal stuffiness. You don't want a nasal problem to stigmatize you with Alzheimer's.

This all boils down to the fact that the diagnosis of Alzheimer's is one of exclusion. There is no specific test that permits you to say, "Aha, this can only be Alzheimer's and nothing else." AD is the diagnosis you're left with when all other possible causes have been ruled out.

Risk Factors for Alzheimer's

Scientists are conducting intensive research in an attempt to identify preventable risk factors for Alzheimer's. Theories abound, but so far there are only *two certain risk factors,* and you can't do much about either of them. The first is *age.* The chances of your developing Alzheimer's increase exponentially with age, so that its incidence doubles every five years after age sixty-five. Then there is *genetic vulnerability.* Several genes have already been identified, some in persons with a family history, and others in the randomly occurring form of the disease. Hopefully, with the mapping of the human genome, we will be able to modify these genes, but we are unable to do so at the present time.

There are, in addition, some very suspect risk factors of which you should be aware:

- Boxers and others who have sustained head injuries earlier in life that have caused loss of consciousness have a higher incidence of the disease.
- More females have Alzheimer's than do men, but that may reflect the fact that they live longer.
- Education appears to be protective. The more formal schooling you've had, the less likely you are to become an Alzheimer's victim.
- The so-called aluminum theory is still held by many. This theory is based on the fact that the plaques and tangles in the brains of Alzheimer's patients contain more than a normal amount of this mineral. Most researchers don't really believe that aluminum is the cause.

After the Diagnosis Is Made

If your memory loss and other symptoms are diagnosed as early Alzheimer's, there are some steps you can take to make life easier for yourself and those around you. Remember that the disease does not progress at the same pace in everyone. It's slow in some, more aggressive in others. Here are some measures to consider:

- Try to sharpen your memory. Seniors with and without Alzheimer's who keep their minds active fare better in the long run. Organize your life. You're less apt to run into trouble if you develop a daily routine. So, for example, shop for your groceries on Mondays, vacuum on Tuesdays, do your washing on Wednesdays, and so on. This frees you from having to make these decisions every day.
- Write everything down. Accept the fact that you can't remember all you should. Make lists of what to do, ap-

pointments to be kept, and whom to call, and refer to them frequently.

- We used to think that estrogen replacement therapy retards or prevents Alzheimer's in menopausal women. Recent studies do not confirm this theory but it is still being tested.
- Testosterone, the male hormone, was recently shown to slow the formation of beta amyloid, the substance present in the plaques of patients with Alzheimer's. Elderly men with AD who were given testosterone improved measurably. It's still too early to recommend this therapy to everyone, but it's worth discussing with your doctor. If the doctor balks, refer him or her to the research conducted by Dr. Gunnar Gouras at Weill Cornell Medical College.
- Antioxidants are the rage these days because they neutralize oxygen-free radicals, the waste products of body metabolism. These radicals have been blamed for almost every human ailment, including Alzheimer's. Recent research suggests that there may be some connection between these radicals and the beta amyloid found in Alzheimer's plaques. Some physicians are therefore giving large doses of vitamin E (1,000 IU and more) as well as vitamin C and selegiline (Eldepryl) to their Alzheimer's patients in the hope of retarding the progress of the disease.
- Certain nonsteroidal anti-inflammatory drugs (NSAIDs) such as ibuprofen, indomethacin, and sulindac were recently found to prevent the formation of beta amyloid in the brains of mice. Aspirin, naproxen, and other NSAIDs did not have this effect. If scientists can determine what it is that has this effect on the abnormal protein, it may conceivably lead to a preventive in humans.
- A lifelong diet rich in folic acid (present in cereals, bread, and leafy green vegetables) appears to protect

the brain in later years. For this and other reasons, I usually prescribe 400 micrograms of folic acid to all my adult patients.

- There are four drugs currently on the market that doctors are prescribing to their Alzheimer's patients. They all increase the level of acetylcholine, in which the Alzheimer brain is deficient. They are marketed as Aricept, Cognex, Exelon, and Reminyl. They may help a little, but frankly, I have been underwhelmed by their effectiveness. Still, they're worth a try.
- Antidepressants, though by no means a cure, help many patients with Alzheimer's who are also depressed.
- I prescribe ginkgo biloba to anyone whose memory is impaired for whatever reason. Several reports in this country have shown that this herb can help a little, and a little can sometimes make a difference.
- The "statins," widely prescribed to reduce elevated cholesterol levels, are now also believed to reduce the risk of AD. Ask your doctor about them.

Alzheimer's is a relentless foe, and ultimately, as patients deteriorate, their loved ones bear a terrible burden. As care becomes more all-consuming—dressing, feeding, medicating, cleaning, dealing with incontinence and irrational, sometimes violent behavior—the stress on the family can become unmanageable. The presence of someone with advanced AD in crowded quarters, especially if there are children at home, severely disrupts a household. Although many families are understandably reluctant and guilt-ridden to send their stricken parents to a "facility," this is often the most reasonable decision and in the best interests of both the patient and the family. The staff in special care units of nursing homes is trained to deal with and protect agitated dementia patients from harming themselves and others. However, when such institutionalization is not feasible or its costs are too great, there are social services that can provide help at home. The high and rising incidence of AD is yet another argument for you to take out long-term health-care insurance while you're still in your fifties in order to cope with the economic burden of this disease should you be stricken.

WHAT TO INSIST ON IF YOU HAVE ALZHEIMER'S

Alzheimer's is the most common of several types of dementia. Like many of the others, it is a disease of the elderly. However, *it is not synonymous with aging.*

The salient point to remember is that there is no specific test for Alzheimer's. At the present time the diagnosis is made by excluding all the other possible causes of dementia. These include multiple small strokes, malnutrition, depression, a variety of illnesses, several neurological disorders, and brain tumors. *If you suspect that a loved one is developing Alzheimer's, do not accept this diagnosis without first insisting on a complete history and physical, a consultation with a neurologist or neuropsychiatrist, and an MRI of the brain.* Remember that cases diagnosed as Alzheimer's are often found at autopsy to be due to some other cause that may be curable.

There are several steps you can take to slow down the progress of the disease, and you should avoid some risk factors. However, the stark reality of AD is that it is neither preventable nor curable. All that a caring family can do is shower the patient with love, attend to the basic needs, and, if necessary, find a humane home in which he or she can live for whatever time is left.

4

ARTHRITIS

How Do I Hurt Thee?
Let Me Count the Ways

If you list "arthritis" as the diagnosis on a disability or insurance claim form, chances are it will be returned for more information. That's because the term "arthritis" by itself refers to a symptom, not a disease. Strictly speaking, it means *inflammation of a joint*—any joint. You'd appreciate this if you knew ancient Greek (not exactly my mother tongue either). "Arthritis" is derived from a combination of *arthros* (meaning "joint") and *itis* (the suffix for "inflammation of"). Anything that can hurt or inflame your joints—injury, infection, a chemical imbalance in the blood, or an immune system that's gone wacky and mistakenly attacks your joints—can give you arthritis. So can too much uric acid in a joint (gouty arthritis); the venerable (oops, sorry, I mean venereal) gonococcus bug can invade a joint and result in infectious arthritis; a virus that hurts the liver can also do so. There are at least one hundred different possible causes of arthritis.

Arthritis reflects a problem with a *joint*—that is, the site where two or more bones meet. To understand what arthritis can do to you and why, let me describe the various components of a joint and what happens to them in most forms of arthritis.

The ends of the bones that form the joint are covered by resilient tissue called cartilage, more than 70 percent of which consists of water. It functions as a cushion that allows the bones to move smoothly against each other. Bones and cartilage are surrounded by a fluid-filled membrane (synovial membrane) covered, in turn, by a tough capsule that protects the joint from injury.

Every time you move your neck, bend, stand, sit, walk, run, put on your coat, or pull up your socks, even crook your finger to beckon someone, there is a dynamic interplay among all these components of the joints—the bones, the cartilage, the fluid, and the capsule. If your joint is normal, it moves smoothly and painlessly. When you have arthritis, the healthy rubbery, smooth cartilage that normally serves as a shock absorber between the bones thins out, becomes stiff and rough, and loses its elasticity; the synovial membrane is chronically irritated and makes an abnormally large amount of fluid; and spurs form on the ends of the bone. And you hurt.

You won't have to wade through all the different conditions that cause arthritis in this chapter. I will describe only the two that account for the vast majority of cases—osteoarthritis and rheumatoid arthritis. Let's start with osteoarthritis, the more common of the two.

Osteoarthritis

Osteoarthritis (OA) is the leading cause of disability in this country, affecting more than 60 million Americans. (I would have expected a higher number, since almost everyone I know over the age of sixty-five—and many younger men and women too—has or complains about osteoarthritis.) This disorder is due to injury or to wear and tear of the joints over the years.

Making the Diagnosis

The location and pattern of the joint pain of OA are usually so typical that you can almost always diagnose it yourself. And if neither you nor your doctor is sure, an X ray or MRI removes all doubt. In fact, were we to X-ray every man and woman over the age of sixty-five, we'd find osteoarthritis at least 50 percent of the time, regardless of whether or not it was causing any symptoms. *There is no specific blood test for OA.* Even though OA is easy to recognize, if there is anything atypical about your joint symptoms, *you should insist on blood tests and X rays to rule out other causes of your pain* (tendonitis, bursitis, rheumatoid arthritis, polymyositis, and any autoimmune disease, all of whose treatments differ from those of OA). It may also be necessary to withdraw a sample of the fluid from the affected joint to confirm the diagnosis. *Insist on a second opinion from a rheumatologist (a specialist dealing in joint disorders), or an orthopedist early on, before it's too late to correct what needs fixing.*

Symptoms of Osteoarthritis

When you have OA, the bones of the joint rub against each other and cause a deep ache or pain, sometimes also creating a crackling sound. Sometimes even just moving them hurts, or they're stiff when you wake up in the morning. When the synovial membrane is irritated, it makes more fluid and leaves the joint swollen, and occasionally red, tender, and stiff. When bony spurs form on the ends of the bones, they distort the shape of the joint.

The symptoms of OA come on gradually. They're usually

one-sided early in the course of the disease, affecting most commonly a hip, a knee, or the spine. Women are more prone to OA of the knees and hands, but the hips are equally affected in both men and women. Other joints such as the fingers and less frequently the elbows and shoulders can also be involved. If your knees are osteoarthritic, they hurt when you walk up and down the stairs; if it's your back, you have trouble bending; if your fingers are involved, you may have problems using your hands or holding a pen. Your arms and legs may also feel weak.

Uncomplicated osteoarthritis does not cause fever, weight loss, anemia, or a generalized lousy feeling. When these symptoms accompany your joint pains, you probably have one of the other hundred causes of arthritis, the most likely being rheumatoid (discussed below).

Who's Most Vulnerable to Osteoarthritis?

Almost every adult has some degree of OA after age forty, and its severity varies: In some it's little more than a minor nuisance; in others it's debilitating. Certain risk factors play a role. For one, heredity can be important. You may have a defective gene that has caused your cartilage to deteriorate. If you were born "double-jointed," you're vulnerable to OA; if you have a congenital spinal abnormality such as a curvature (scoliosis), you're also prone to osteoarthritis.

There are several important nonhereditary factors. Overweight can hasten and aggravate OA, especially in the knees and other weight-bearing joints. Athletes who use anabolic steroids to augment their performance leave themselves vulnerable to OA, as do football and soccer players, who injure or repeatedly stress their knees. If you've broken a bone near its joint, its cartilage can be affected. Ballet dancers often develop OA of the feet and hips.

Don't conclude from any of this that the best way to prevent OA is to reduce your level of physical activity. That's not protective. Couch potatoes also develop stiff and painful joints. The fact is, you can't win because *in most cases even if you just live normally and do everything right, you can still develop osteoarthritis.* Although there is much you can do to minimize its symptoms and even slow down its progression, I don't know of any way to *prevent* it.

Managing (and Living) with Osteoarthritis

Although OA won't kill you, it can impair the quality of your life. Its management requires a team effort. *Physiotherapy or occupational therapy helps most people with OA. Insist on referral and access to these specialists.* Although your family doctor can prescribe painkillers to make you more comfortable, you need experts to design a physical therapy program.

There are five key approaches to the treatment of osteoarthritis:

- Weight loss
- Exercise (including physiotherapy)
- Heat and cold
- Pain medication
- Surgery

Weight loss helps relieve the symptoms of OA. Overweight leaves you more vulnerable to OA and worsens its symptoms because it puts extra pressure on the joints. I have not seen any specific diets that help OA other than those that cause weight loss. I prescribe vitamins C and D to my patients because there is some evidence that their lack may increase the risk of osteoarthritis.

Exercise is extremely important for several reasons: It promotes weight loss, strengthens the muscles that support the diseased joints, makes it easier for them to function, and increases joint flexibility. Finally, the right exercise can be fun and emotionally uplifting. After all, how sick can you be if you're able to exercise?

It's not enough to be told that exercise is good for you. You need to be evaluated to determine how much and what kind to suit your particular needs and limitations. Should it be anaerobic (stretching, strengthening, and weight lifting) or aerobic (walking, swimming) or a combination of the two? What level of exercise should you perform and for how long? The wrong kind of physical activity at the wrong time for the wrong duration can make matters worse. *Insist on a qualified specialist to instruct you after your joint problem has been assessed.*

Here are some basic rules concerning exercise and OA:

- Do it when you have the least pain and your joints are most flexible. Any exercise that makes you uncomfortable is not good for you.
- Exercise several times a day for shorter periods rather than for prolonged sessions that leave you exhausted.
- In the morning take a hot shower or bath to limber up joints that tend to be stiff just after you wake up.
- Avoid jogging and high-impact aerobics. Walk regularly on flat surfaces and swim whenever you can.

Both *heat and cold* are important. Deciding which is better for you is often a matter of trial and error, but don't use either for longer than twenty minutes at a time. And always let your skin temperature return to normal before reapplying either heat or cold.

As a rule, heat (from compresses, hot packs, heating pads, a hot shower, or languishing in a hot tub or pool) should be used to *relax your muscles before exercising.* Cold, on the other hand, is a *pain reliever.* Ice or a cold pack from your freezer applied directly to your skin can burn it. Always wrap it in a towel.

Analgesic lotions are helpful too. However, a word of caution. Since they numb the pain (which is what you want them to do), you might unknowingly burn yourself if you use them in combination with heat or cold therapy.

You'll probably need *medication* at some point in the course of your disease—not to cure it, but to relieve the pain. *But remember these two cardinal rules: First, there's nothing noble about enduring pain. Insist on something to control it. Second, if you decide that you do "need something," start with the weakest medication and proceed step by step to stronger preparations as necessary.*

The first painkiller to choose is one that you can buy over-the-counter. But make no mistake: These drugs are potent even though they do not require a prescription. If you're using them on an ongoing basis, let your doctor know, because they may interact with some other preparation you're taking. If you're over sixty, I suggest you start with *acetaminophen* (Tylenol). It doesn't cause as much stomach irritation as do aspirin and the nonsteroidal anti-inflammatories (NSAIDs). However, it often takes days for Tylenol to relieve the pain of OA. Taking a couple of tablets now and then isn't likely to be effective. The usual dose is one or two tablets, three or four times a day. It reduces pain, but doesn't do much for redness, warmth, and swelling because, unlike aspirin and the NSAIDs, Tylenol is not an anti-inflammatory agent. Don't take it with alcohol, and avoid it if you have any chronic liver or kidney problem.

If acetaminophen doesn't provide enough relief, move on to one of the over-the-counter NSAIDs. They not only lessen pain but also reduce inflammation. The most widely used preparations are ibuprofen and naproxen, although there are many more on the market. Both ibuprofen and naproxen are more effective than aspirin, but, like aspirin, they can cause stomach irritation, ulcers, and bleeding. Stop them at the first sign of heartburn, indigestion, or the appearance of black stools (indicating that you're bleeding). (If you're on aspirin, make sure it's the enteric-coated variety, which dissolves in the intestine and not in the stomach.) If you're using NSAIDs for any length of time, you should also be on an acid-blocking medication such as omeprazole (Prilosec) to prevent gastric complications. Remember, too, that these drugs should not normally be taken with anticoagulants (blood thinners).

More and more physicians are prescribing the new COX-2 inhibitors, the best known of which are *Celebrex and Vioxx.* They are as potent as the other NSAIDs and are much more expensive. Celebrex, for example, costs twenty times as much as any of the older generic NSAIDs, yet it is one of the most widely prescribed drugs in the United States. According to early marketing claims, both Celebrex and Vioxx were said to result in a much lower incidence of stomach ulcers than the other NSAIDs. For this reason, the manufacturers of these two medications petitioned the FDA to remove the statement on the labels that warned patients of this risk. However, a government advisory panel found that although reduced, the risk of gastric bleeding is still high enough for the FDA to refuse to remove the warning label. Gastric complications are highest when you combine any NSAID with aspirin, as is done by many older people who require pain relief from arthritis and also wish to reduce their risk of heart attack and stroke. In such cases, always use low dose (81 mg) aspirin and use the full strength preparation. Another problem with NSAIDs is that they cause retention of salt when taken in higher doses than recommended. This can cause swelling of the feet, raise blood pressure, and worsen heart failure. There is yet another ongoing controversy between some doctors and the manufacturers of the COX-2 inhibitors. Researchers at the Cleveland Clinic published a report in the *New England Journal of Medicine* calling for additional studies of the safety of these drugs. After analyzing the data reported in all English-language scientific papers between 1998 and February 2001, they concluded that their use is associated with an increased risk of vascular events due to an increased clotting tendency of the blood. This is apparently not the case with the older NSAIDs. Until the matter is clarified, it would seem wise to stay with the ibuprofen family of drugs, especially if you already have some vascular problems in your heart or brain, or are at increased risk for developing them.

Here's the bottom line: If you're careful with their use, NSAIDs are the best drugs available for the relief of chronic pain due to arthritis.

What about *narcotic drugs,* such as codeine or oxycodone? Although they are more effective against pain than any of the others discussed above, avoid them for as long as you can. They are habit-forming and osteoarthritis is a chronic condition.

The natural supplements *glucosamine and chondroitin* are very popular for the treatment of arthritis. In a recent three-year study of more than two hundred arthritis patients, glucosamine reduced symptoms and cartilage damage in up to 25 percent. They're worth a try.

Corticosteroids can be injected directly into the involved joint. The oral preparations are dangerously seductive and should not be taken by mouth. They make you feel great; they eliminate pain and inflammation. However, their chronic use can cause such serious side effects as gastric ulcers, osteoporosis, hypertension, the resorption of cartilage, vulnerability to infection, impaired healing, and avascular necrosis of the hip (in which the blood supply to the hip is reduced, requiring it to be replaced). When injected into the joint, very little of the hormone is absorbed. Still, such injections should not be done more than a few times a year.

Hyaluronic acid is one of the newer developments in the treatment of OA of the knee. It is a constituent of joint fluid, a synthetic version of which can be injected directly into the joint. The literature on the subject is conflicting. Several of my patients have tried it with only mediocre results. However, there probably isn't a major downside to it before having your knee replaced.

There is also *topical therapy,* the application of lotions, sprays, creams, and ointments to a painful joint. You can buy almost all of them at pharmacies and health food stores without a prescription. Bengay is perhaps the best known. Some of these products do provide temporary relief and are worth trying. They contain a variety of ingredients such as salicylates, menthol, skin irritants that distract from the painful joint, and *capsaicin.* In my opinion the latter is the most effective of the lot. Capsaicin, derived from chili peppers, prevents the transmission to the brain of pain messages from the nerve endings on the surface of the skin. Apply it three or four times a day. It may take three or four weeks to work, so be patient. Capsaicin has no significant side effects but may sting and burn for the first few days when you sweat or wash with hot water. I recommend it for any skin condition that hurts (including shingles). Remember not to use any of these topical preparations while applying heat or cold; their analgesic affect may prevent you from realizing that you're being burned.

Acupuncture, though still controversial, is gaining wider acceptance for pain control in various situations, especially arthritis. I am not aware of any downside to its use and encourage anyone with chronic pain to try it. Make sure, however, that your acupuncturist is qualified. Check his or her credentials with your local medical or acupuncture society.

Transcutaneous electrical nerve stimulation (TENS) is a noninvasive technique that sends electrical stimulation to the local nerves through a small battery-powered stimulator. This probably blocks pain signals to the spinal cord. It can be very effective, but don't use it if you have a pacemaker or are pregnant. For some reason, TENS is not as popular as it once was.

Your doctor may also recommend *arthroscopy.* This procedure permits a direct look into the joint and repair of whatever damage there is, or removal of pieces of cartilage and gunk inside the joint. Arthroscopy can be done in a hospital outpatient clinic, and you go home the same day.

Finally, there's *surgery.* If your arthritis is painful, crippling, or deforming, and the joint has been destroyed and is resistant to any of the therapies mentioned above, it may have to be fixed or replaced. *Always insist on a second opinion before accepting such surgery.* However, having had a hip replaced myself, I can tell you that these procedures, though far from trivial, are now almost always successful. It's important to remember that once any joint is replaced, you must take antibiotics for the rest of your life whenever you're having dental work done or undergoing an invasive procedure that can release bacteria into the bloodstream and infect the artificial joint.

Here are some additional practical tips for living with osteoarthritis. You'd be surprised how much they can improve the quality of your life:

- Squatting and kneeling stress your hips and knees. If there's something to be picked up off the floor, ask someone else to do it or buy one of those grabber canes. Whenever you bend, do so at the knees, keeping your back and legs as straight as possible.
- Avoid slippery floors. Don't have loose throw rugs or anything you can trip on lying around. Install wall-to-wall carpeting.
- Wear sensible low-heeled shoes with good arch supports. If you have arthritis in your fingers or have trouble bending, wear slip-ons rather than shoes that lace.
- Sit in chairs with arm supports and backrests, and not in low, soft seats that are hard to get out of.
- If you have knee or hip problems, use a cane. It's elegant. Don't be embarrassed by crutches or a walker if you need them to get about. They're better than being housebound.

- If your fingers are arthritic and you find it hard to write, buy a thick pen that you can grab hold of instead of one of those spindly little things.
- Apply a no-slip finish in your bathtub or use a nonskid rubber mat. Install handrails to help you get in and out.
- A raised toilet seat is much more convenient than one of conventional height.
- Don't hesitate to ask for help when you need it. And make sure that that teenager gives you his or her seat on the bus or subway. Sometimes a dirty look is all you need for compliance!

Rheumatoid Arthritis

If you think OA is bad, thank your lucky stars that you don't have rheumatoid arthritis (RA). But if you do, read on, because there's been lots of progress in the treatment of this crippling disorder.

More than 2 million Americans have RA. Unlike OA, which affects specific joints that may have been excessively used (or abused), injured, or stressed over the years, and in which patients usually feel well except for their joint symptoms, rheumatoid arthritis affects the entire body (doctors call it a "systemic" disorder). In addition to the joints, other organs of the body are inflamed—the lungs, skin, eyes, blood, nerves, kidneys, and even the heart. You feel lousy all over.

There doesn't appear to be any rhyme or reason why RA hits some joints and not others. Nor does it have anything to do with how you've used them over the years. It's a crapshoot as to whether it will be large joints such as the knees or smaller ones such as the hands, or both. Also, unlike OA, you may have a fever, you're apt to be tired, and your joints not only hurt but also are usually red, inflamed, swollen, and deformed. Another distinguishing characteristic of RA is that the joint involvement is symmetrical—that is, both sides of the body are similarly affected. For example, if your right knee is hot, swollen, and painful, your left one will be too. Although OA usually develops gradually, worsens slowly, and never clears up, RA often appears out of the blue, waxing and waning, abruptly going into remission. There are age and gender differences, too, between these forms of arthritis. OA is a complication of aging; the years take their toll on the joints. RA strikes younger people, usually twenty to fifty years of age, and sometimes even children. It's also three times more common in women than in men.

What is the process that makes your joints and the rest of you so miserable? Malfunction of the immune system. Something, whether it's genetic, environmental (possibly a virus or a bacterium), or hormonal, affects the immune system. So now, instead of protecting you, this defensive system gets its signals crossed and attacks your joints and other organs of the body. Stimulated perversely in this way, the immune system, instead of attacking hostile invaders and cancer cells, sends its "troops" into the joints. This irritates and inflames them, causing all the other problems that occur with RA. The cartilage is worn down (until the bones eventually rub against each other), the synovial lining makes more fluid, and the joint becomes red, swollen, painful, and, ultimately, deformed.

Diagnosing Rheumatoid Arthritis

The diagnosis of RA is not a difficult one. In addition to the symmetrical involvement of joints and their characteristic appearance and deformity, little bumps (nodules) may appear under the skin over bony areas such as the elbow and even in internal organs. Other evidence consists of an elevated sedimentation rate of the blood, a typical X-ray appearance of the joint, and a positive blood test called the *rheumatoid factor.* The latter isn't always present, and it can be detected in other conditions such as lupus and sarcostosis, but when your doctor strongly suspects RA, a positive rheumatoid factor supports the diagnosis. Sometimes fluid must be obtained from the swollen joint and analyzed to confirm the diagnosis. *If there is any question as to why your joints are diseased, insist on being tested for the rheumatoid factor and, if necessary, on fluid aspiration from a joint.*

Treating Rheumatoid Arthritis

Although they suffer from totally different conditions, RA and OA patients obtain pain relief from many of the same measures: rest and exercise, physiotherapy, and surgery. The same medications afford relief in both conditions. However, there is one big difference in the treatment of OA and RA. Whereas the basic medications for someone with OA are painkillers, which do nothing for the disorder itself, there are drugs for RA that modify the underlying disease process. Many of these are new and potentially toxic. Your doctor must be expert at dealing with them. *If you are diagnosed with rheumatoid arthritis, insist on being referred to a rheumatologist for this treatment.*

Specific Medications for Rheumatoid Arthritis

The following drugs fall into the category of *disease-modifying antirheumatic drugs* (DMARDs). They act on the immune system. When successful, they cause the disease to go into remission. They include:

- Oral corticosteroids, such as prednisone, should be avoided in osteoarthritis, but are often necessary in RA because they improve the underlying disease process. Take only the smallest effective dose for the shortest time possible. Remember that steroids have serious potential complications, including hypertension, diabetes, susceptibility to infection, impaired healing of wounds, osteoporosis, gastric ulcers, and mood changes, among many others.

- Antimalarial drugs such as hydroxychloroquine may control whatever it is that causes RA and put it into remission.

- Gold injections are not quite as popular as they once were because of the availability of other drugs that are less toxic and more effective. However, gold remains a reliable standby when other treatments have failed.

- There are three anticancer drugs currently prescribed for RA, and all of them are somewhat effective. Methotrexate (Rheumatrex) is the most widely used; the other two are azathioprine (Imuran) and cyclophosphamide (Cytoxan). They are given in smaller doses for RA than for cancer, and so do not produce the severe side effects usually associated with them. In doses used to treat cancer, these drugs kill the malignant cells. When prescribed for RA, they modify the behavior of the cells in the immune system but do not kill them. Methotrexate is usually taken once a week; azathioprine and cyclophosphamide are administered daily. Even in lower doses all these drugs can cause anemia, reduce the number of your white blood cells, and decrease your platelet count, making you vulnerable to bleeding. They can also damage the liver, lungs, and other organs. *Do not take these medications unless they're prescribed by someone experienced in their use. Also insist on the necessary examinations and blood tests to make sure they are not harming you.* But don't let these warnings scare you off and don't abandon these drugs before you've given them a chance to work. They are not painkillers, whose effect is apparent in minutes or hours. It may take several weeks before their full benefit is apparent.

However, don't take them for longer than four months if they haven't helped you by then. But if you do feel better, and you're able to tolerate them, you can continue them indefinitely.

- If you are unable to tolerate methotrexate or its results are not impressive, here's some good news. You can try leflunomide (Arava), approved by the FDA in 1998. Although it's not clear how this medication works, it appears to be at least as effective as methotrexate (and even better, according to some studies) in preventing erosion of the joints. Start with a loading dose of 100 milligrams a day for three days, then drop it to 20 mg per day. (You can even go as low as 10 mg if side effects force you to do so). Don't be impatient. It usually takes 4–8 weeks for Arava to work. This drug can hurt your liver, so be sure to have a blood count and liver function tests done every month, and don't take it if you're pregnant. If the liver is affected, it returns to normal after Arava use is stopped. This is an expensive drug, and some carriers may balk at providing it. *Insist on it if you need it.*

- The most exciting breakthrough in the fight against RA is the observation that tumor necrosis factor (TNF), a naturally occurring substance, is found in large quantities in affected joints where it causes inflammation. A number of drugs are now available that limit the production of TNF and have a beneficial effect on the course of RA. Their long-term safety is not yet established, and they can cause serious side effects such as pneumonia and other infections in vulnerable individuals. Overall, however, they present a major breakthrough. Again, they are expensive and insurers may not make them available to you. *If your RA is progressing and resistant to the other treatments insist on these new agents.*

- The most widely used TNF inhibitors at the time of writing are etanercept (marketed as Enbrel) and infliximab (Remicade). Etanercept (Enbrel), a human substance that binds TNF protein, can be used if other RA therapy has failed. When injected under the skin twice a week (most patients can do it themselves), it has been shown to cause improvement in more than 50 percent of patients with active RA (including children with the juvenile form of the disease). What's more, the benefit lasts for many months and can be documented on X rays of the affected joints. There is no increase in side effects when Enbrel is added to methotrexate. Infliximab (Remicade) is an injected monoclonal antibody that also binds TNF. Originally used in the treatment of inflammatory bowel disease, specifically Crohn's disease, it works well in RA, especially when combined with methotrexate, with which it should always be used. All TNF-blocking agents can cause serious infections especially among the elderly and those with a history of recurrent infection.
- Vitaxin is another antibody that may prove useful in the treatment of RA. It is being evaluated at the time of writing. Ask your doctor about it.
- Finally, an expert panel has recommended to the FDA that Kineret, a naturally occurring chemical called interleukin-1 receptor, be approved. In preliminary trials of more than 2,000 patients with RA, this drug significantly reduced joint pain and stiffness in a substantial number. Again, it may cause serious infection when combined with the TNF inhibitors.
- Another agent available to your doctor is penicillamine, a chelating agent (that is, a chemical that binds to other substances in the body and is excreted with them). It's most useful in eliminating excess copper, but also helps RA. However, it's not used much anymore because of its toxicity. Other agents are sulfasalazine (also prescribed

for inflammatory disease of the bowel), cyclosporine (widely used to prevent organ rejection), and minocycline, an antibiotic effective against mycoplasma that some doctors think may cause RA. Most rheumatologists don't agree, and this is a fringe drug at the moment.

- Sulfasalazine (Azulfidine) is also effective in several forms of arthritis because of its anti-inflammatory action. Do not use it if you're sensitive to sulfa.

No one can predict with certainty which of these medications will help you. You may have to try them one by one until you find what's best. In my own experience, prednisone and methotrexate are most effective.

Some practitioners prescribe antioxidants—especially those found in green tea and tart cherries—for anyone suffering from rheumatoid arthritis. Their polyphenols inhibit the COX-2 enzymes that trigger inflammation. (Black tea also contains polyphenols, but in smaller concentrations.) According to some researchers, twenty tart cherries have the same anti-inflammatory power as one aspirin. (When I read this report, I bought some tart cherries. Ugh! Very sour. I couldn't wait to take an aspirin.)

WHAT TO INSIST ON IF YOU HAVE ARTHRITIS

The term "arthritis" means "inflammation of a joint." There are about one hundred different kinds of arthritis, including those due to injury, infection, and gout. However, the two most common forms are osteoarthritis (OA) and rheumatoid arthritis (RA).

OA occurs mostly in older people and is basically the result of wear and tear and chronic injury to the joints over the years. However, genetic vulnerability probably plays a role as well. *If you have disabling osteoarthritis, insist on the proper tests and X rays to confirm the diagnosis; then insist on a referral to a physiotherapist or occupational therapist to prescribe the proper exercises that can permit you to continue to function (and work) as normally as possible.* If your physician is having difficulty in confirming a diagnosis, *insist on a second opinion from a rheumatologist or orthopedist.* Once the diagnosis is confirmed, treatment consists of the appropriate balance of rest and exercise, hot and cold preparations, physiotherapy, and painkillers, the most important of which are the anti-inflammatory drugs. There is no cure. *If surgery is recommended, insist on a second opinion before accepting the treatment.*

Rheumatoid arthritis has nothing to do with wear and tear. It's a disease of the immune system. No one knows what causes it, but there are many theories. The same therapy to obtain relief for OA is appropriate for RA. In addition, there is a group of drugs that can modify the underlying disease process. *If you have RA, insist on the appropriate blood tests and X rays to confirm this serious diagnosis. Once it's made, insist on a referral to a specialist in RA, a rheumatologist.* That's because the special medications now widely used in RA, and which in many cases can slow down the progress of the disease and put it into remission, are potentially toxic and dangerous. They do work, but they need to be carefully monitored by a specialist.

5

ASTHMA

When You Aim to Wheeze

Seventeen million Americans of all ages are asthmatic. Although most of them are over sixty-five, asthma also makes more kids sick than does any other illness, and accounts for more than 10 million lost school days every year. A third of all pediatric emergency room visits are from wheezing, breathless children with asthma. Both genders are equally affected, but asthma that begins after age twenty is more likely to occur in women.

To appreciate what an asthmatic *feels* like, do this: The next time you're outside on a very cold day, take a deep breath, hold it, and then try to inhale some more. You can't, and it feels terrible, which is why 2 million asthmatics rush to emergency rooms for relief every year.

What Is Asthma?

The term "asthma" comes from the Greek word for "panting." Asthmatics pant because their air passages, which start in the throat and end up in the lungs, become narrowed and sometimes almost completely obstructed. This is because they have become hypersensitive to certain "triggers" that inflame them, throw them into spasm, and fill them with mucus. Mucus is made by the lungs and is normally present in small amounts in the air passages. Its function is to trap tiny particles and bacteria and prevent them from getting into the lungs. Although small amounts of mucus are good for you, the massive globs that form in asthmatics are not. The muscles that surround the air passages further aggravate matters by going into spasm, compressing the already constricted airways even more. So asthmatics wheeze because their airways are narrowed, and they cough in order to try to get rid of the excess mucus.

Oxygen in the air we inhale enters little air sacs in the lungs called alveoli, from which it is transferred to the blood. These same alveoli receive carbon dioxide, a waste product of oxygen metabolism. When we exhale, the alveoli get rid of the stale carbon dioxide from the lungs. Asthmatics, whose airways are narrowed by spasm and mucus, can't expel all the waste air from their alveoli. Some remains trapped and as a result the alveoli become distended. Also, since the carbon-dioxide-rich air in the alveoli can no longer move freely out of the lungs and just sits there, the increased amounts of carbon dioxide back up into the blood. When they reach toxic levels, they are a major threat to health and life.

The *good* news about asthma is that we now have a better understanding of what causes it. There are many new drugs that can prevent attacks, and others to treat them. The *bad* news is that between 1982 and 1994 the prevalence of asthma increased 42 percent in men, 81 percent in women, and 160 percent in children. The annual death rate from asthma is now five thousand, almost twice what it was in 1979. I can only assume that's because many asthmatics are unaware of what can be done for them. However, the good news may be spreading because recently the mortality rate in kids has begun to drop slightly.

Asthma Triggers and How to Deal with Them

- Most cases of asthma are due to respiratory infections, especially in children and the elderly whose immune systems are weak. These infections may be viral (the flu) or bacterial (sinusitis). However, the kind of asthma they cause is usually short-lived and does not as a rule become chronic. I can't tell you how to prevent "catching a cold," but you can sharply reduce the chance of getting influenza by being vaccinated. The best time is in the fall just before the annual flu season starts. Get your shot even if you're not at "high risk." Just because you're not likely to die from the flu is no reason to not be vaccinated. But if you are at special risk (over sixty-five or suffering from some chronic disease), *insist* on being vaccinated. You should also receive a pneumonia shot every seven or eight years before age sixty-five, and only once after that. If you or your child does contract any respiratory illness, treat it vigorously, especially if there is an underlying allergy.

- Most asthmatics are allergic to something—mostly airborne particles such as pollens (which cause hay fever) and animal dander from pets. The prevalence of asthma in the inner cities is probably due to dust mites (which live in bedding, carpeting, upholstered furniture, and clothes), molds, and cockroach debris. Fifteen percent of asthma cases among adult males are due to exposure to industrial chemicals and contaminants. Find out what you're allergic to and, if possible, eliminate it from your environment. (Exposure can trigger an attack within twelve hours and sometimes in minutes.) Make your environment "user-friendly." For example, keep your windows closed during the pollen season and stay inside as much as you can. Don't use any strong scents, such as perfumes or aromatic candles. Keep your dogs outdoors if you can and certainly out of your bedroom. Put filters in the bedroom air vents to trap any dander that might otherwise get in. Wash your animals weekly to get rid of skin flakes and dried saliva. Since dust mites live in carpets, leave the floors bare in bedrooms. Ask someone to vacuum carpets for you so you don't subject yourself to the dust it stirs up, and have them cleaned every few months. Wash the kids' stuffed toys in hot water every week and keep them out of their beds. Cockroaches are a problem too, even dead ones. Get rid of them with traps or poison. Encase your pillows and mattresses with plastic to reduce the accumulation of dust. Try electronic devices that purify the air in your home and remove particles that may induce an attack. Some patients swear by them; others swear *at* them because they say they are costly and don't work very well.

- Chemicals in foods can also trigger an allergic reaction. The most important are sulfites added to prevent spoilage. Sulfites leave salads looking crisp and fresh even after they've been sitting around for hours. The FDA has banned their use on salad greens, peeled fruits, and guacamole. However, they are permitted in a wide variety of other foods, drinks, and even some medications. One of the great therapeutic ironies was that epinephrine, used in the treatment of a life-threatening asthmatic attack, often contained sulfites! I think they have all been removed, but to play it safe, whenever the doctor is preparing to give you an injection to relieve the symptoms of an acute asthmatic attack, ask what's in the syringe. If it's epinephrine, have someone double-check whether or not it contains sulfite. Sulfites may also be present in some antibiotics. Make sure that whatever drug you're being given to save your life doesn't end it! Read the labels carefully on all food products, especially wine, beer, and other beverages.

- Irritants such as smoke (from tobacco, fireplaces, aromatic candles, and industrial sources), gases, fumes, and a host of strong odors can induce asthmatic attacks. (A child growing up with a smoker in the house is at much greater risk of becoming asthmatic and is twice as vulnerable if a parent smokes ten cigarettes per day.) Ask your guests not to smoke. Get rid of wood-burning stoves and fireplaces.
- Exercise, especially in cold weather, can bring on an asthmatic attack by drying and cooling the airways, especially if you breathe rapidly through your mouth. Such attacks usually start within five or ten minutes, and symptoms peak about ten minutes after you've stopped exercising. If you must exercise in cold weather, cover your mouth and nose with a muffler or wear a face mask. Whenever you work out, get into the habit of breathing through the nose; this humidifies and warms the air to the respiratory passages. If you know that exercise makes you wheeze, there are medications (bronchodilators) you can take beforehand (more about specific therapy later).
- Sudden weather fluctuations can cause an asthmatic attack, especially if the change is from warm and sunny to cold and windy. Keep a scarf handy to cover your mouth. Wear clothes that can maintain your body's warmth. Temperature is not the only villain. A sharp increase in humidity can stir up dangerous air pollution and result in asthma. In summertime, children are especially vulnerable to abrupt increases in humidity that raise pollution caused by ozone, sulfur dioxide, or nitrogen oxide.
- A variety of painkillers ranging from aspirin to anti-inflammatory drugs (naproxen, ibuprofen, indomethacin, and the many others you probably know by such names as Advil, Aleve, Motrin, Voltaren) are an important cause of asthmatic attacks. Ten percent of asthmatics, especially those who have nasal polyps, get a wheezing attack

when they take even a single aspirin. So be sure to look carefully at the label of any product that might contain aspirin, such as many cold tablets, headache remedies (Fiorinal, Percodan), or products for the relief of menstrual cramps. The most recent products in this group, the COX-2 inhibitors, marketed as Vioxx, Celebrex, and a related drug, Mobic, may have less asthma-producing effects than the original NSAIDs. If you're at all vulnerable, use a nonaspirin painkiller such as aceteminophen, (Tylenol). If that's not strong enough, you may need a narcotic such as codeine or one of its derivatives. Beta-blockers (used in the treatment of heart disease, migraine, high blood pressure, and as drops for glaucoma) can also worsen asthma. Take one of the calcium channel blockers, such as verapamil, diltiazem, or nifedipine instead.

- Stomach reflux, acid backing up into your food pipe, can bring on an asthmatic attack. Reflux attacks occur mostly during the night while in bed. If this is happening to you, take your main meal at lunch, eat lightly at dinner, and have no food, tobacco, or liquids for two hours before you go to bed. (Caffeine helps prevent asthmatic attacks, but don't have it at night.) If you experience reflux, and especially if you also have a hiatus hernia, raise the head of your bed by putting blocks or a couple of big city telephone directories under the headboard posts. An antacid or an H_2-blocker such as ranitidine (Zantac) at bedtime can reduce the amount of acid reflux.

- Excitement and stress can bring on an asthma attack, probably by changing the normal breathing patterns. Thank goodness for "stress" and "viruses," though—the diagnostic scapegoats doctors use when they can't explain your symptoms. Stress probably does worsen asthma, but most doctors don't believe it actually causes it. A strong emotional reaction can affect the way you breathe, and presumably trigger an asthmatic attack.

- If one of your parents has asthma, there's a 25 percent chance that you will too. A positive family history also leaves you more vulnerable to other allergies even if you don't actually develop asthma.
- Premature infants are at great risk for asthma because their lungs are not yet functioning normally.

Symptoms of Asthma

Several warning signs often precede the full-blown asthmatic attack by a few hours. Here's what to look for:

- Unusual fatigue
- Tight feeling in the chest
- Dry mouth
- The need to breathe through your mouth
- Sudden coughing
- Rapid heartbeat
- Anxiety and irritability for no special reason
- Itchy throat
- Perspiration even when the room temperature is comfortable

Once an asthma attack starts, breathing (especially exhaling) becomes difficult; you're short of breath; you cough, sometimes in "fits," as you try to spit up the mucus (a losing battle); you may break out into a sweat; your chest feels tight; your pulse rises; and you're anxious.

The first fifteen minutes of the attack are the worst, after which the symptoms usually subside within a couple of hours. However, they sometimes start up again within eight hours, and may last for days. This "late asthmatic response" is due to chemicals released by the allergic process.

Confirming the Diagnosis

You don't have to be a genius to recognize an asthmatic attack. The wheezing, coughing, and labored breathing are
giveaways. Still, *every asthmatic should have pulmonary function tests to determine the severity of the condition and the best
treatment for it. Insist on them.* No matter how experienced
your doctor, a physical exam alone is not enough. That's why
the National Heart, Blood and Lung Institute's (NHLBI) guidelines call such testing essential.

Evaluating lung function is as simple as it is important. The
easiest way to do it is with a *peak flow meter*—a simple plastic
cylinder with a mouthpiece at one end and a hole at the other.
It is calibrated along its side and contains a movable marker.
You take a deep breath and then blow into the mouthpiece as
hard and as fast as you can. This shifts the marker's location on
the scale, indicating the peak expiratory flow rate (PEF) and
how well you're moving air through the air passages. It can
also assess the effectiveness of your medication. You can buy
one of these little devices and test yourself after your doctor,
the nurse, or a pharmacist has taught you how to use it.

A *spirometer* is more sophisticated than a peak flow meter.
It's what doctors use. These units are connected to a graph or
even a computer to measure and analyze the different phases
of respiration.

If you're asthmatic, it's as important for you to check your
peak flow regularly as it is for a diabetic to monitor the blood
sugar or for someone with hypertension to keep track of
blood pressure. You should do it in the morning before taking your medication, and again during the day. This tells you
how effective your treatment is and can also predict an attack
even before symptoms develop.

Preventing the Attack

Always be on the alert to control or eliminate the various triggers that can precipitate an asthmatic attack. That's often not possible, but *if you're allergic to something in your environment that you simply can't avoid, insist on being desensitized to it by an allergist.* It takes time and money, but it's worth it. Ask your doctor to refer you.

You may have to take medications even when you're symptom-free in order to prevent an attack. The most widely used drugs for this purpose are:

- Inhaled corticosteroids (beclomethasone, flunisolide, fluticasone, budesonide) not only treat acute asthma, as you will see below, but are the most effective preventives and are often used on an ongoing basis when the condition is persistent, whether mild, moderate, or severe. They reduce inflammation within the air passages. However, they can cause hoarseness and yeast infections of the throat. *So rinse your mouth* and *gargle after every inhalation,* and don't swallow the water; spit it out.
- Salmeterol (Servent) is a long-acting beta-agonist, a bronchodilator that keeps the airways open by relaxing the muscles surrounding them. Beta-agonists are also widely used to *prevent* attacks caused by an allergy or by exercise, not to treat them. They work too slowly. They are usually inhaled twice a day. If your asthma is triggered by exercise, it's a good idea to take a bronchodilator (see below) *before* you start.
- Cromolyn (Intal) a "mast cell stabilizer" was once more widely used than it is these days. Here's how it works: When you're exposed to something to which you're allergic, mast cells present in certain tissues release histamine, a chemical that makes you itch and wheeze, gives

you a runny nose, and constricts the airways. Cromolyn can prevent the release of histamine. And here's an important practical tip: Rinse your mouth immediately after inhaling cromolyn and then drink a few sips of water. This will prevent the cough that cromolyn sometimes causes. It may take six weeks before cromolyn works. If you're using it with an inhaled beta-agonist, take the latter first.

Cromolyn and salmeterol are strictly preventives. Never use them to treat an acute attack.

Treating the Attack Itself

Every asthmatic attack is a potential emergency. Have all your medications with you at all times and use them the moment you get any of asthma's warning signs. If they don't seem to be working, and especially if your breathing becomes difficult, or you have trouble walking or talking, or your lips and fingernails are turning blue, *call your doctor and insist that he or she see you immediately.* If it's after office hours, go to the nearest hospital emergency room. And when you get the bill, *insist that your insurance carrier pays for it.*

Drugs to treat the acute attack fall into several different categories, each of which targets a different symptom. Bronchodilators break the spasm and widen the airways when you're wheezing; if you're choked up with mucus, there are drugs such as guaifenesin and glyceryl guaiacolate (Robitussin, Humibid) to loosen the mucus so that you can bring it up and spit it out. (But don't take codeine to suppress the cough. That will make it difficult to get rid of the mucus. What's more, codeine, present in many cough preparations, can make you sleepy and reduce the depth of your breathing.) Drugs that decrease the inflammation in and around the air passages afford relief too. Finally, if you have an underlying respiratory infection, you should take the appropriate antibiotic.

Bearing these categories and actions in mind, here are the various asthma treatments at your disposal. Keep in mind that no two asthma patients respond to treatment in the same way, even to the same drug. It's often a matter of trial and error. At the very onset of an asthma attack, you should follow these steps:

1. Take a short-acting *bronchodilator* in a "whiffer" or nebulizer or spacer to reduce the constriction of the airways. (A nebulizer contains pressurized air that converts a liquid into a fine mist to be inhaled. A spacer, which I prefer, is a holding chamber into which you insert the mouthpiece of the nebulizer. The contents of the nebulizer go into the chamber instead of directly into your mouth. This prevents the medication from ending up on your tongue and causing yeast infections. You inhale the contents of the spacer in two or three deep breaths.) I prefer the short-acting beta$_2$-agonist albuterol (Ventolin). It takes from five to fifteen minutes to work. Two puffs usually last four to six hours. The main side effects of albuterol are nervousness, a rapid heart rate, and insomnia. Ventolin is probably all you'll need for a mild attack. The newest entry in the field is Advair Diskus, inhaled twice a day. It consists of a combination of a steroid and a bronchodilator. Beta-agonists (albuterol), theophylline, and ipratropium (Atrovent) are the main bronchodilators. They are most effective when inhaled because they go right to the lung, work within five minutes, and their effect persists for about three hours. In liquid or tablet form they take about thirty minutes to work, but they last for up to six hours. Don't take theophylline on an empty stomach or with hot food. It comes in tablets, liquids, or capsules and you need a dose every eight to twelve hours. If you miss one, don't double up on the next one. If you take any of these preparations too often, or in higher doses than recommended, they can all cause rapid heartbeat, headache, nervousness, and nausea.

2. If the attack is really severe, you may have to resort to *anti-inflammatory agents* such as steroids, and the more recent leukotriene receptor antagonists. High doses of oral steroids can be effective. Don't take them casually because they can cause high blood pressure, diabetes, osteoporosis, skin problems, reduced growth in children, fluid retention, weight gain, gastric ulcers, and hip problems over the long term.

Leukotriene modifiers or receptor antagonists (zafirlukast, zileuton, montelukast) are the latest addition to the antiasthmatic armamentarium. They block the action of leukotrienes, chemicals produced by the immune system during an acute asthmatic attack. They are not usually as effective as inhaled steroids and are usually combined with other drugs.

After the asthmatic attack, take inhaled steroids two or more times a day for a couple of weeks to reduce the inflammation.

WHEN YOU'RE PREGNANT AND ASTHMATIC

If you're asthmatic and become pregnant, there's no way to predict how your chronic asthma will behave—it may worsen, remain unaffected, or clear up for the duration. The safest medications, if you need them, are the inhaled corticosteroids and albuterol. However, their repeated use does raise the possibility of premature birth, low birth weight, and even stillbirth. Nevertheless, failing to end the attack as quickly as possible is a greater threat to your baby than almost any medication needed to do so.

WHAT TO INSIST ON IF YOU HAVE ASTHMA

Asthma affects 17 million Americans. Attacks can occur suddenly and without any real warning. There are preventive strategies you can follow if you are diagnosed with asthma. If you have asthma, *insist on the following:*

- An annual flu shot
- Pneumonia vaccine (the frequency depends on your age)
- Pulmonary function tests once the diagnosis is made. A doctor listening to your chest with a stethoscope is not enough to assess the severity of your asthma or how it should best be treated.

Most family practitioners and internists can manage your asthma. However, you should *insist on being referred to a specialist when:*

- You've been rushed to the hospital with a life-threatening attack.
- The attacks continue despite all the treatment plans prescribed by your doctor.
- There is any question about the diagnosis or the cause of your asthma.
- You need allergy shots or desensitization from an allergist.
- You have chronic sinusitis or nasal polyps that should be treated by a nose and throat specialist.

6

ATRIAL FIBRILLATION

When in Your Heart You're Not a Regular Guy

This may come as a surprise to you, but the heart has nothing to do with romance. It's a pump whose sole function is to keep us alive, whether or not we're in love. Normally, it beats regularly, like a metronome, anywhere from sixty to one hundred times a minute (usually between seventy and eighty). Each time it does so, it squeezes out its blood, whose oxygen and other nutrients supply every organ and tissue in the body. The term "arrhythmia" means that the rhythm of the heart is abnormal—too fast, too slow, and/or irregular.

There are many different kinds of rhythm disturbance. Some develop for no apparent reason. You may be completely unaware of them, or they may be annoying and simply make you a little uncomfortable, they may be very troublesome, or they may cause sudden death. However, they are usually innocent and not a threat to your life. The most common example of a harmless variation in rhythm is one that we all experience from time to time, the so-called extra beat. (It's not really extra; it occurs earlier than it should, and so feels like an additional contraction.) The troublesome and dangerous arrhythmias are usually due to disease of the heart or some other organ. In such cases, the heart may beat much too quickly, so that there isn't enough time to rest between beats and fill up again with blood. Or it may beat too slowly, in which case vital body organs aren't nourished adequately.

Atrial fibrillation (AF) is best described as an irregularly irregular heartbeat, in which the irregularity does not follow a pattern. It is the most common significant cardiac arrhythmia reported to doctors. More than 2 million Americans are "fibrillators," more men than women. The older you are, the more vulnerable you become to it, so that about one person in ten over the age of eighty has a fibrillating heart. Although regular vigorous exercise is good for you, people who do so are more likely to develop AF. (But don't let this keep you from working out. The benefits of exercise far outweigh this relatively small risk of its causing fibrillation). It's interesting that a recent celebrity fibrillator, former Senator Bill Bradley, was a basketball star. One important point: Don't confuse atrial fibrillation with *ventricular* fibrillation. The former is a chronic condition which, if treated properly, allows you to live an essentially normal life; the latter can be fatal within minutes.

AF becomes news when someone famous is reported to have it. For example, in addition to Bill Bradley, Presidents George H. Bush and Richard Nixon were also treated for it. You may not know you have AF until it's diagnosed during a routine exam, or it produces very troublesome symptoms. It may be due to serious disease of either the heart or some other system of the body, or it may develop for no apparent reason; it may be chronic and continuous, or it may come and go. *No matter into which category your AF falls, it must be thoroughly evaluated to determine what treatment is indicated. Insist on it.*

In order for you to understand why this is so, and the logic behind the treatment of AF, I need to remind you of some basic cardiac anatomy.

The heart has four chambers—two upper ones called *atria* and two lower ones, the *ventricles*. The atria contract only gently, just enough to move the blood that flows through them into the ventricles, which do the main pumping (the right ventricle sends blood to the lungs; the left supplies the rest of the body).

An electrical sequence of events that begins in the right atrium initiates each heartbeat. A signal (doctors call it an impulse) spreads along an electrical network from the right atrium to the ventricles, causing them to contract. However, in someone with AF, instead of producing a single impulse in a regular manner and at a reasonable rate, the atria beat wildly and rapidly, almost quivering, hundreds of times a minute, helter-skelter, without any pattern. The network of specialized tissue that is designed to carry the signal down to the ventricles in an orderly way is so overwhelmed by the sheer number of these impulses that it can't conduct all of them to the ventricles. However, too many do get through, and the pumping chambers respond by beating much too rapidly, thus reducing the amount of blood ejected with each beat. Also, when the atria beat so rapidly, they don't have time to empty completely. The residual blood within them stagnates, forming clots. When one of these clots slips down into the left ventricle and leaves it during a contraction, it can end up in any part of the body, blocking an artery to a vital organ and cutting off its blood supply. In the brain this causes a stroke. In fact, atrial fibrillation is the leading cause of embolic stroke (the brain is damaged by a traveling blood clot, or embolus) and accounts for some 75,000 strokes in this country every year. Twenty-three percent of these people die, and almost half are left disabled, much more so than from stroke due to other causes, in which the mortality rate is only 8 percent. So atrial fibrillation is dangerous on several accounts: It can exhaust the heart, cause a heart attack, and produce traveling clots in arteries anywhere in the body, most critically the brain.

Here's one scenario of how you might discover that you have atrial fibrillation. You wake up one morning and your heart is going a mile a minute. You may feel weak, dizzy, light-headed, or faint; you may be short of breath or experience chest pain or pressure. If you know how to take your pulse, you find that it's fast—possibly too fast to count—and totally irregular; some beats are stronger than others. You have the feeling (and if you don't, you will after reading this chapter) that this is something you should see your doctor about.

In another common presentation, your doctor surprises you with the diagnosis of atrial fibrillation during a routine checkup.

In either case, your doctor will proceed to investigate what caused it and how best to treat it.

Causes of Atrial Fibrillation

Evaluation of your atrial fibrillation will lead to one of its following causes:

- No apparent reason. Of course, there's always a reason why someone develops atrial fibrillation, but we sometimes can't find it. When that happens, we call it lone atrial fibrillation. I remember being consulted many years ago as to whether one of our astronauts should be allowed to go into outer space despite his lone atrial fibrillation. Other cardiologists and I agreed that he should, and he did—uneventfully.

- Heart disease of some kind or another, the most common causes being coronary artery disease, long-standing high blood pressure, valvular disease (most frequently involving the mitral valve on the left side of the heart), or an abnormality of the heart muscle (cardiomyopathy). Other less common cardiac disorders can also result in atrial fibrillation, as can any form of heart surgery. In the latter case, the arrhythmia is usually transient.

- An overactive thyroid gland. This gland sets the body's metabolism level (see Chapter 38). Too much thyroid hormone makes everything hyper, including the heart rate. This sometimes include atrial fibrillation.

Regardless of why the fibrillation came about, it is a threat to health and life and is a number one treatment priority. Left alone, it can cause heart failure, stroke, and in some cases death.

Treatment of Atrial Fibrillation

Treatment of atrial fibrillation requires a simultaneous two-pronged approach. The doctor must first determine the underlying cause and deal with it. At the same time, he or she must slow the heart rate, attempt to normalize rhythm, and thin the blood (anticoagulation) so as to prevent clots from forming.

If there is no obvious reason for the fibrillation—that is, if you have lone atrial fibrillation—treatment consists of the various drugs and electrical techniques described below, all of which are calculated to terminate the abnormal rhythm and/or slow the heart rate. However, regardless of the reason, and even if one is not apparent, *everyone who is fibrillating must have an echocardiogram in addition to the blood tests including thyroid function, and an electrocardiogram. Insist on it.*

- Your AF may be due to too much coffee, alcohol, excessive amounts of thyroid hormone, weight-control medications, decongestants, or other cardiac stimulants.

If so, you must stop them, or at least reduce their dosage.

- If one or more of your heart valves are diseased, and the overall situation warrants it, you may be advised to have the valve repaired or replaced if it is affecting your health in other ways. If you have some other form of heart disease that may be causing or contributing to your arrhythmia, it should be treated.
- If you have an overactive thyroid gland (see Chapter 38), and it is corrected by drugs (propylthiouracil), radioactive iodine, or surgery, the AF may disappear.

The first treatment priority in all cases is to terminate the fibrillation, especially if it is causing chest pain or shortness of breath. *The longer the arrhythmia is allowed to continue, the less likely it is to be successfully converted to regular rhythm.* So rule number one is to see your doctor as soon as you're aware that your pulse is irregular.

Here is the treatment sequence I usually follow in my own practice:

If my patient and I are both absolutely certain that the fibrillation has been *present for no longer than forty-eight hours,* and especially if the heart can't tolerate it (severe chest pain, dangerously low blood pressure, heart failure, excessive fatigue, loss of consciousness), I perform electrical "cardioversion" (electroconversion) in the hospital. You're given a very short-acting anesthetic (from which you awake in a few moments), and two paddles on the chest wall deliver a synchronized electric shock to the heart. Most patients can go home the same day. I then prescribe one of the medications discussed below to prevent the fibrillation from recurring.

If you prefer to try medication rather than electroconversion (a reasonable choice if the arrhythmia is not too troublesome, since many cases convert to normal rhythm spontaneously within twenty-four hours), any one of the following drugs can be used: flecainide, propafenone, quinidine, dispyramide, procainamide, sotalol, amiodarone, and two newer ones, ibutilide and dofetilide. The right one for you should be decided by a cardiologist experienced in treating rhythm disorders because some should not be used if you have a structural disorder of the heart (flecainide, propafenone) and others can induce an even more serious arrhythmia. You should be hospitalized if they are used (quinidine, procainamide, disopryamide, dofetilide, sotalol).

If your AF is of recent onset, there is a 60 to 90 percent chance of regaining normal cardiac rhythm with these drugs. However, when the arrhythmia has been present for longer than forty-eight hours, that likelihood drops to 30 percent. What's more, all these rhythm-normalizing drugs have potentially dangerous side effects that range from making it difficult for you to urinate to causing malfunction of the lungs, liver, and thyroid. However, their most serious threat is inducing a life-threatening abnormality in the ventricle. So you must be carefully monitored as long while you're taking them.

If the fibrillation has been present *for more than two days,* immediately restoring normal rhythm can dislodge a blood clot (embolus) that may already have formed in the atria and send it on its way to the brain. In such cases, I first thin the blood (anticoagulation) with warfarin (Coumadin), which the patient continues for about three or four weeks, after which it is safe to perform the electroconversion. During this waiting period, I prescribe drugs that reduce the heart rate to an acceptable level. The best agents for this purpose are verapamil (a calcium channel blocker), a beta-blocker such as propranolol, metoprolol, or atenolol, and digoxin.

If the situation requires immediate electroconversion because the patient simply can't tolerate the arrhythmia, and we can't wait three or four weeks for the anticoagulant to provide the necessary protection against an embolus, we can actually look into the heart to see if a clot is present in the atria. This is done by means of a *transesophageal echocardiogram.* This differs from the usual echocardiogram in that you have to swallow a probe attached to a string. It is lowered into the food pipe to lie adjacent to the heart, and from this vantage point the interior of the heart can be viewed more accurately. If there is no clot, one can proceed with the conversion attempt.

Some patients are resistant to every treatment and continue to fibrillate. In such cases, they usually have to live with their arrhythmia. I have many such patients, one of whom was Herbert Lehman, the former governor and senator from New York. He developed AF when he was fifty-four years old and lived an active, normal life until his death at age eighty-six. However, when AF is chronic, one must ensure that the heart does not beat too quickly. Some patients are so sensitive to these heart-slowing drugs that the dosage required to prevent it from racing can also leave it beating too slowly. You're then between a rock and a hard place. The only solution is to implant a pacemaker that will prevent the heart rate from falling too low yet at the same time making sure it doesn't go sky-high.

In addition to controlling the heart rate, the blood must be thinned as long as the fibrillation persists. The most effective blood thinner is warfarin. If you can't tolerate warfarin, aspirin is your next best choice, but no drug prevents embolism as effectively as does warfarin. The downside to using warfarin is that you need to have your blood checked regularly, usually every three to four weeks, to make sure that, like Goldilocks, the dosage you're taking is not too much, leaving you vulnerable to internal hemorrhage, or too little, allowing clots to form.

Several invasive approaches are also now available to help control the rapid rate of atrial fibrillation. Basically, they all interfere with the transmission of the stimulus from the atria to the ventricles. This requires interrupting the pathways between the upper and lower chambers of the heart (the atria and the ventricles) in some way. This can be done by an open-heart surgical procedure (called the maze operation) that cuts into the right and left atria and creates scar tissue in these chambers, isolating them electrically. I never recommend this operation because I feel it's much more risky than leaving things alone.

The electrical pathways along which the impulses travel from the atria to the ventricles can also be "ablated"—that is, rendered incapable of transmitting the signal. This is done by directing radio waves at them by a thin flexible wire introduced through a vein at the groin. This is a nonsurgical approach and the one that's most widely used at this time. However, you should know that you will need to have a pacemaker implanted in the event that your heart ends up beating too slowly. If your fibrillation comes and goes, you can have an atrial defibrillator implanted that detects the arrhythmia and sends low-level shocks to the atria to restore normal rhythm. However, in the real world of cardiology, most chronic fibrillators are simply maintained on drugs that control that heart rate along with anticoagulants. In my experience, you can lead a virtually normal life with this irregular cardiac rhythm.

WHAT TO INSIST ON IF YOU HAVE ATRIAL FIBRILLATION

Atrial fibrillation is a common disturbance of cardiac rhythm in which the upper chambers of the heart, the atria, beat rapidly and irregularly. The ventricles, the main pumps of the heart, receive too many of these impulses and beat too quickly. This may weaken the heart and cause it to "fail." Blood within these "quivering" atria may stagnate and form clots, which, if expelled from the heart, can result in a stroke.

If you develop atrial fibrillation, insist on a thorough evaluation to determine its cause. This should include

*an echocardiogram, in addition to the standard car-
diac examination. If the arrhythmia is of very recent
onset (within a day or two), insist on an attempt to convert it to normal rhythm. Do not accept a laissez-faire
attitude to this condition, and make sure that everything has been done to correct it. You must insist on a
consultation with a cardiologist, preferably one who
specializes in rhythm disorders.*

Regardless of the cause of the fibrillation, this rhythm
disorder can have serious consequences and must be
treated. *Insist on it.* The therapy consists of restoring
normal rhythm either by electric shock (electroconversion) or with medications. The latter do not always
"convert" the arrhythmia and are associated with a high
incidence of side effects. You must therefore be carefully monitored while taking them. There are several
other procedures for controlling the rate of the fibrillation, but they are currently being performed in only a
minority of patients.

When atrial fibrillation becomes chronic, the blood
must be thinned to prevent clots from breaking off and
traveling to various organs, notably the brain. Such anticoagulation must be continued as long as the heart is
fibrillating. *Insist on it.*

It is possible to lead a virtually normal life with atrial
fibrillation as long as the rate at which the ventricles respond to the rapidly beating atria is controlled.

7

CHRONIC FATIGUE SYNDROME

Give Me Your Tired, Your Poor, Your Huddled Masses

The most common health complaint I hear from adults of both genders (other than why their insurance carrier won't pay for a particular test or treatment) is "Why am I so tired and what can I do about it?" Most healthy people feel "wiped out" now and then—usually for an obvious reason such as lack of sleep, perhaps because of a large prostate that has nature calling them too often during the night, a hangover, anxiety, depression, or jet lag. Once the cause is identified and corrected, energy is restored.

However, if you remain exhausted day in, day out, for weeks on end for no apparent reason, no matter how much you rest or how long you sleep, your body is telling you that something is wrong. Don't ignore that signal! There are many possible reasons for the way you feel, and a careful, thorough workup will almost always reveal the answer to your problem. *If it's not forthcoming, insist on such an evaluation.*

There is a unique kind of fatigue—a bone-breaking tiredness that keeps you in bed even after a good night's sleep;

wears you out no matter how much you rest; depletes you of the energy you need to work or play.

You want some explanation from your doctor for the way you feel. However, after scores of tests at a cost of thousands of dollars, he or she has no answer. Every conceivable exam is "normal."

You can't believe there's no medical reason for the way you feel. Under pressure and embarrassed, your doctor is apt to fall back on one or more of the popular wastebasket diagnoses, the most common being "a virus of some kind" that will run its course, and you're likely to be given "potent" vitamins; if you're sick enough, you'll get them by vein. But vitamins don't help either. Hypoglycemia (low blood sugar) is another favorite diagnosis of desperation. You're given a low-carbohydrate, high-protein diet. You feel no better. Now it's time to implicate *Candida* (a yeast infection) and treat you for that. Still no results. By this time, you've probably changed doctors. Your new physician reviews your record very carefully and proudly points out something that was obviously missed by his predecessors and that explains everything. You have Epstein-Barr antibodies in your blood. Nonsense! These antibodies are present in 95 percent of Americans and merely reflect the fact that at some time in the past you had infectious mononucleosis. A third doctor may conclude that you suffer from "total allergy" (whatever that is) and that you must be desensitized to virtually everything. If you're foolish (or desperate) enough to go that route, you'll be disappointed. Finally, after all leads are exhausted, you may well be referred to a psychiatrist for your "depression."

The truth is that none of these diagnoses is accurate and none of the treatments for them will help you one iota. I'm not being critical of these doctors. They're desperate for a label, any label, because they honestly believe that a real "condition" would have yielded some detectable abnormality in one or more of the multiple tests they performed. The fact that none of them were positive raises the possibility that the problem is all in your head.

The scenario of a severely and chronically tired patient who tests normal to everything is so common that in 1988 in this country, some doctors decided to give it a name—chronic fatigue syndrome (CFS) and designated it a "real" illness. However, American-trained physicians have always been hesitant to name something they don't understand. Many of us resisted accepting CFS as a viable diagnosis. I was one of them. But I've changed my mind. I'm now convinced that CFS does exist and is probably due to some derangement of the immune system, possibly triggered by an as-yet-unidentified virus, or is an allergy, or the result of some hormonal imbalance. Despite the dissenters, the medical establishment officially legitimized CFS in 1993, although its cause or causes remain a mystery.

Symptoms of CFS

Although there are no reliable statistics concerning the incidence of CFS, I suspect that hundreds of thousands of Americans suffer from it. It can strike anyone at any age, but is two to four times more common in women of childbearing age, most of whom are white and middle-income.

CFS often sets in after some infection such as the flu, a stomach virus, or a bout of diarrhea. In some patients it follows an emotional crisis.

CFS causes more than just profound exhaustion. There are other symptoms too. For example, most of these patients are depressed (and who can blame them, feeling the way they do?). But their depression is the result and not the cause of the symptoms. They are often achy with a low-grade fever and feel like they have the flu; their blood pressure is apt to be low; their memory poor; they have trouble thinking clearly; they tend to be irritable; they complain of headaches, frequent sore throat, and tender, enlarged glands in the neck and armpit. Some also suffer joint and muscle pain, and may be diagnosed with fibromyalgia, an equally mysterious disorder (see Chapter 12), or Gulf War syndrome—both of which many believe have some relationship to CFS.

Making the Diagnosis

There is no specific test for CFS. It's not like diabetes that's diagnosed by a high blood sugar, or hepatitis with its abnormal liver function tests, or heart trouble by changes in the ECG. Your doctor takes a detailed history, performs a thorough physical exam, and obtains a battery of blood tests looking for evidence of a number of diseases. Specifically, you'll be checked for sleep apnea (which leaves one tired the next day because sleep is so disturbed during the night), a major depression, an underactive thyroid gland, adverse reaction to some medication, a hidden cancer, massive obesity (Dickens first described the sleepiness due to excessive fat in his Pickwick papers, a condition doctors still call the pickwickian syndrome), chronic alcohol or substance abuse, HIV infection, or some immune disorder. If all these tests come back normal, you are said to have chronic fatigue syndrome, a diagnosis of exclusion.

The formal requirements for the diagnosis of CFS are:

- Fatigue that persists or recurs for at least six months
- The exclusion of any other condition that might account for the fatigue
- The distinct onset over a period of hours or days of at least four of the following symptoms that persist for at least six months: severe exhaustion, low-grade fever, sore throat, painful lymph nodes, generalized muscle

weakness and aches, prolonged fatigue after exercise, joint pains, generalized headaches, disturbed sleep, nervous system complaints such as memory loss, inability to concentrate, and irritability.

I've heard it said that CFS is a "yuppie" disease, something peculiar to this generation and to our society. Yet many CFS equivalents are described in the medical literature of yesteryear. For example, in a medical textbook published in 1750, an English doctor named Sir Richard Manningham described what he called "febricula" (little fever) characterized by unusual tiredness, low-grade fever, but few objective findings. Other doctors have reported malaise and indisposition due to the "vapors" (whatever that was supposed to mean). Soldiers unable to cope with the stress of battle were said to have "the effort syndrome" or "soldier's heart." When you read some of these descriptions, they sound remarkably like what today we refer to as chronic fatigue syndrome.

What's the course of a typical case of CFS? Some patients recover completely; others get better for a while and then relapse in cycles. In several studies some did recover within five years, but most did not.

Possibly Effective Measures

Despite what some entrepreneurs would have you believe, there is no proven treatment for CFS. However, there are some measures that may alleviate your symptoms:

- Eliminate any food or medication to which you are allergic.
- Avoid any activity that tires you except gentle home-based exercises prescribed by your doctor or a qualified physiotherapist.

- If you have flulike symptoms (headache, low-grade fever, joint and muscle aches) take aspirin, Tylenol, or one of the nonsteroidal anti-inflammatory agents (NSAIDs).
- Antidepressants may improve sleep and reduce fatigue and muscle pain.
- Some doctors have claimed success using Tagamet, an antiulcer drug in an attempt to strengthen the immune system, but this therapy is still experimental.
- Intravenous gamma globulin has been tried with questionable success. But it's worth looking into.
- Make sure you're eating "healthy." This is no time for fad diets. Emphasize whole grains, beans, rice, fish, fresh fruits and vegetables, and take it easy on alcohol and high-fat foods. I advise my patients to have liberal amounts of garlic (either fresh cloves or the commercial extracts), because garlic is said to stimulate the immune system. There is no proof that it does so, but it can't hurt to take it.

Complementary Medicine

Since conventional medicine has so little to offer in the way of specific treatment for CFS, a number of alternative approaches have been suggested. You should try them, but let your doctor know you're doing so.

Acupuncture and acupressure are said to be successful in some cases. There's no harm in trying them.

Various herbs have been reported to improve CFS, but the evidence is anecdotal. The most popular ones are echinacea, goldenseal, milk thistle, and ginseng. Chinese herbalists have their own concoctions that they say help. Try them if you're desperate.

Various mind-body approaches have been used, including tai chi, meditation, relaxation, guided imagery, qigong, and yoga. They increase your energy level by reducing stress, and I recommend them.

WHAT TO INSIST ON IF YOU HAVE CHRONIC FATIGUE SYNDROME

Chronic fatigue syndrome is a real disease whose cause is unknown and for which there is no specific treatment. As a result, many insurance companies refuse to pay for its care. *Insist that they do!* Although the medical establishment has formally listed the criteria for diagnosing CFS, it remains a diagnosis of exclusion. That means that every other possible cause of the profound fatigue and other symptoms described above must be ruled out. *Insist on such a complete evaluation before accepting the diagnosis.*

Some doctors take advantage of the frustration felt by patients with CFS and exploit them with a wide variety of expensive but worthless therapies. *Here is one instance when you should not insist that you be reimbursed for them.*

If your doctor is unable to reach a diagnosis or does not believe that CFS is a real condition, insist on a second opinion by another physician or a specialist.

8

DEPRESSION

When There's No Light at the End of the Tunnel

Depression is the "common cold of mental illness." Thirty million Americans are chronically "sad"—twice as many women as men, rich and poor alike. Although depression occurs more frequently in older people, children are also plagued by it, and suicide is the leading cause of death among teenagers and young adults in this country.

Most depressed people, when they finally decide to seek help, first consult their physician rather than a psychotherapist. Your doctor can determine whether your problem is due to a physical disorder or is of purely psychiatric or emotional origin. In the latter event, there is a plethora of effective new medications with which to treat depression, regardless of its cause. Your doctor will refer you for psychiatric care if you need it.

Although there are elaborate classifications of depression, for practical purposes there are basically two main types. In the first, there is some obvious reason for your melancholy, but you may be overreacting to it—and for too long. For example, you may have lost a loved one or are in the midst of a nasty divorce. Perhaps you are out of a job and in financial straits, or you may be very sick and fearful of dying. You may recently be menopausal, have a drug or alcohol problem, or be suffering from seasonal affective disorder (SAD), in which the darkness of winter precipitates depression. Or your depression may be due to the most treatable of all reasons—a drug you're taking, anything from an antibiotic to a birth control pill to a blood-pressure-lowering agent. The problem, whatever it is, appears to you to be insurmountable.

A depression with such an identifiable cause is obviously the best kind to have. Most people eventually "snap out of it" with or without professional help. The cause of their sadness may have cleared up, or they've learned to cope with it, or they're responding to an antidepressant that their doctor prescribed.

The other kind of depression comes on for no apparent reason. You may be sitting on top of the world as far as everyone else is concerned, but for you, the future is bleak. There is no light at the end of the tunnel—and you don't know why. This type of depression may be part of a cyclical manic-depressive disorder that's full of ups and downs. One day you're wildly stimulated, full of energy, and things couldn't be better. You're sure that Sophia Loren loves you and you plan to fly to Europe to visit her. But then your mood swings to the other end of the spectrum—you're so down that all you can think about is suicide.

Depression isn't always obvious to others. Some people can hide the way they feel. But even if they appear to be functioning normally, their depression stifles spontaneity and creativity; it hurts interpersonal relationships with family, friends, and coworkers. If it persists long enough, it almost inevitably causes physical symptoms such as weight loss or weight gain, a poor appetite or an insatiable one, fatigue, irritability, stomach problems, impotence and lack of libido, insomnia—you name it. If it's bad enough, you'll harbor suicidal thoughts or even try to end it all, as sixteen thousand succeed in doing every year in the United States.

Are You Depressed?

How do you know if you're seriously depressed and not just temporarily down in the dumps? According to the latest edition of the American Psychiatric Association's *Diagnostic and Statistical Manual,* you have a *major* depression if you've had any *four* of the following symptoms for at least two weeks:

- Sleep is a big problem. You either have severe insomnia, tossing and turning all night, or you're sleeping all the time.
- Either you have no appetite or you can't stop eating.
- You have no interesting in doing anything or seeing anybody.
- You feel worthless and guilty, and you know there's no hope for you.
- You have trouble concentrating, and you can't make decisions.
- Suicidal thoughts run through your mind, and you've even tried to end it all.
- You realize that you're sad, but you just can't snap out of it.
- You're pessimistic about your future and life in general.

It doesn't take a professional to recognize these major symptoms. However, here are some others that should also ring a warning bell:

- You've started writing things down because your memory has become so poor, even though you're not yet fifty.

- You're not doing nearly as well as you used to at school or at work because none of it really interests you anymore.
- You don't enjoy anything anymore, not even sex (besides which, you can't even "perform" even if you wanted to).
- You're always too tired to do anything, even watch TV.
- You always seem to have a headache, bellyache, or backache. (You may be depressed, but be sure to tell your doctor about these symptoms).
- You're restless and irritable.
- You're drinking a lot and taking more tranquilizers than ever.
- You've developed a "what difference does it make?" attitude about almost everything. You don't even use a seat belt anymore.
- You can't be bothered with people, even old friends. Crowds bother you.
- You've rushed to make a will, and have even been thinking about your funeral.

Treating Depression

All right. It's begun to dawn on you that this isn't you. Something's wrong. You're depressed. What now? Well, here's what *not* to do. Don't adopt a "this too shall pass" attitude. It's time to get help. Start by sharing how you feel with someone who's close to you—*and with your doctor.* If you think he or she is too busy or doesn't really care, now's the time to switch to someone who does. You should be carefully examined to make sure that a physical problem or medication you're taking isn't in some way responsible for the way you feel. Many diseases cause depression—thyroid malfunction (especially an underactive gland), rheumatoid arthritis and any other pain-producing disorder, heart trouble, cancer, lupus, hormonal imbalance (menopause is a classic example), and any chronic condition such as multiple sclerosis or Parkinson's disease. If there is no discernible physical cause, then you need to have your depression treated with either pychotherapy, or drugs, or both.

Modern therapy for depression still includes several older antidepressants such as the *monoamine oxidase (MAO) inhibitors and tricyclics* (of which Elavil is the best known). I don't prescribe these as much as I used to because even though they are effective, they have more unpleasant side effects than the newer generation of *SSRIs (selective serotonin reuptake inhibitors)*. The first and still the best known of these is Prozac, but there are several others. Depressed persons have less serotonin than do normals. These medications act by increasing the concentration of serotonin, a neurotransmitter, in the brain. Although many patients do well with Prozac, others prefer Paxil, Effexor, Celexa, or Serzone, to name but a few of the many that have swept into pharmacies. They all differ a little from one another. Find the one that's right for you. Although they're generally well tolerated, they can all reduce your sex drive, increase your appetite and weight (or cause nausea), and leave you constipated. They're potent medications that your doctor should prescribe and monitor, so don't run out and "borrow" one of these drugs from a friend.

There's been a great deal of interest in the antidepressant properties of an herb called *St. John's Wort*. I used to prescribe it for many of my patients with mild depression. I no longer do because it has recently been determined that this herb speeds up the excretion of a wide variety of medications, including heart drugs, cholesterol-lowering pills, oral contraceptives, HIV drugs, and others. All of these drugs become less effective when taken together with St. John's Wort.

There has also been a great deal of interest and enthusiasm for a "natural" agent called *SAMe (S-adenosylmethionine)* in the treatment of depression. SAMe is formed in the body by the combination of methionine (an essential amino acid) and ATP (adenosyl triphosphate). It was discovered in Italy in 1952, and most of the research on it has been done in that country. Levels of SAMe are decreased in the elderly, in patients with liver disorders or osteoarthritis, or when there is a deficiency of folic acid or vitamin B_{12}—and in depression. So some doctors have been using it to treat osteoarthritis, fibromyalgia, liver disorders, migraine headaches, and depression. It is said to work in depression by increasing the level in the brain of important neurotransmitters such as serotonin and dopamine. The usual oral dose is 400 milligrams two to four times a day. I suggest you start with 200 mg twice a day and work your way up gradually to 1,600. There have been reports that SAMe is particularly effective in women who are depressed after childbirth and in persons who are in emotional turmoil during drug rehabilitation. SAMe appears to be safe and without serious side effects other than occasional nausea and stomach upset. It's worth a try.

If antidepressants fail, and your depression is so severe that you're having suicidal thoughts, don't hesitate to consider *shock therapy*. It doesn't deserve its scary reputation and is not nearly as bad as it sounds. Newer techniques are well tolerated and can lift you from the abyss of despair.

Self-Help

In addition to all the things that can be done for you, there are some lifestyle changes you can make. For example:

- Pace yourself. Learn to relax. How long has it been since you've had a vacation?
- Start exercising regularly. Working out releases a variety of cortisone-type hormones that can lighten depression.

It will also improve your appetite, help you sleep, and raise your interest in sex.

- Don't look to alcohol, or depend on it to drown your sorrows. You're better off avoiding it for the duration.
- Certain foods—the most important of which appear to be chocolate (that shouldn't be hard to take) and fish—may make you feel better.
- If your diet is less than optimal because you have no appetite, take a multivitamin. Deficiencies of the vitamin B group, folic acid, and C can worsen depression.
- Music, especially Mozart (the "Mozart effect"), can improve your mood. Get yourself a CD player and listen to your heart's content.
- Until your memory improves, you can relieve anxiety that you'll forget something important by writing things down. As Confucius said, "The weakest ink lasts longer than the strongest memory." If that embarrasses you, put it in a Palm Pilot. Look around you. Many people have one and are constantly making notations.

WHAT TO INSIST ON WHEN YOU'RE DEPRESSED

Depression is the "common cold of mental illness." For many who feel sad, there is an obvious reason, some bad luck or bad news to which they are unable to adjust. In others, there is no apparent cause. In both situations, sympathetic understanding from family, friends, and their doctor can help matters. Most insurance plans do not cover psychiatric care. Remember that there's no shame in being depressed. You're one among at least 30 million people in this country who are also chronically depressed. You can cut the doldrums short if you get the right help. If you are depressed, it may very well be for nonpsychological reasons. Several "physical" diseases and certain medications can affect your spirits. *See a doctor and insist on a complete physical if you're down in the dumps. Insist that all physical diseases or reactions to medications be ruled out before any treatment is prescribed.*

Even if there is no physical basis for your sadness, your family physician may be able to help with one of the new antidepressant drugs. *Insist on being informed of all your treatment options before beginning any drug treatment.*

9

DIABETES

When Life's Too Sweet

Men and women everywhere are increasingly aware of the symptoms of diabetes and the importance of recognizing them. There's an old joke about three men who were lost in the desert and had run out of drinking water. After two days in the blazing sun, they were seriously dehydrated. One of the men, an Englishman, said in desperation, "I am so thirsty, I must have some ale." The second, a Frenchman, complained, "I am so thirsty, I must have some wine." The third fellow, an Ashkenazi Jew, moaned, "I am so thirsty, I must have diabetes."

The ancient Greeks knew as long ago as 1500 B.C. that some people have too much sugar in their blood. They called the condition diabetes mellitus (the Greek word *diabetes* means "to flow"; *mellitus* is Greek for "honey"). During the 1800s a scientist named Paul Langerhans discovered that certain cells are dispersed in the pancreas, which were subsequently shown to produce a hormone named insulin. (Those cells are called either the islets of Langerhans or beta cells.) In 1921 two researchers in Canada injected insulin into diabetics and found that it lowered blood sugar.

Sixteen million Americans have diabetes mellitus (DM), but

only half of them are aware of it. Despite a better understanding of what causes this disease and how to manage it, the incidence of diabetes is increasing dramatically as more Americans live longer and grow fatter. Although many diabetics lead normal lives except for the considerable inconvenience of having to keep track of calories, insulin, and other sugar-lowering drugs, the disease can leave you chronically sick, and in this country alone its complications kill 160,000 people every year. It is the leading cause of blindness, kidney failure, and leg amputations (other than from accidents).

Why does diabetes have such dire effects? It's all about sugar and insulin. *Glucose* is the "fuel" (other than pure fat) that provides the energy for most of the body's processes. All food digested in the stomach and intestines is ultimately converted into various sugar molecules, one of which is glucose. (This conversion happens more quickly with carbohydrates than with protein and fats.) The gut absorbs the glucose and passes it into the bloodstream. Its final destination is the cells, mostly in the liver and muscles, which either burn it as fuel right then and there or store it to be used later when needed.

But here's the catch: Glucose can't get into the cells if there's no *insulin* available. So think of insulin as the key that unlocks the cell door for glucose to enter and be burned to provide energy.

In nondiabetics the increased blood sugar level after eating signals the pancreas to make more insulin so that the sugar can get into the cells. The pancreas obeys, delivers the extra insulin, and the glucose moves out of the blood and into the cells. The blood sugar level drops, canceling the order for more insulin.

There are two forms of diabetes, and this simple sequence of events does not occur normally in either one. In the first, called type 1 diabetes, there is too little insulin because the pancreas can't make it (there's no key to open the cell lock); in the other, type 2, the insulin is there, but the cell doesn't react to it (the key doesn't fit the lock). So in both types 1 and 2 diabetes, blood sugar rises because it is not being burned.

Despite the fact that both forms of the disease result in abnormally high blood sugar and similar symptoms, they have different causes, affect different age groups, require different treatment, and differ in their severity and long-term outcomes.

Type 1 Diabetes

Only 10 percent of all diabetics in the United States, roughly 1 million men and women, have type 1 diabetes. Thirty thousand cases are newly diagnosed every year. It's most common among persons of northern European descent and is rare among Asians and African Americans. These patients lack insulin because some process begins to destroy the pancreatic beta cells very early in life. However, enough beta cells are spared early on so that the disease does not usually become apparent until after ten years of age, although it occasionally begins during infancy or is delayed until thirty years of age.

Causes of Type 1 Diabetes

The cause of type 1 diabetes was recently discovered to result from an abnormal autoimmune reaction. Here's what that means: When a bacterium, virus, or cancer cell attacks us, our immune system dispatches its killer T cells to eliminate it. But the body sometimes gets its signals crossed and destroys its own perfectly normal cells as if they were hostile invaders. In some children who are infected with an otherwise harmless respiratory virus, their immune system, instead of attacking the virus, directs its T cells to infiltrate and destroy the beta cells in the pancreas—a totally pointless and irrational action that ends up causing type 1 diabetes! Fortunately, this abnormal autoimmune response often burns itself out before too many beta cells are killed, and the child remains healthy. However, kids who lose at least 80 to 90 percent of them become diabetic.

In their efforts to conquer type 1 diabetes, researchers are trying to identify the various viruses that can provoke this abnormal autoimmune process in the hope of preparing a vaccine against them. They are also searching for the specific antibodies made by the deranged immune system so they can neutralize them. Another goal is to discover why some kids infected with a virus develop this abnormal autoimmune response and others do not. To date, suspicion focuses on genetics, since there is a 10 percent risk of becoming a type 1 diabetic if a first-degree relative, such as a brother, sister, mother, and especially father, has it.

Here's yet another puzzling observation about type 1 diabetes: children fed cow's milk in the first eight days of life are twice as likely to develop this disease as those who were breast-fed. The current explanation is that cow's milk contains a protein similar to that of the beta cells and that these kids develop antibodies to this protein that later mistakenly attack and destroy the pancreatic beta cells.

Symptoms of Type 1 Diabetes

Always suspect diabetes in an infant or child who, for no apparent reason, suddenly begins to urinate more often, or wets his or her bed after having been toilet-trained. Also look for unusual fatigue, muscle weakness, weight loss, disturbance of vision, and irritability, all of which are due to the failure to convert sugar into energy. These kids don't do as well in school as they used to, and they are sometimes mistakenly diagnosed with attention deficit disorder or other behavioral problems when the real villain is diabetes. A fasting blood sugar of 200 mg confirms the diagnosis.

Treating Type 1 Diabetes

Medication: All type 1 diabetics *must* have insulin every day in order to survive! That's because they don't have the beta cells to make it. So although diet and exercise are important, the key to therapy is insulin.

Diet: Whereas the main treatment in adult diabetes are caloric restriction and weight loss, a diabetic youngster's diet must provide the kind of nutrition that permits normal growth and development. This requires coordinating insulin dosage and caloric intake in order to keep the blood sugar normal, no matter what kind of food is eaten or how much.

Exercise: Physical activity reduces blood sugar levels. The number of calories a youngster consumes and how much insulin he or she needs to burn them off must take into consideration his or her level of physical activity.

Additional Treatment Options

Many diabetics have already benefited from pancreatic transplants that improve the diabetes and arrest some of its long-term complications. Because type 1 diabetics also frequently have kidney disease, these organs are often transplanted along with the pancreas. The ten-year survival rate among such patients is greater than 75 percent.

The main downside to transplantation is rejection. Several drugs can suppress the immune system and stop it from rejecting the transplanted organs, but they may cause severe side effects. If you need a transplant, add your name to a waiting list. Transplantation is expensive and your carrier may balk at paying for it. *Insist on your rights.*

More recently, researchers have successfully transferred pancreatic beta cells, rather than the entire organ. These, too, are taken from cadavers, and several pancreases may be necessary to provide enough cells for one patient. The procedure does arrest the progress of the disease, and as with the whole organ transplant, you will need antirejection drugs for the rest of your life. If you or a loved one is in dire diabetic straits, *insist that you be considered for this procedure.*

Both nicotinamide (a derivative of vitamin B_3) and vitamin E may protect the beta cells from the harmful effects of antibodies in type 1 diabetes. Some specialists recommend that either or both of these vitamins be taken along with insulin as soon as the disease is diagnosed. Trials to test this hypothesis have not been completed at the time of this writing. Ask your doctor for news about them.

Virtually every diabetic must have a home monitoring device to check the blood sugar as often as necessary. This permits you to adjust and coordinate your medications with your diet and level of physical activity. Such control of the sugar level is the best way to prevent progression of diabetes and the onset of symptoms.

An endocrinologist specializing in diabetes should establish the guidelines to be followed by the primary physician and the family of every diabetic child. Insist on it. In addition, there must be ongoing consultation with a trained dietitian. Insist on that too. The truth is that most doctors still do not know enough about the nuts and bolts of nutrition to provide such counsel—they're the first ones to admit it. *If during the course of the illness, blood sugar levels swing wildly and symptoms come and go, consultation with an endocrinologist specializing in diabetes is a must. Insist on it.*

It's extremely important to teach young diabetics how to control their sugar levels. Although all diabetics are vulnerable to the complications of this disease, youngsters are at a special risk for: visual problems that can lead to blindness, eating disorders (a third of young diabetic women have anorexia, bulimia, and other eating problems), ketoacidosis, and coma (described below). They also frequently harbor suicidal thoughts. *If a type 1 diabetic is having any such problems, referral to the appropriate expert is essential. Insist on it.*

Type 2 Diabetes

Ninety percent of all diabetics are type 2. There are 16 million of them and half don't know that they have it because the disease remains silent for years. Type 2 diabetes primarily affects adults over age forty, although more and more people under thirty are developing it as a result of eating more, getting fatter, and exercising less. Their number has more than tripled in the past seven or eight years. The risk of developing diabetes increases as you get older, so that you have a 20 percent chance of being diabetic at age eighty-five.

Unlike type 1 diabetics, in which the insulin-producing beta cells in the pancreas are destroyed, these cells are usually intact and making enough insulin in the type 2 form of the disease. However, the cells in the muscle and liver are unable to utilize the insulin that's produced, and the glucose does not enter them. It just sits there. This situation can sometimes be improved if the beta cells can be stimulated by certain oral diabetic medications to make more insulin, helping it to penetrate some of the cells.

Causes of Insulin Resistance in Type 2 Diabetes

Type 2 diabetics are almost always overweight, although there are exceptions. Overweight people have three substances in their blood that may be responsible for abnormal glucose metabolism: free fatty acids that are formed when fat is broken down; leptin, a protein made by fat cells; and tumor necrosis factor, a constituent of the immune system. Obesity has several shapes. If you're built like an apple, with your excess fat concentrated in your abdomen and upper body, you are at greater risk for diabetes than if you look like a pear— fat in the hips and flanks.

Your genes are important too. One-third of type 2 diabetics

have a family history of the disease. Scientists have identified several genes that make cells resistant to insulin, but are still unable to modify them. Additional proof of the importance of genetics is the fact that half of all Pima Indians have type 2 diabetes.

As if causing cancer and heart disease weren't enough, smoking also increases your chances of developing type 2 diabetes. And once you do, you're much more prone to suffer from some of its serious complications.

Symptoms of Type 2 Diabetes

When blood sugar remains chronically high, regardless of what kind of diabetes you have, it will ultimately cause great thirst, frequent urination, weight loss, fatigue, and impaired vision. It may also leave you vulnerable to all kinds of infections—overgrowth of yeast in the groin (of both genders), under the breasts, and in the vagina. Gums are also frequently inflamed. Nor are you apt to heal nearly as quickly. Men become impotent, and both men and women may experience generalized pain, numbness, and tingling of the extremities because the nerves are involved. More about these complications later.

Diagnosing Type 2 Diabetes

Because diabetics do not always have typical symptoms, especially early in the course of their disease, everyone should be routinely screened for this disease. That's especially important if you:

- Are overweight (20 percent or more beyond ideal weight)

- Have a "bad" blood fat profile (high cholesterol, low HDL, elevated LDL, and an increased triglyceride level)
- One or more of your close relatives have the disease
- Are in a high-risk ethnic group such as African American or Native American
- Are pregnant between the twenty-fourth and twenty-eighth weeks
- Previously became diabetic while pregnant

These are the risk factors of diabetes. You can only establish the diagnosis by having your blood tested for sugar, preferably after you have fasted for at least eight hours.

The acceptable upper limit of fasting sugar in most laboratories is 110 mg; readings between 110 and 126 are borderline; a result greater than 126 on two different days is abnormal. If the fasting sugar is borderline, you should have a *glucose tolerance test*. Here's how it's done: After the fasting sugar has been obtained, you drink a measured amount of glucose solution. You then wait around the doctor's office reading old magazines for the next two hours, after which your blood is drawn again. In normal persons, blood sugar may be elevated initially, but it returns to normal two hours after drinking the glucose solution. In diabetics, the two-hour reading is more than 200. Some doctors continue the test for three or four hours to see how high the readings go and how long it takes for them to return to the baseline.

Glucose attaches itself to and modifies the hemoglobin molecule, which carries oxygen in the blood. This is the basis for the more sophisticated diagnostic blood test for diabetes, the glycolated hemoglobin (also known as hemoglobin A_{1c}). An elevated hemoglobin A_{1c} reflects poor diabetic control.

Treating Type 2 Diabetes

The goal of treatment is to keep the blood sugar level as close to normal as possible—and below 140. Such strict control is the best way to minimize the risk of developing the complications of diabetes that kill and cripple.

Only a third of type 2 diabetics require insulin. In fact, if you're overweight and lose enough pounds, you can often control your diabetes through diet and regular exercise alone. If these don't normalize your blood sugar, the next step is an oral blood-sugar-lowering agent.

Oral diabetic medications work in one of two ways. Either they stimulate the beta cells in the pancreas to make more insulin so that some gets into the cells, or they act on the cells, twisting their arms, so to speak, to get them to utilize whatever insulin is available. The most widely prescribed oral diabetic drugs are the sulfonylureas and metformin. They are used either alone or along with low doses of insulin.

Sulfonylureas stimulate the pancreas to make more insulin. However, after about ten years, the cells usually become exhausted and no longer respond to this prodding. At this point you either add insulin or take one of the other oral agents described below. (Available brands of sulfonylureas include Glucotrol, Amaryl, Micronase, and Diabeta, as well as several newer ones.)

A sulfonylurea is taken about a half hour before meals. It's less likely than insulin to cause hypoglycemia, but when it does, the sugar stays low for a longer time. Don't use any of these drugs if you're allergic to sulfa, are pregnant, or are nursing. Although sulfonylureas decrease sugar levels, there is some question as to whether this makes a difference in mild diabetics who have no symptoms. I prescribe them anyway because their side effects are minimal, and my patients and I both feel more comfortable knowing that sugar levels are normal.

Metformin (marketed as Glucophage) is not a sulfonylurea.

It lowers blood sugar by making cells, especially those in the liver, more receptive to insulin. It is especially effective when combined with one of the new drugs that either stimulate the secretion of insulin (repaglinide [Prandin]) or that block the breakdown in the intestine of sugars and starches such as potatoes, pasta, and bread (acarbose [Precose, Glucobay], or meglitol [Glyset]). Acarbose may also be combined with the sulfonylureas or insulin. Although it doesn't cause hypoglycemia when used alone, it can do so when taken with these other drugs. Prandin acts in much the same way as do the sulfonylureas, but it goes well with metformin and is less likely to result in hypoglycemia. Take it just before eating.

Diabetics who are overweight do well with metformin. Unlike insulin, this drug doesn't cause weight gain. In fact, patients who take it may lose a few pounds. Metformin also lowers cholesterol a little, something that's important for diabetics. But don't use this drug if you have kidney or liver disease. *I do not recommend combining sulfonylureas with metformin. There is evidence that doing so may lead to a higher incidence of heart disease.*

A new study suggests that metformin, given prophylactically to vulnerable individuals, can reduce the risk of developing diabetes by 31 percent, probably by improving sensitivity to insulin and decreasing glucose production by the liver. The dosage is 850 mg of metformin a day for two weeks and then twice a day. The therapy appears to be more effective for younger overweight individuals than for older ones. If you have a family history of type 2 diabetes, discuss taking prophylactic metformin with your doctor.

There is one further complication of metformin of which you should be aware: It reduces the absorption of vitamin B_{12} and can result in its deficiency. Taking supplemental calcium along with the B_{12} can prevent this from happening.

The newest antidiabetic drugs are the *glitazones* (Avandia, Actose). They are successors to Rezulin, which was withdrawn from the market because of its toxicity. Like metformin, they reduce cellular resistance to insulin. Have your liver checked at regular intervals when taking any of them.

Insulin, the ultimate treatment for diabetes, comes in many forms and from several sources. However, all of them need to be injected because they are inactivated in the stomach and not absorbed when taken orally.

There has been a big (and convenient) change with regard to how insulin is injected. In the past, patients were told always to clean the skin with an alcohol swab. This was often inconvenient in a public setting. However, according to a recent large study, you may safely inject insulin through your clothes (but obviously not a sheepskin coat) without risk of infection. So now diabetics can surreptitiously take their insulin at the table in a restaurant instead of having to do so in the rest room. The availability of pen injectors eliminates the need to carry a syringe and vials of insulin.

Insulin preparations are derived from pigs or cows, or made in a laboratory from genes. They vary in how quickly they reach peak effectiveness and for how long they continue to lower blood sugar. One of the newest insulin products, lispro insulin (Humalog), works faster than the older ones, so you should eat within fifteen minutes after taking it. Regular insulin is also fast-acting and it, too, is taken before meals. Its sugar-lowering effect persists anywhere from four to twelve hours. The longer-acting preparations, referred to as NPH or Lente, are usually taken later in the day or at night. The newest form of insulin, glargine (Lantus), works continuously for twenty-four hours.

The kind of insulin you use, when and how often, as well as its relation to food and exercise, are important decisions that should be made by an expert. Insist on having such a consultation before you start this therapy.

If you're needle-shy, you'll be happy to know that researchers are working on a portable inhaler from which you can take a puff of insulin into your nose—and it will hopefully work as quickly as an injection. It's not ready yet, but it's only a matter of time.

A fungus with an insulin-like action that you can take orally is also in the works. The days of the insulin needle are truly numbered.

Some diabetics wear an external insulin pump that is programmed to deliver insulin at given intervals into the abdominal wall through a catheter. These pumps are more expensive than insulin needles, but some patients find them convenient. However, they are not without their problems, as, for example, when the catheter becomes blocked.

Before leaving the subject of medication, let me remind you to check with your doctor regarding any other drugs you're taking along with your antidiabetic medications. For example, beta-blockers increase the risk of hypoglycemia, and so does alcohol.

Lifestyle Changes That Every Diabetic Should Practice

Diet

No single diabetic diet suits everyone. *Each patient must be evaluated individually by a qualified dietitian. That's an absolute must on which to insist.* That's why diabetes specialists often enlist the services of a dietitian.

There are many misconceptions about what someone with diabetes is allowed to eat. *It's not the kind of food but the total number of calories that's important.* The best diet for you depends on your age (growing children have very different needs and levels of physical activity than do overweight fifty-year-olds). When coordinating diet and insulin dosage, make allowance for your level of physical activity, your nutritional and caloric needs, and your food preferences.

Remember that much of what you eat is eventually converted into glucose. The main difference among the major food groups is the speed with which this happens. It takes protein that contains fat six to eight hours after a meal to convert; protein in lean meat and fish requires three to four hours; most carbohydrates appear as glucose within minutes. As far as pure sugar is concerned, the big change in our thinking is that it's no different from any other carbohydrate except it gets into the blood much more quickly.

Here are the general dietary guidelines for diabetics: 50 percent of daily calories should come from carbohydrates, 30 percent from protein, and 20 percent (less if possible) from fat. No more than 10 percent of this fat should be saturated; this fat is especially bad because it promotes hardening of the arteries and vascular disease. Plenty of fiber and fresh vegetables are a must.

The timing of your meals is as important as what you eat. If your medication acts within a specific time frame, you don't have the luxury of dining when you happen to feel like it. For example, if your insulin preparation peaks within half an hour, you mustn't wait an hour before eating. Whenever possible, dine and snack at the same time each day, don't skip meals, and try to consume the same number of calories every day in order to stabilize your therapy.

Exercise

You won't lose weight over the long term just by dieting. You should exercise regularly three to four times a week for at least twenty minutes. That means brisk walking (not window-shopping pace), biking, swimming, dancing, jogging, skiing, or any other activity *you enjoy*. Before setting out, drink plenty of liquids, preferably water, and no caffeine. Check your blood sugar and urine too. If your glucose level is higher than 250, or there are ketones in the urine, don't exercise. On the other hand, if your sugar is less than 100, have a snack rich in carbohydrates, because exercise will further lower it. Consider reducing your insulin dosage just before you exercise. If your sugar is normal, a glass of skim milk before you begin is a good way to keep it high enough to prevent a serious drop without increasing the level too much.

Here's a useful tip of which many diabetics are not aware: Don't inject the insulin into a muscle that you will be using during exercise, because that speeds up its absorption.

Don't exercise when your legs hurt, or your blood pressure is high, or if it's either very hot or very cold. If you become unusually winded while working out, or feel faint and dizzy, sit down and rest and check your sugar level. Don't start at a high intensity of exercise if you've always been a couch potato. Ease into it; build it up gradually over several days or weeks. Warm up before each session and cool down afterward. Always check your feet for cuts, scrapes, blisters, or other signs of injury before and after exercising. Be careful to avoid resistance or high-impact exercises if you have any evidence of vascular disease, because these can injure blood vessels that have been weakened by the diabetes.

Foot Care

More amputations are due to diabetes than to any cause other than trauma. The legs in particular have decreased blood supply, and their perception of pain is also apt to be impaired. Examine your feet carefully before you put your socks on in the morning. Look at their color; inspect them for sores; feel them to see whether they're hard, firm, too warm or too cold. Don't wash your feet in very hot water because your blood vessels may not be able to dilate in response. Dry your feet thoroughly and wipe between the toes to prevent fungal infections. Use a moisturizer on dry skin, but don't let any of it get between the toes. If you have corns or calluses, pumice them gently with an emery board; don't shave them with a blade. Avoid high heels, sandals, and thongs (even though they are sexy-looking) and never walk barefoot. Wear sensible low-heeled shoes with enough room for you to wiggle your toes. Check for pebbles before you put your shoes on; walking all day on a little stone can cause an abrasion of the skin and infection. Socks should be seamless so as not to irritate the skin. Finally, don't further reduce an already compromised circulation to your legs by wearing tight stockings.

Vascular Disease

Adult diabetics should take a baby aspirin (81 mg) every day to protect against heart attacks and strokes, especially if they already have evidence of vascular disease (except, of course, if they have a bleeding problem). I also have them come to the office for regular cardiac exams.

Diabetes thickens blood vessel walls, leaves them less elastic, and clogs them with cholesterol plaques. The organs and systems of the body that are affected when their blood supply is compromised in this way are the brain (25 percent of diabetic deaths are due to stroke); the heart (heart attacks account for 60 percent of the deaths among diabetics); the eyes (diabetes is the most common cause of blindness in the United States); the kidneys (their involvement results in high blood pressure, which further accelerates vascular disease). When the kidneys eventually stop working (renal failure), dialysis becomes necessary. When the blood supply to the legs is reduced, walking becomes difficult.

Diabetes results in the need for about 54,000 leg amputations in this country every year. You should suspect that the circulation in your legs is impaired when they itch, the skin becomes shiny, the hair is lost, and your calves hurt when you walk. Later you may develop leg ulcers that don't heal. If that happens, there are new and effective antibiotics as well as potent drugs that stimulate healing. If none of them work and the ulcers remain open, you may need a skin graft. The most exciting news in this area is the development of bioengineered tissue grown from human skin that appears to speed healing of diabetic foot ulcers. This product, called Dermagraft, was not on the market at the time of writing, but, you should ask your doctor about it. Some centers use hyperbaric oxygen chambers and with apparently good results. However, this therapy is still experimental and not universally available.

Erections become difficult or impossible when the blood supply to the penis or nerve function is compromised. Thank goodness for Viagra.

Since diabetes often damages the nerves, diabetics may lose the ability to perceive pain. Someone who might ordinarily experience chest discomfort on exertion because his or her coronary arteries are significantly narrowed may not have any symptoms. The ECG taken when you are at rest often fails to show any abnormalities, so *insist on a stress test as part of a cardiac workup*.

Since elevated cholesterol and blood pressure are important contributing factors to vascular disease, I recommend the following:

- Every adult diabetic whose total cholesterol is over 200 and whose LDL is higher than 100 should be treated with diet and, if necessary, one of the "statin" drugs.
- Blood pressure should be no higher than 130/80. (We used to think that a diastolic of 90 was acceptable; it is not.)
- Whenever possible, avoid beta-blockers (atenolol, popranolol) for treating high blood pressure, because these drugs may obscure the symptoms of hypoglycemia. I prefer ACE inhibitors such as captopril (Capoten), because they also delay or prevent kidney and eye disease.

Monitoring Your Sugar Level

Check your blood sugar level whenever you want to know whether you need extra insulin or think that a "low" sugar is coming on. Buy a blood sugar monitor at a pharmacy. They are easy to use and relatively inexpensive. Your insurance will reimburse you. Aim for a pre-meal sugar level of 80 to 120 and between 100 and 140 at bedtime.

If an illness or infection has raised your blood sugar, check your urine for the presence of ketones (high levels of which may herald ketoacidosis and diabetic coma—see below). Also test your urine from time to time for the presence of albumin, an early marker of diabetic kidney disease.

Acute Complications of Diabetes

Ketoacidosis is the most serious acute and life-threatening complication of diabetes. It can develop in patients with both forms of the disease but is more common in type 1. Here's how it happens: When diabetics develop a high blood sugar because they forgot a scheduled dose of insulin, or failed to adjust the amount when they "pigged out," or developed an infection and did not take extra insulin, the body can't use it for energy. Other sources such as the fat stores must therefore be tapped, and when large amounts of fat are burned, they produce fatty acids that in turn are converted into toxic ketones.

Suspect ketoacidosis if you are nauseated and vomiting for no apparent reason, begin to breathe rapidly (the lungs are trying to eliminate the toxic acid), and your heart rate increases. Kids often complain of a bellyache. Unless you receive enough insulin quickly (intravenously), along with fluids to correct abnormalities of sodium and potassium, you may go into coma. Two percent of such cases end in death.

A special word of caution: If you're asthmatic and taking terbutaline regularly, you are at increased risk for ketoacidosis and should monitor your sugar levels especially carefully.

Low blood sugar (hypoglycemia), in which the blood sugar drops too low, is a much more common acute complication of diabetes than is ketoacidosis. These attacks are more frequent these days because diabetic patients are trying to maintain near-normal sugar levels so as to delay or prevent the long-term complications of this disease. Hypoglycemia usually occurs when you've taken insulin (or one of the glucose-lowering drugs) and haven't eaten enough to "cover" it, or if you've exercised too much and lowered the blood sugar, took too much insulin, or have a drinking problem (alcohol drops sugar levels).

Children with type 1 diabetes are especially vulnerable to hypoglycemia, especially during the night. To avoid that possibility, if your child's sugar levels tend to swing wildly, give him or her a snack at bedtime. It's better for the sugar to be a little high than to allow the attack of hypoglycemia to go unrecognized and untreated during sleep.

You'll usually have enough warning that your sugar is dropping so you can correct matters before the situation becomes serious. You feel hungry, tremulous, and sweaty; your heart pounds and you may develop a headache. If you don't recognize the typical warning symptoms or ignore them, a train of neurological symptoms sets in. These are especially dangerous for older persons whose cerebral circulation may already be compromised by vascular disease. You become confused, disoriented, weak, and irrational. Unless you take some sugar right way, you may slip into a coma. That's why diabetics, young and old, should always carry with them, wherever they are, little packets of sugar or glucose tablets (available at the drugstore), or some hard candy.

You should also wear a visible bracelet or necklace indicating that you are diabetic. If you're brought comatose to an emergency room, you don't want anyone thinking you're a drunk, or have the doctors lose valuable time evaluating you for a stroke, head injury, or overdose, instead of measuring the blood sugar forthwith and correcting it.

My wife is diabetic. Even though she's never had a serious attack of low blood sugar, she always keeps glucagon at home and in her travel kit. Glucagon is a hormone made by the alpha cells of the pancreas (the beta cells are the ones that produce the insulin). It has an anti-insulin effect that raises blood sugar by causing the liver very quickly to release stored glucose into the bloodstream. Glucagon takes effect within one minute after being injected into the muscle. Every home in which a diabetic is living should have this medication handy in the event of a low blood sugar emergency. Someone in the family should know how and when to use it.

The best way to prevent hypoglycemia is to monitor your sugar three or four times a day so that you can anticipate when you're vulnerable to precipitous and dangerously low sugar levels.

Long-Term Complications of Diabetes

Prolonged or frequent elevations of blood sugar over the years can lead to devastating complications that affect blood vessels and nerves everywhere in the body and shorten the life span of diabetics.

Neuropathy. Long-standing poorly controlled diabetes damages the nerves (neuropathy) in half of all diabetics who have the disease for twenty-five years or more. Neuropathy causes a variety of symptoms: numbness, tingling, loss of sensation, or severe pain in the upper and lower extremities, and inability to sense the location of the feet when walking.

Neuropathy is difficult to treat. I recommend antidepressants such as sertraline (Zoloft), not because of their effect on the emotions, but because they can reduce pain. Topical capsaicin (derived from hot peppers) is useful too, because it dulls the nerve signals from the skin. Try to avoid morphine-type drugs for the pain of neuropathy, because diabetes is a chronic disease and narcotics can leave you addicted.

When the nerves of the autonomic (involuntary) nervous system are involved, bowel and bladder control may be lost, along with the ability to have an erection. The penis needs intact nerves as well as adequate blood flow in order to "perform."

When its nerves are damaged, the stomach doesn't empty quickly enough, a condition called *gastroparesis*. The best treatment for this condition is cisapride (Propulsid), a drug that was mainly used for the treatment of heartburn. However, it was withdrawn from the market after some cases of fatal cardiac arrhythmia were attributed to its use. Gastroparesis may also respond to the antibiotic erythromycin or to metoclopramide (Reglan). If you're troubled by this gastric problem and other therapy doesn't help, your doctor can obtain Propulsid for you from the manufacturer. *Insist on it, but remember to have your cardiac status monitored carefully while you're taking it.*

One of the major complications of neuropathy is the inability to perceive pain. That may sound good, but it's actually quite dangerous, because pain is nature's way of warning you that something is wrong. If you're diabetic, learn to recognize the other symptoms of a heart attack—abnormal sweating, sudden fatigue, palpitations, dizziness, and shortness of breath. As mentioned earlier, *every adult diabetic should have a stress test to detect "silent" heart disease. Insist on it.*

Visual problems. Diabetes is the leading cause of blindness in adults aged twenty to seventy-four; more than 24,000 new cases are reported every year. Most type 2 diabetics have some degree of visual impairment, even though only a minority lose all vision. Sight is impaired when the blood vessels in the eye rupture and leak, especially into the central

portion of the retina. Early signs of trouble are blurred or double vision, spots or floaters before your eyes, the inability to
see from the outer border of the eyes, difficulty reading even
after you're changed your glasses, and pain or a feeling of
pressure in your eyes. The best way to treat leaky blood vessels is to seal them with laser photocoagulation. Vitrectomy,
in which blood and scar tissue are surgically removed, is also
effective. Diabetics are more vulnerable to glaucoma and
cataracts. *Every diabetic should be examined by an eye specialist at least once a year. Insist on it.*

Kidney problems. A third of all type 1 diabetes patients
have renal problems, the greatest cause of death and disability among them. The normal kidney filters the blood, retains
what the body needs, and excretes the waste in the urine. In
diabetics with kidney disease (diabetic nephropathy) the kidney also eliminates substances that the body should be retaining, as, for example, protein, and holds on to toxic
products such as urea that are normally eliminated. So you
end up with swollen feet, anemia (healthy kidney normally
makes a hormone that stimulates the bone marrow to make
red blood cells; this hormone may be lacking in diabetics),
and are unusually tired. In the final stages of nephropathy,
you may need dialysis (a machine that does the filtering job
for the kidney) or a kidney transplant. Diabetic nephropathy
may not cause any symptoms until it reaches an advanced
stage. *Every diabetic should have frequent and regular blood
and urine tests. Insist on them.*

Lowered resistance to infection. Bacteria and all infectious
agents thrive on sugar. That's why cuts and sores take so long
to heal in diabetics and must be treated early and vigorously.
Urinary tract infections by bacteria or fungus are especially
common in diabetic men and women. Since vulnerability to
infections of the mouth and gums is also increased, diabetics
must pay special attention to their oral hygiene. That means
flossing after every meal, using a soft toothbrush twice a day,
and having your teeth examined every six months. Influenza

is especially dangerous for diabetics. You must be vaccinated against it every year. It's also a good idea to ask for a pneumococcal pneumonia vaccination every seven or eight years before age sixty-five, after which only one shot suffices.

Increased risk of cancer. Diabetic men and women have a higher incidence of cancer of the colon and rectum than does the rest of the population. *Insist on a routine colonoscopy* every three years after the age of fifty and more often if there is a family history of colon cancer or if you had a polyp removed in the past.

The Pregnant Diabetic

One in every 200 pregnant women develop type 2 diabetes during their pregnancy, a condition called *gestational diabetes.* It's most likely to happen if you have gained anywhere from eleven to twenty-two pounds after the teen years or just before you became pregnant, or if you have a family history of the disease, smoke, or are African American, Hispanic, or Asian.

When blood sugar levels are elevated, glucose crosses the placenta to the fetus, which responds by making extra insulin. This combination of extra sugar and more insulin increases the baby's birth weight. It also poses for the mother the risk of preeclampsia, a dangerous elevation of blood pressure. Babies of diabetic mothers are at increased risk too of being born with a birth defect of some kind.

Every pregnant woman should have a glucose tolerance test between the twenty-fourth and twenty-eighth week to rule out the possibility of gestational diabetes. Her sugar should not be higher than 165 mg two hours after eating, and no more than 145 after three hours.

The best treatment for gestational diabetes are diet and insulin. In many cases blood sugar returns to normal after delivery, but one-third to one-half remain diabetic. If you're nursing and taking an oral contraceptive, make sure it does not contain high levels of progestin. This hormone raises the risk of type 2 diabetes.

It is very important that you and your unborn child have optimal blood sugar levels when you're pregnant. You should have the counsel of a specialist. Insist on it.

WHAT TO INSIST ON IF YOU'RE DIABETIC

There are two types of diabetes, 1 and 2. Both result in high blood sugar and several potentially life-threatening complications. In type 1 the insulin-producing cells of the pancreas are destroyed very early in life, and these children need insulin to survive. Type 2 diabetes is most commonly found among overweight adults and usually responds to weight loss, oral blood-sugar-lowering drugs, and insulin, when necessary.

The key to a long and healthy life for any diabetic is sustained normalization of the sugar. This involves teamwork among your health-care providers. Your primary-care physician should coordinate your care, but cannot manage the entire spectrum of disease when complications of diabetes develop.

Throughout this chapter I've emphasized all the services necessary to keep your diabetes under control. In summary, *insist on:*

- The availability of a specialist in diabetes to monitor your progress, and to define your diet, exercise, and treatment regimens
- Instructions from a dietitian with regard to your diet

- Consultation with an expert before beginning insulin therapy
- Transplantation of your pancreas or kidney, or the injection of insulin-producing beta cells, if these are your only chance of survival
- The expertise, whenever you need it, of a specialist in every area in which diabetes can present problems—the heart, brain, kidneys, emotions, sexual activity, the legs, eyes, and nerves

10

DIVERTICULAR DISEASE

Forbidden Fruit?

We had some friends for dinner one night and my wife served delicious fresh raspberries for dessert. One of our guests, a woman in her fifties, looked longingly at the dish but turned it away. As a host, I normally wouldn't comment on that, but being a doctor, I felt I should try to make her feel better about it.

"I have many patients who are allergic to raspberries," I said. "It's not at all unusual."

"Oh, I'm not allergic to them. I love them. Ate them all my life." She looked wistfully at everyone else enjoying the plump, juicy berries.

I was puzzled. "Then why aren't you eating them now? Is your stomach upset?"

"No, I'm fine. It's just that I had a routine colonoscopy last month. I'm over fifty and I thought it would be a good idea. I'm glad I did because my doctor found that I have diverticulosis, and he warned me about eating anything with seeds: raspberries and strawberries, nuts and grapes—that kind of food. He told me that if a seed gets stuck in one of these little pouches in my colon, it could make me very sick. So I'm being careful, that's all."

I've heard this story so many times, and it's all wrong! This woman was depriving herself of delicious, healthful, high-fiber food because of a theory that was never proved in the first place, and has now largely been abandoned. In fact, the very foods that are "prohibited" happen to be exactly what most people with diverticulosis need! My dinner guest was my friend, not my patient. I didn't feel I had the right to tell her that what she had been told was nonsense. I did, however, suggest that she get another opinion (and I'm sending her a copy of this book).

More than half the men and women over the age of sixty in this country have diverticulosis. It usually doesn't cause symptoms. You're apt to find out that you have it after undergoing some examination of the colon such as a colonoscopy, barium X ray, or sigmoidoscopy. If you have the wrong doctor, that examination can change your life—for the worse—if you're advised to avoid foods that you enjoy and that are good for you.

What Are Diverticula?

You will better appreciate what diverticulosis is all about and the problems it does (and doesn't) cause by reviewing the anatomy of the intestinal tract.

The stomach leads into the small intestine—the long, thin segment of bowel whose loops end at the large intestine (colon) in the right lower part of the abdomen. The colon then courses up the right side of the belly, across to the left side, descends as the sigmoid colon, and ends up as the rectum.

Diverticula are outpouchings the size of large peas that develop in the colon over the years, usually in someone who is chronically constipated and tends to strain at stool. (The Latin word *diverticulum* means a "small diversion from the normal path.") The incidence increases with age. Some 5 to 10 percent of people in their fifties have diverticulosis, and the number climbs to 50 percent among those in their seventies. By the time you're eighty-five, you're virtually certain to have them.

Repeatedly forcing hard stool down weakens areas of the bowel, causing them to bulge. Although diverticula can occur anywhere in the colon, 80 percent of them are found in the sigmoid on the left side of the abdomen, because that's where the colon is narrowest and pressures are highest.

Diverticulosis was first recognized in this country early in the twentieth century, coincident with the introduction of processed food from which roughage had largely been removed. This condition is prevalent in other developed countries where most people eat predominantly low-fiber foods. By the same token, it's relatively uncommon in Africa and Asia where the diet is rich in fiber.

Symptoms of Diverticulosis

Diverticula don't usually cause any symptoms unless they become inflamed, infected, or leak into the abdominal cavity. However, if you have enough of them, they can thicken and narrow the sigmoid, resulting in chronic constipation and pelletlike stools, sometimes diarrhea, or intermittent spasm and pain in the left lower portion of the belly.

Prevention of Diverticulosis

You can help prevent diverticulosis by moving your bowels regularly. The best way to do that is to drink at least eight glasses of water a day and eat plenty of fiber. The roughage keeps your stools soft, bulky, and passed easily without straining. To obtain the necessary bulk, eat whole-bran cereal at breakfast and add more whole grains to your diet. Lots of fruit such as berries, apples, and peaches, as well as vegetables such as broccoli, spinach, carrots, squash, and asparagus, are also important. Beans and cabbage are controversial; some doctors believe they're a good source of roughage; others say they cause gas and bloating. Try them and see who's right. Be careful to increase your fiber intake very gradually to the desired level of 35 grams a day, because fiber can cause gas and takes getting used to. And drink lots of water because the fiber sucks out the water in the bowel like a sponge and can leave you constipated.

Diverticulitis

Although uncomplicated diverticulosis doesn't usually cause problems, 10 to 25 percent of cases do become infected, at which point you have *diverticulitis.* No one knows why that happens. It's not the result of seeds invading the pouches, as is commonly believed, although every now and then a patient will blame raspberries! A more likely explanation is that bacteria normally present in the bowel seep into the diverticula, whose walls are thinner and more easily penetrated than those of the rest of the bowel. Some scientists also speculate that the diverticula become inflamed as the result of an autoimmune reaction.

The diagnosis of diverticulitis is fairly straightforward, especially if you are aware that you have underlying diverticulosis. Your belly is tender when the doctor presses on it, especially in its left lower part. The doctor will often want to look into the interior of the bowel by means of a colonoscopy or sigmoidoscopy just to make sure of the diagnosis.

Diverticulitis may cause nothing more than pain or tenderness in the lower abdomen, or it may produce vomiting, chills, cramping, fever, bleeding (when a blood vessel in the pouch ruptures—this happens in less than 5 percent of patients), perforation and tears of the infected, distended diverticulum, and obstruction of the bowel. When a pouch bursts, its bacteria spread into the interior of the belly, where they can cause a generalized infection called peritonitis or a localized abscess. In such cases you may need an operation to clean things up.

Treatment of an acute attack of diverticulitis usually consists of bed rest, a liquid diet to ease the burden on the gut, painkillers, antispasmodic medication, and the appropriate antibiotic (usually doxycycline) continued for seven to ten days. If attacks recur and affect the quality of your life, you may need to have the portion of the colon that contains the diverticula removed. That, I suppose, makes you a semicolon! (Sorry, I couldn't resist that pun.)

Chances are you can keep your diverticulosis from becoming diverticulitis by eating more fiber (at least thirty grams a day) or if that's not possible for any reason, take a stool-bulking agent such as psyllium (Metamucil, FiberCon, Perdiem, and others) or methylcellulose (marketed as Cologel and Citrucel). Drink at least eight glasses of water a day and respond promptly when you "have to go."

WHAT TO INSIST ON WHEN YOU HAVE DIVERTICULOSIS

Diverticula are fingerlike outpouchings of the bowel commonly present in persons with chronic constipation. Half the population over the age of sixty has them, and they usually do not cause any symptoms. However, these pouches can become infected and/or bleed, requiring dietary restriction and antibiotics. When they leak or burst into the abdominal cavity, you may need surgery. The best way to prevent diverticulosis is to eat a high-fiber, high-residue diet and drink enough water.

If you're found to have diverticulosis in the course of a routine examination, but do not have any symptoms, *do not accept a low-roughage, seedless diet. Insist on a second opinion.*

If you have diverticulosis and develop abdominal pain and fever, *do not accept the diagnosis of diverticulitis without an appropriate evaluation. Insist on it.* There are many other causes of such symptoms.

ENDOMETRIOSIS

Not Tonight, Dear, I Have Endometriosis

Endometriosis is a disorder in which tissue that normally lines the cavity of the uterus is also found in other locations where it has no right to be—most commonly on the ovaries (in 75 percent of cases) or in the fallopian tubes (through which the egg travels down from the ovaries to the uterus), elsewhere in the pelvis, between the rectum and the vagina, in the rectum itself, the appendix, the urinary bladder, and occasionally the stomach. It has even been discovered in the gallbladder, spleen, liver, and lungs.

This peripatetic tissue, wherever it happens to be or by whatever route it got there, sometimes behaves in all these areas as if it were still in the uterus. In other words, it menstruates! So every month women with such endometriosis develop a host of symptoms, the nature of which depends on where their misplaced uterine tissue is located. That's why no two women with endometriosis have the same complaints. Unlike menstruating tissue in the uterus, these aberrant endometrial cells usually don't have any way of getting out of the body. They remain where they are, eventually forming scar tissue and irritating the area in which they are located. Even when the aberrant tissue doesn't menstruate, it forms scars or adhesions. These adhesions attach themselves to nearby structures. They can then cause symptoms all month long, not only during the week or so of the menses. It's as if some of your heart muscle settled down in your knee, or there was lung tissue in your elbow joint, or pieces of brain in your nose. You'd then have a beating knee, a breathing arm, and an intellectual schnoz.

An estimated 7 percent of American girls and women of reproductive age (that's more than 5 million) have endometriosis (more whites than blacks, more Asians than Caucasians). This disorder becomes apparent right after the menses begins and continues until menopause. It's one of the most common, complex, and poorly understood gynecological conditions. Some women have no symptoms and only become aware of the diagnosis in the following circumstances: During a routine examination, the doctor may find thickened areas in the pelvis, or limited motion of the uterus and pelvic structures similar to a pelvic infection—but without fever or changes in the blood count. Or, the doctor sees the tissue—on the fallopian tubes or somewhere else in the belly—during some type of unrelated abdominal surgery; the woman tries to have a baby and can't because the misplaced tissue distorts the anatomy of the reproductive tract or interferes with the passage of the egg.

However, most women with endometriosis do have symptoms. They are usually intermittent but sometimes constant, when they are related to menstruation. One or two days before the onset of the menstrual flow and continuing for the duration, patients experience abdominal discomfort that interferes with sleep and results in chronic fatigue and mood swings. Intercourse is painful when there is endometrial tissue behind the uterus and the walls of the pelvis. Urination and bowel movements are uncomfortable too; there may be premenstrual spotting, lower backache, blood in the urine, and rectal bleeding. Regardless of its pattern, endometriosis can leave women feeling so miserable that the last thing on their mind is lovemaking, which is why this condition is sometimes referred to as "husbanditis."

If your doctor suspects endometriosis because of the symptoms and the physical findings, the diagnosis is confirmed by laparoscopy. This can be done at any time during the cycle. You are given an anesthetic, after which the doctor makes a small incision (about a quarter inch long), usually just below the navel. He then inserts a telescope-like thin, rigid tube about twelve inches long with a lens at the end attached to a light source that permits a direct look at the uterus, ovaries, fallopian tubes, and other pelvic structures. If endometrial tissue is present, it is biopsied. Treatment should not be started until the tissue in question has been looked at under a microscope and identified with certainty. If it is indeed endometrial and not too widespread, it can be surgically removed or lasered away. In any event, it can be debunked (reduced in size). The small incision in the abdominal wall and the anesthesia are well worth the trouble if they lead to a positive diagnosis and successful treatment.

You can also have a vaginal ultrasound to help make the diagnosis. This procedure can detect endometrial tissue in the ovaries. It is less expensive than laparoscopy but not nearly as revealing. *If you're in pain, insist on the definitive laparoscopic procedure and biopsy.*

How uterine tissue ends up in all these strange places and why it does so in some women and not in others is a puzzle, as is the reason why women with endometriosis usually start their periods at a younger age, and have menses that are more regular, with a shorter interval (less than twenty-seven days) between them. It would seem that the more menstrual cycles there have been, the more endometriosis. So female athletes are also more likely to develop it, presumably because strenuous exercise reduces the number of periods. The fact that women who have their children later in life have a lower incidence of endometriosis also supports this conjecture.

Here's one piece of news that will surely startle you, as it did me. Endometriosis has been diagnosed in men! Yes, men! It appears that very rarely, men who are treated with high doses of estrogen for their prostate cancer may actually form endometrial tissue in their prostate glands. However, I'm not suggesting that if you're male and have abdominal cramps that you be investigated for endometriosis.

There is a genetic component to endometriosis. If your sister or mother has it, there's a greater chance that you will too. However, some gynecologists think that this disorder is due to an abnormality of the immune system that allows uterine cells not only to migrate but to survive where they don't belong. There are other theories too. It is speculated that the endometrial cells migrate throughout the body in the bloodstream or in the lymphatic system, or that fluid containing these cells leaks out of the uterus; or that during menstruation, in addition to flowing out of the uterus, some blood backs up into the fallopian tubes, onto the ovaries, and into the pelvis. That's what the doctor who delivered my children and who reviewed this chapter thinks.

Toxic chemicals have also been implicated in the causation of endometriosis. These include dioxin (a group of chemicals that may also produce cancer), as well as environmental contaminants such as PCBs and other "endocrine disrupters" that act like hormones in the body and upset the normal hormonal balance. For example, monkeys deliberately exposed to high concentrations of dioxin have developed endometriosis—and the greater the exposure, the more severe the disease. The experimental data are sufficiently convincing for us to do everything necessary to remove these pollutants from our environment.

There is no cure for endometriosis, but there are several treatments that can reduce pain, restore fertility, and shrink the size of the wandering tissue. The benefits of medical therapy are usually transient. The best treatment option is to have the aberrant tissue removed if possible. *Insist that this be considered.*

The most effective medications for pain relief are the

prostaglandin inhibitors such as aspirin and the NSAIDs (ibuprofen, naproxen), although Tylenol might also help. The earlier you start taking them, the more effective they are. If the pain is very severe, you may need a prescription painkiller.

Anything that stops your periods will usually ease the symptoms of endometriosis. However, this is not a satisfactory long-term solution for many women. The hormone progestin used to be popular but has been abandoned because the high doses required resulted in bloating, weight gain, depression, and irregular vaginal bleeding. It may also sometimes cause a prolonged effect on ovarian function even after it is stopped.

The most popular agents for the treatment of endometriosis are the GnRH agonists (gonadotropin-releasing hormones). They decreased the hormones (LH and FSH) produced in the brain that stimulates the formation of estrogen. (Remember that estrogen makes the endometrial implants grow.) GnRH, which takes about a month to start working, is marketed as a nasal spray (Synarel); it can be injected into the muscle once a month (Lupron) or under the skin (Zoladex). The side effects of the GnRH drugs are what you would expect when there is no estrogen around, the kind of symptoms menopausal women have: hot flashes, insomnia, mild depression, breast tenderness, vaginal dryness, and reduced sex drive. Pregnant women should not take any of these hormones.

Finally, there is surgical or laser removal of the wandering tissue. *If it's possible to remove enough to make a difference, that's the route to go.* How extensive the procedure needs to be will depend on the amount of wayward tissue and its location. If it's localized to a small area, it's no big deal. But sometimes the surgery must be extensive.

Any disorder whose cause is not clear and whose treatment is not always entirely satisfactory spawns misconceptions. For example, some of my patients have told me that they suspect that intercourse during menstruation results in endometriosis (presumably by causing the flow of blood up into the fallopian tubes). There is no basis for this belief. Others think that tampons and douching cause endometriosis. Again, unlikely and unsubstantiated.

WHAT TO INSIST ON IF YOU HAVE ENDOMETRIOSIS

Millions of women suffer from endometriosis during their reproductive years. The condition is due to the abnormal presence of tissue that normally lines the interior of the uterus elsewhere in the body, usually in the pelvis, abdomen, or rectum, but in other exotic locations as well. These far-flung islands of endometrium may menstruate every month, sometimes behaving as if they were still inside the uterus. This causes a wide variety of symptoms, the most common of which are infertility, pain, and malfunction of the organ on which they happen to be attached.

Your doctor should suspect endometriosis if your symptoms are cyclical—that is, they occur at the time of menstruation. If the diagnosis of endometriosis is likely, *insist on its confirmation by laparoscopy.* The most reliable way to diagnose this condition is by laparoscopy and biopsy, which permits the doctor to visualize the pelvic and abdominal cavities and to look at the tissue under the microscope. Laparoscopy also makes it possible to remove or vaporize by means of lasers any abnormal tissue so detected. Ultrasound is another widely used method of diagnoses. However, it is not as reliable as laparoscopy. *Insist on the definitive procedure.*

The most effective treatment is surgical removal of the offending tissue if possible. *Insist, too, that this option be considered if medical management does not provide the necessary relief.*

12

FIBROMYALGIA

It's Not "All in Your Head"

When doctors encounter a disorder whose cause they cannot determine and whose treatment is unsatisfactory, they may blame it on the patient. Those unfortunate enough to suffer from such a mysterious ailment may be stigmatized as neurotics. Fibromyalgia fell into that category until fairly recently, and still remains there in the minds and attitudes of some physicians.

Fibromyalgia affects more than 6 million Americans, more than 75 percent of them women, most of whom are in their forties or fifties. It's rare in children. Their main complaint is severe deep aching or burning muscular pain anywhere (and sometimes everywhere) in the body. It usually occurs during physical activity but sometimes also at rest. These people not only hurt but they're also chronically and seriously tired. That's because night after night they sleep so poorly—they toss and turn, awaken often, and never really enjoy deep slumber. Many of them are also depressed and are apt to suffer from a "nervous stomach," with bouts of diarrhea or constipation.

The curious thing about fibromyalgia is that despite all these miserable symptoms, these patients don't *look* sick. They have no fever; their appetite is good and they don't lose weight. Their joints are not arthritic despite the pain; there is no evidence of any connective-tissue disease such as lupus despite the multiplicity of symptoms; thyroid function is normal and does not account for their fatigue; and every conceivable test comes back normal! In short, fibromyalgia leaves no physical evidence of its presence. Patients go from doctor to doctor, desperately looking for an explanation, trying to understand why they feel so lousy. After a thorough and careful workup reveals no abnormalities, most of them are told, "There's nothing wrong with you" or "It's all in your head."

The symptoms of fibromyalgia were first described in 1816, and over the years it has been given a number of different names such as "chronic rheumatism," "fibrositis," and "fibromyositis." None of these are correct: It's not "rheumatism," because the joints are not involved and none of the tests for arthritis are ever abnormal; nor is it or "fibrositis" or "fibromyositis," because muscles and tendons show no evidence of inflammation or disease.

Fibromyalgia occurs worldwide, it does not discriminate among ethnic groups, and although it begins most frequently between twenty and fifty-five years of age, it can develop at any time during adult life.

We do not know what causes fibromyalgia, and there is no specific test available to diagnose it. However, a list of criteria defined by the American College of Rheumatology was formulated in 1990, establishing the fibromyalgia syndrome (FMS) as a distinct and separate medical entity.

Symptoms of Fibromyalgia

If you've had most of the following for at least three months, you probably have FMS:

- Deep, aching pain in various parts of the body: the neck, between the shoulder blades, the shoulders themselves, the hips, the knees. This is the sine qua non of fibromyalgia. *You must have pain to qualify for this diagnosis.*
- Inordinate fatigue for no apparent reason, worse in the morning than later in the day
- Trouble falling asleep and then waking frequently during the night
- Joint pain
- Chronic headache
- Urinary frequency
- Restless legs and/or leg cramps
- Anxiety/depression
- Painful menstrual periods (premenstrual syndrome)
- Attacks of diarrhea and constipation
- Sensitivity to heat, cold, and changes in humidity
- Chronic sore throat
- Difficulty in concentrating and impaired memory
- Mottled skin
- Sensitivity to bright light, odors, and loud sounds

A key diagnostic finding shared by all fibromyalgia patients is their "trigger points"—discrete, painful little knots in the muscles that really hurt. These trigger points are located above and below the belly button; in the neck (where they may be mistaken for a tension headache); on the hips or buttocks; around the knees and elbows—indeed, in any muscle. They are generally paired—that is, when present on one side of the body, they have a similar distribution on the other.

Patients with chronic fatigue syndrome (see Chapter 7) have many of the same complaints, and they, too, test normal for everything. However, their main symptom is pain, not fatigue.

If you have FMS, chances are that some other blood relative does too, although no specific inheritance pattern or gene has been identified. Most patients cannot relate the onset of their symptoms to any specific event or illness, although there does seem to be some relationship to acute stress. Several different theories have been proposed to explain FMS, all of which have their passionate advocates but none of which are universally accepted. Blood tests may reveal a deficiency of tryptophan, the precursor of serotonin, a chemical in the brain that transmits nerve messages, inhibits pain perception, and induces deep sleep. The problem is that serotonin levels are also low among those suffering from depression without FMS. Some researchers believe that FMS is due to a viral or other infection, but the responsible agent has not been identified. Others suspect that FMS is a disorder of the immune system, but again they have not been able to prove it.

Although the multiple symptoms of FMS when they occur together are typical, you should not accept this diagnosis until other possible and treatable causes have been ruled out. These include thyroid dysfunction, a number of neurological disorders, connective-tissue diseases such as scleroderma, certain forms of arthritis, and even malignancy. However, none of these conditions alone ever mimic FMS closely. Still, *insist on a consultation with a rheumatologist,* who can exclude the possibility of some arthritic or muscular disorder that may resemble FMS. Such an opinion can save you a great deal of repeated and unnecessary testing as you travel from doctor to doctor in search of an answer.

Treatment of Fibromyalgia

There is no cure for FMS. Its symptoms wax and wane but almost never clear up. However, there are several things you can do to feel better.

Regular exercise is extremely important, not so much for relief of pain, but because it promotes sleep—and sleep is the key to this disorder. The body needs stage 4 sleep, the deepest level, in order to repair damaged and aging tissue, produce antibodies, and make enough hormones, neurotransmitters, and immune system chemicals. The kind of exercise you do is not important as long as it's aerobic, includes stretching and flexibility exercise, and you do it every day. In my experience, most patients prefer walking, cycling, or exercising in water. I don't recommend jogging or weight lifting. In order for it to be effective, exercise should cause some sustained increase in your heart rate. Start with five minutes a day and gradually increase it to thirty minutes over several weeks. Whatever exercise you do is most likely to be beneficial when done in the late afternoon or early evening. Just before bedtime it interferes with sleep. Several studies have shown that most patients who perform such exercises along with relaxation therapy (described below) do feel better. Remember not to do too much too soon. I usually refer patients with FMS to specially trained physiatrists (medical doctors who specialize in physiotherapy) for advice on an appropriate exercise regimen.

There are other steps you can take. Moist heat relieves pain. Try hot packs, warm baths, heating pads, or whirlpool baths at a physiotherapy clinic. Gentle massage is beneficial too. Some patients are helped by TENS, transcutaneous electrical nerve stimulation (electrodes applied to the body stimulate nerves and relieve pain). I encourage patients with FMS to try anything that reduces stress such as meditational yoga, biofeedback, and various relaxation exercises, the best known of which is Herbert Benson's Relaxation Response, described in his books. Try acupuncture (or acupressure) too.

You may obtain temporary relief by having your trigger points injected with a local anesthetic such as lidocaine and then stretching the involved muscle. However, there are too many of these trigger points for this technique to be of much help over the long term.

Anyone suffering from a chronic and incurable disorder

such as FMS is a target for unscrupulous promoters of any product that sounds reasonable. The Internet is full of such remedies, most of which are ineffective supplements and herbs. My advice is to eat a well-balanced whole-food diet. Cut back on sugar, too much of which can reduce your energy level. I also tell my patients to avoid acid-forming foods, red meat, carbonated drinks, and caffeine. Saturated fats are harmful for everybody, including patients with FMS. On theoretical grounds you should avoid any food to which you are allergic. Make sure you consume enough protein necessary for tissue repair.

Essential fatty acid supplements may be an exception to my warning about supplements. Adding gamma linolenic acid (GLA) was reported to improve symptoms in some patients.

DHEA, a steroid produced by the adrenal glands (which the body later converts to estrogen, testosterone, and cortisone), declines with age. Small amounts of DHEA (25 and 50 mg/ day) improved symptoms in one study. Discuss its use with your doctor. It may be worth a try given the paucity of other options.

There have been several reports and at least two books written about the use of guaifenesin for the treatment of FMS. You may know guaifenesin as Robitussin, a popular cold remedy that helps loosen mucus in the respiratory system. It is said to work by reducing calcium phosphate deposits in muscles and other tissues of the body. The proponents of guaifenesin claim that it acts on the kidneys so that they eliminate these deposits from the body. Unfortunately, I have never seen a properly documented scientific study to substantiate this theory. What's more, I'm not aware of any sophisticated diagnostic techniques that detect the presence of such deposits. A double-blind study on twenty-three patients revealed that guaifenesin did not increase phosphate excretion and was no more effective than a placebo.

There are medications that can improve the quality of life in those suffering from FMS. Unfortunately, the usual painkillers such as aspirin or the NSAIDs are not really effective. Avoid the use of narcotics and barbiturate sleeping pills, which can only lead to habituation or addiction. The most effective agents in the management of FMS raise the level of serotonin. The most widely used is amitriptyline (marketed as Elavil) in a dose of 25 to 75 mg taken at bedtime. Antidepressants such as Prozac are also useful. I have obtained the best results by prescribing Elavil at night and Prozac in the morning. Some patients hesitate to use these medications because they think they are being prescribed to cure depression, which they know is not their primary problem. I recommend them because they promote deep slumber by prolonging stage 4 sleep and raising the serotonin levels in the brain. Other helpful drugs are Tofranil and Desyrel, as well as newer selective serotonin reuptake inhibitors (SSRIs) in the Prozac family.

WHAT TO INSIST ON IF YOU HAVE FIBROMYALGIA

Fibromyalgia is a common and disabling condition whose victims, mostly women in the prime of life, suffer from a serious sleep disorder, chronic generalized muscle pain, and a host of other seemingly unrelated symptoms. Because there are no specific tests to diagnose this condition, and since its cause remains unclear, doctors call it a "syndromic diagnosis"—one that's subjective. Such patients are sometimes accused of being malingerers, depressed, or hypochondriacs. The depression that many of them do experience is the result of, and not the cause of, their symptoms. Although there are measures to reduce the severity of the symptoms, they can persist. However, one quarter of them go into remission within two years, and many more simply adjust to their disease and just cope.

Tell the world that it is not all in your head. There is no reason to be ashamed of your illness. *Insist on active medical care* even though the cause of your disease remains unknown and there is no specific curative treatment for it. Do not allow yourself to be deprived of any intervention that can help you. You are not a hypochondriac; you are not a neurotic. You are entitled to receive whatever (little) medicine can do for you at the present time. So *insist on seeing a physiatrist to help you with an exercise program; insist on a thorough evaluation of your symptoms to exclude some other disease that might possibly account for your misery; insist on access to the various therapeutic agents that can ease your suffering.* Be careful about seeing a "fibromyalgia specialist." There's no such thing. The best you can hope for, and insist on, is a doctor who believes you, who knows that fibromyalgia is a real disorder, and who will leave no stone unturned to help you.

13

GALLBLADDER DISEASE

When You're 5F, Not 4F

You may have been 4F in your army physical because of flat feet or asthma, but you're 5F if you have pain in the right upper portion of your abdomen. 5F stands for "fertile, female, fat, fiftyish, and flatulent"—the hallmarks of many people with gallbladder disease with or without gallstones.

Twenty million Americans (about 9 percent of the population) have gallbladder disease, and 500,000 of them undergo surgery for it every year. Even if you have no reason to suspect a gallbladder problem, read on anyway. You may be one of the million people in this country who are newly diagnosed annually.

What Are Gallstones?

What are gallstones, why do they form, what symptoms do they cause, what can (and should) you do about them, and when?

Let's review some human anatomy. The healthy gallbladder is a pear-shaped sac between three and six inches long and one inch wide. It's located in the right upper part of the abdomen under the liver and near the pancreas. Its job is to store the bile, a greenish-yellow fluid made by the liver. We need bile in order to digest the fat we eat and to absorb several vitamins and minerals in our diet. Bile leaves the liver through two ducts: One empties directly into the small intestine, where it breaks up the fat that you've eaten; the other branches off from this one and leads back into the gallbladder.

The liver makes as much as three cups of bile a day regardless of whether or not it's needed at any particular time. But if you haven't eaten any fat, and there's nothing in the small intestine to be digested, the bile has nowhere to go and nothing to do. So it comes down from the liver and backs up into the second duct (cystic duct) into the gallbladder where it's stored. Since the gallbladder can only accommodate one cup, it stores as much as it can and concentrates the rest. When you do eat fat (and I hope that that isn't too often), the gallbladder squirts back into the intestine the bile that it stored.

Bile consists mainly of water, cholesterol, lipids (fats), bile salts (these are natural detergents that break up fat), and bilirubin, a pigment that gives bile its greenish-yellow color. After the bile has finished its job of digesting the fat in the small intestine, some of it is excreted in the stool (giving it the normal brown color) and the rest is reabsorbed from the gut back into the bloodstream, which returns it to the liver to be used again.

Two ingredients in the bile, cholesterol and pigment can crystallize in the gallbladder. (Eighty percent of all gallstones are made up of cholesterol. Pigment stones are especially common in persons with liver disease and sickle-cell anemia.) The resulting crystals fuse to form stones that range in size from a tiny speck no bigger than a grain of sand to a rock the size of a golf ball. However, most gallstones are less than one inch across. Some never get any bigger, others do, and depending on their size, there can be hundreds of them.

When the crystals simply accumulate but don't fuse, they form sludge in the gallbladder. This is especially likely in someone who fasts for any length of time. However, sludge can form stones at any time—especially if you're overweight.

A poorly functioning gallbladder that fails to squeeze out all its bile, allowing it to stagnate and become abnormally concentrated, also contributes to stone formation.

Who's Vulnerable and Why

If you fall into any of the following categories, start taking steps to reduce the risk of developing gallstones:

- Men and women who weigh too much are three to seven times more likely to form gallstones, probably because their bile contains more cholesterol and their gallbladder is sluggish.
- Men and women aged sixty or older are more vulnerable. By the time they reach eighty, 10 percent of men and more than 20 percent of women have gallstones.
- Females between the ages of twenty and sixty are at least twice as vulnerable as are their husbands, boyfriends, or lovers.
- Pregnancy is associated with increased gallstone formation due to some mechanism that is not fully understood.
- Diabetics with high triglyceride levels are more vulnerable to gallstones.
- Birth control pills and estrogen replacement therapy raise the risk of gallstones because estrogen increases the cholesterol level and decreases contractility of the gallbladder.
- Certain drugs, such as clofibrate, that lower cholesterol increase its concentration in the bile, raising the risk of

gallstones in both men and women. This does not apply to the cholesterol-lowering "statin" drugs.

- Most Native American men have gallstones by the time they're sixty; 70 percent of female Pima Indians from Arizona develop gallstones by age thirty; and Mexican-Americans of any age and both genders are also vulnerable because their bile is very rich in cholesterol.

- The liver secretes extra cholesterol and tends to form cholesterol stones in someone who has been following a very low-calorie diet (less than 800 calories per day for twelve to sixteen weeks). Stones may also form after the gastric bypass operation to reduce stomach size in order to lose weight. (In one study, 38 percent of those who underwent such surgery developed gallstones within a few months.) Women who lose between nineteen and twenty-two pounds over a two-year period are 44 percent more likely to develop gallstones too.

- Fasting slows down the contractions of the gallbladder, as there is no need for bile in the gut. If this continues for long enough, the bile contains too much cholesterol and forms stones.

When You Have Gallstones

Eighty percent of all gallstones are silent. They're usually detected serendipitously by an abdominal ultrasound or CT scan done for some other reason. If the stones don't bother you, leave them alone. Doctors didn't always give this advice. We used to assume that gallstones would inevitably cause problems in the future, so the sooner you got rid of them, the better. After all, the reasoning went, you don't want to have an emergency gallbladder operation while you happen to be having a heart attack. It stood to reason that you were a better operative risk today than you would be when you were older. That suggestion would make sense if gallstones inevitably acted up. The fact is that only 2 percent of them do so each year. It would take about twenty-five years for gallstones to cause symptoms in most people. And by that time . . .

When the Gallbladder Acts Up

Gallbladder attacks can occur from time to time. The presence of stones indicates that the gallbladder may not be concentrating the bile properly, so that crystals, sludge, and stones form within it. Or it may not contract normally and fails to deliver the bile needed to digest fat in the intestine. Undigested fat can give you the classic symptoms of gallbladder disease: chronic indigestion, nausea, bloating, and lots and lots of burping after a fatty meal. (Many people go through life with these symptoms in the mistaken belief that they were born that way. If you're one of them, get yourself tested for gallstones.)

Gallstones can irritate the lining of the gallbladder leaving it chronically inflamed and/or infected. This causes pain, sometimes severe, in the right upper part of your abdomen, often radiating to the chest, the right shoulder, and through to the back.

Gallbladder disease can lead to digestive symptoms that come and go, often after a fatty meal. Then there is the acute gallstone attack that occurs when the gallbladder, contracting to deliver bile, also squeezes one or more of its stones into the gallbladder outlet. If the stone gets stuck there, the gallbladder muscles keep contracting to move it down and out. These contractions cause the severe colicky pain that is so typical of a gallbladder attack. If the stone moves into the bile duct that connects directly with the liver, no bile can get into the gut. That leaves the stool clay-colored because there is no bile pigment to make it brown. The blocked bile backs up into the liver and ultimately into the bloodstream. Too much bile in the blood leaves your skin and eyes yellow (jaundiced). If this obstruction continues for hours or days, the ducts become inflamed and infected (cholangitis). In addition, a stone in the bile duct can obstruct the opening into the adjacent pancreas and cause pancreatitis.

In addition to severe pain and jaundice, an acute gallbladder attack can result in fever, chills, nausea, and vomiting. Occasionally, a stone that's made its way from the gallbladder through the ducts and into the bowel can cause intestinal problems.

There is another complication of gallstones one doesn't hear much about. Statistically, a single large stone in your gallbladder may predispose you to cancer of that organ. I tell my patients about this possibility, and together we decide what to do. I usually recommend removal of the gallbladder in such cases even if there are no symptoms and despite the fact that the risk of cancer is low.

Diagnosing Gallstones

The acute gallbladder attack is usually fairly typical and easy to diagnose. Characteristically, patients with gallbladder pain often prefer to move around and rub their abdomen, whereas someone with pancreatic or ulcer pain stays put! There are several laboratory tests that are diagnostic too. The white blood cell count is often elevated, there is an increased bilirubin level in the blood, and various liver and pancreatic tests may also be abnormal.

In the "old days" we would get a cholecystogram to confirm the diagnosis. You swallowed some iodine pills the night before; the iodine was absorbed and made its way to the liver, which excreted it along with the bile. An X ray was then taken that showed the dye and the stones in the gallbladder or the ducts.

The modern way to clinch the diagnosis of gallstones is with an echo test (ultrasound) of the abdomen. This painless and noninvasive procedure detects stones or sludge in 98 percent of cases. There's no dye to take and no chance of an allergic reaction. You lie on the table while a technician moves a handheld device over your abdomen that directs sound waves (you can neither hear them nor feel them) to the gallbladder area. These waves bounce off the gallbladder, liver, pancreas, and everything else in the area. The resulting impulses create an image on a video screen of stones, sludge, the organs themselves, and even an occasional cancer.

Some doctors prefer the CT (computerized tomography) scan of the abdomen when they suspect not only gallstones but the possibility of some other cause of the symptoms such as a pancreatic tumor. This type of X ray is more revealing than the echo with respect to all the structures in the area of the abdomen where the gallbladder is located, but it is less sensitive for gallstones than ultrasound.

A radionuclide scan of the gallbladder is a third method of determining what's going on in the gallbladder, liver, and pancreatic area. It's probably the best way to detect inflammation of the gallbladder (cholecystitis) and assess its function (whether or not its contracting normally), with or without stones. This technique employs radioactive tracers instead of dye.

If the stone is lodged in one of the bile ducts, your doctor may want to have an ERCP (endoscopic retrograde cholangiopancreatograhpy) examination. This is more complicated and invasive than the other procedures described. You swallow a long, thin, lighted flexible tube that's connected to a computer and TV monitor. It passes from the stomach into the area of the small intestine where the ducts deliver their bile. The doctor then injects a special dye that "lights up" the ducts. He looks through the tube and can remove any stones that are present.

The same information can be obtained by means of another

test if for some reason the ERCP can't be done. A thin needle is passed through the abdominal wall and the dye is injected through it into the ducts. This procedure is called PTC (percutaneous transhepatic cholangiogram).

Living with Your Gallstones

If you have gallstones that don't bother you and have wisely decided not to rush to surgery, here's how to live with them: Avoid fat in your diet. Every time the fat globules (in butter, bacon, cream, marbled steak) reach the small intestine, they send signals calling for more bile. That means more gallbladder contractions, and the risk of dislodging a stone into a duct. And even if this doesn't happen, a fatty meal (as well as spicy food) will usually result in gas, bloating, and indigestion.

When your gallstones act up, here are some medications to have on hand to relieve your symptoms:

- An antispasmodic such as dicyclomine (Bentyl) relaxes the muscles of the gastrointestinal tract. The usual dose is anywhere from 10 to 40 mg taken orally three or four times a day. But avoid Bentyl if you have glaucoma, active angina, ulcerative colitis, or a big hiatus hernia with lots of acid reflux. This is a prescription drug and your doctor will know when it is not safe for you to take it. Glycopyrrolate (Robinul), one tablet three times a day, acts in much the same way.
- For nausea, I prefer Compazine (prochlorperazine) in a dose of 5 to 10 mg every four hours as necessary. But be careful with it if you have heart disease or narrow angle glaucoma. Promethazine (Phenergan) is also effective in doses of 12½ to 25 mg by mouth. Avoid it if you have active heart disease, asthma, or impaired liver

function. You'll need prescriptions for both these medications.

- There are various analgesics for pain relief, ranging all
the way from Tylenol and aspirin to narcotics such as
Demerol. The best one for you depends on many factors, including how often you need it. If your attacks are
frequent, consider surgery.

Getting Rid of Your Gallstones

Your decision to do something about your gallstones is often
elective (that is, when it's convenient for everybody concerned). You then have the luxury of choosing the method,
time, place, and surgeon. If you're fed up with all your symptoms, find the best doctor, decide when it most suits you to
have the operation, and schedule it. By contrast, in an emergency situation, you're suddenly sick and develop severe un-
relenting belly pain, fever, chills, nausea, vomiting, and
jaundice that demand immediate intervention.

Here are your treatment options in both circumstances:

- If there's no hurry, there is a pill you can take to dissolve
the stones. I haven't seen this therapy work very often,
although other doctors have found it effective. The medication is called ursodeoxycholic acid (Ursodiol). It's a
natural bile salt that cuts down the amount of cholesterol that the liver adds to the bile. If it's going to work,
it will dissolve small stones in six to twelve months. But
several of my patients have taken it without success for
more than two years. Also, even if the Ursodiol does dissolve the stones, there's no guarantee that new ones
won't form in the future. In fact, they actually do in
about half the patients so treated.

- A few medical centers use shock wave lithotripsy to shatter single stones that are less than an inch in size. The shock waves break the stones into smaller pieces, after which Ursodiol is prescribed. I first became aware of this technique some fifteen years ago when I visited the medical center in Austria where it was developed. The shocks fragment the stones, but at a high price! The smaller pieces get down into the ducts, where they can cause more trouble than did the one large stone, at least over the short term. The recurrence rate after lithotripsy is 10 to 40 percent, another reason I give this procedure a thumbs-down.

- When time is of the essence, or you've decided that your gallstones must go, surgery is the most predictable and effective course to follow. Removing gallstones, in effect, means taking out the gallbladder. Can you live without it? Absolutely. I don't mean to denigrate the gallbladder, but let's face it: It's not vital like the brain, heart, liver, or kidneys. When it's removed, its ducts are left behind and are able to deliver bile from the liver to the gut. An occasional problem after gallbladder surgery, and it's not a major one, is chronic diarrhea. Since the liver continues to make bile, it now goes directly into the gut in larger amounts, frequently causing loose movements.

Until just two decades ago, in performing the standard "open" gallstone operation, the surgeon always made a five-to-eight-inch cut into the muscles of the abdomen. This required a hospital stay of several days and more weeks at home to recover. Although it was a relatively safe operation, it was a miserable one. That became history with the availability of laparoscopic surgery. The surgeon makes four incisions in the abdomen, each only about half an inch long. A tiny video camera is then introduced into one of the incisions. It sends back a magnified image on a video monitor of what it sees inside the belly. The surgeon then inserts various instruments through the other incisions and, provided with the close-up view of the abdominal interior, separates the gallbladder from the liver and ducts and then removes it through one of the other incisions. You leave the hospital after a day or two and rest at home on restricted activity for another few days. Eighty percent of the nearly 500,000 gallbladder operations done each year are performed this way. *Insist on a second opinion if you're offered the old procedure.* In about 5 percent of cases the camera reveals scarring or infection that make the "open" operation necessary.

After the gallbladder is removed, however it's done, your pain will clear up, but you may have persistent gas, bloating, and indigestion after eating fatty foods for several months until your body adjusts.

WHAT TO INSIST ON IF YOU HAVE GALLBLADDER DISEASE

You're most vulnerable to developing gallstones if you have the 5Fs—fat, flatulent, female, fiftyish, and fertile. Gallstones occur more frequently as you get older—more commonly in women, especially those taking estrogen, Native Americans, Mexican Americans, and people who yo-yo their weight with crash starvation diets.

Most gallstones consist of cholesterol present in bile and to a lesser extent of bile pigments.

Gallstones do not usually cause symptoms. Right-sided abdominal pain, fever, and jaundice are the hallmarks of an acute attack.

Several noninvasive diagnostic tests are available to make the diagnosis.

The best way to deal with gallstones, when it becomes necessary to do so, is to remove them. This can now be done laparoscopically, a minimally invasive technique. You should *insist on it*. The older major operation is now done only when laparoscopy is not possible due to scarring or infection in and around the gallbladder.

There are nonsurgical ways to treat gallstones, but these are neither as predictable nor as effective as surgery.

The key fact to remember is that the mere presence of gallstones does not mean that you need an operation. If such stones are found "accidentally," and you're advised to have surgery, *insist on a second opinion*.

$\boxed{14}$

GOUT

A Royal Pain

Does this scenario sound familiar? You're a man in your fifties, a little overweight, and you love to eat. And I mean *eat*! You enjoyed an exceptionally gratifying meal last evening—a three-pound lobster washed down with a couple of beers and topped off with a great banana split. Delicious! It made you kind of sleepy and you couldn't wait to hit the sack, hoping to double your dining pleasure by dreaming about all that wonderful food. You fell asleep soon after your head hit the pillow, but before you could begin to dream, you were awakened by a terrible pain in your right big toe. This was no ordinary pain; it was so excruciating you couldn't even bear to have the bed sheet touch it. You'd never experienced anything like it before and couldn't imagine what was going on. You hadn't hurt your toe; you hadn't fiddled with an ingrown toenail; your shoes are not too tight. But then, suddenly, now fully awake, you remembered your father—and his attacks of gout. Like father, like son!

What is gout? Why did it happen to you? How can you relieve the pain? What can you do to prevent another attack? Does this mean that you will never be able to enjoy great meals again? Or quaff some beer? Or savor wine? Or sip a cocktail or two? Here are the answers you're looking for.

Men (and a few women) have suffered from gout over the centuries. It has often been referred to as "the disease of kings and the king of diseases." Its incidence varies from country to country. England is considered by many to be the mother country of gout. Remember the stereotype of a fat, old Englishman with a paunch and bulbous nose resting his foot and its swollen big toe on a footstool? That may be justified because while the incidence in the United States is 2.7 in every 1,000 adults, in England that figure is 19.3! (Gout is even more common among the Maoris of New Zealand and Pacific Islanders, 10 percent of whose men suffer from it.) Despite the image of gluttony, booze, and obesity, gout is not usually caused by lifestyle; it's in the genes.

These days, however, gout is no longer viewed as an exclusively English disease or a "complication" of wealth, dietary indiscretion, and age. Given a life expectancy well into the seventies in this country, and the affordability for most people of food and drink that can provoke gout among the vulnerable, it's everyone's disease. However, it's much more common in men over the age of forty-five or fifty, with a male-to-female ratio of 9 to 1. It virtually never occurs in premenopausal women.

How Gout Develops

Here's how your attack of gout that unforgettable night happened to you—and your father.

We all have a small amount of uric acid in the bloodstream. Its source is purine, the by-product of normal cell death that occurs constantly in the body, and is present in certain foods. Uric acid is a waste material without any function. Since it is constantly entering the blood stream, we'd be in big trouble if there were no way to get rid of it. Happily, there is. Most animals have an enzyme that breaks down uric acid, but humans don't. We depend on our kidneys to excrete it—and they do it so that we normally maintain a level in the blood of between 2 and 7 milligrams. That number increases when the body makes more uric acid than the kidneys can eliminate, or we eat far too many purine-containing foods, or the kidneys are diseased and can't get rid of even normal amounts.

Whatever the cause, high uric acid levels result in the formation of needlelike crystals in several different joints, most commonly in the big toe, but also in the foot, ankle, heel, knees, elbow, wrist, or fingers. When uric acid crystals develop in the joint, the immune system tries to get rid of them by unleashing a barrage of defense mechanisms. Swarms of white blood cells attack and engulf them, and as they do, they also release enzymes that cause inflammation. It's this vigorous counterattack against the crystals, and not the crystals themselves, that cause the painful, hot, red, swollen joint characteristic of gout. As it turns out, all this posturing by the immune system is for naught. The gout attack persist until the immune system has abandoned its fruitless countermeasures.

Although you're most apt to develop gout if you have too much uric acid circulating in the bloodstream, that only happens to one person in twenty. What's more, you can also have an attack even if your uric acid level is normal. So remember this: *If you have all the typical symptoms of gout but the diagnosis is dismissed because your uric acid isn't elevated insist on seeing an arthritis specialist (rheumatologist), who may withdraw some fluid from the affected joint and look for the presence of the diagnostic uric acid crystals under the microscope. By the same token, if you have joint pains that don't really look like gout, but are given that diagnosis because your uric acid level is high, also insist on a consultation with a rheumatologist.*

Gout usually begins in middle age. I have never seen a

case in anyone under thirty, and women rarely have it before menopause. If you have never had an attack, but are predisposed to it because of a strong family history of the disease (one in four people with gout has a close blood relative with gout), try to keep your uric acid level as close to normal as possible, either by diet or by medication (see below).

When You Have Gout

Ten percent of patients with gout have too much uric acid either because of their diet or because their bodies make too much. In the remaining 90 percent, uric acid is not being adequately eliminated from the body due to some kidney problem.

Overproduction of Uric Acid

Here are some of the more important circumstances in which there is overproduction of uric acid:

- Various forms of leukemia in which there are too many white blood cells
- Polycythemia vera (too many red blood cells)
- Severe psoriasis
- Paget's disease of bone
- Dehydration
- Alcohol excess
- Obesity
- Diet rich in purine

- Vitamin B_{12} supplements in patients being treated for pernicious anemia

---

AN EXCESS OF THESE PURINE-RICH FOODS CAN RAISE URIC ACID AND RESULT IN GOUT:

- Meat: veal, venison, bacon
- Turkey
- Animal organs: sweetbreads, liver, beef kidneys, tripe, tongue
- Seafood: shellfish, scallops, fish roe (no more caviar!), sardines, anchovies, herring, mackerel, salmon, codfish, trout
- Nuts
- Dried legumes: soy, peanuts, peas, lentils, beans

If you've had gout, you should theoretically avoid or limit your intake of all of the above to keep your uric acid level down. I say "theoretically" because in this day and age there are effective medications that can lower uric acid despite what you eat. Because these drugs are inexpensive and have few if any side effects, they have liberated gout patients from the need to follow such a diet strictly. In fact, dietary management is no longer an important part of preventing or treating gout.

Decreased Excretion of Uric Acid

You can develop gout when the body doesn't get rid of enough uric acid under the following circumstances:

- Kidney disease (of which there are many types)
- High blood pressure

- Down's syndrome
- Starvation (producing ketosis)
- Underfunction of the thyroid gland
- Hyperparathyroidism. (An excess of parathyroid hormone made by the parathyroid gland near the thyroid gland in the neck. This hormone controls calcium metabolism.)

Various drugs can also interfere with uric acid excretion and cause gout. These include:

- Low-dose aspirin
- Diuretics (water pills)
- Alcohol
- Levodopa-carbidopa (Sinemet) for the treatment of Parkinson's disease
- Nicotinic acid (to lower elevated cholesterol)
- Cyclosporine (for the prevention of rejection of transplanted organs)
- Tuberculosis medications (pyrazinamide, ethambutol)

The Acute Gout Attack

The typical gout attack usually comes on during the night and is often precipitated by a sudden rise in uric acid levels after binge drinking and/or the excess consumption of purine-rich foods. It can also follow an injury, even a minor one, an operation, an unrelated illness, and unusual stress or fatigue. Initially, only one joint, usually the big toe, is affected (90 percent of persons with gout have it in the big toe sometime during the course of their disease). The onset of pain is sudden and without warning. At first, it's not bad, but as the affected joint becomes swollen, red or purplish, and warm, it ends up exquisitely tender even to the lightest touch. The skin is shiny and tight; you can't bear to have anything touch it. Even the vibration of a slammed door makes it hurt! Some patients develop a slight fever, occasionally accompanied by chills, and they feel sick all over.

The legs are more often affected than the arms because the temperature of the legs is lower than that of the arms. Cooler temperature favors the formation of the crystals. The attacks typically come on during the night because that's when fluid in the joints is reabsorbed, increasing the concentration of the crystals. The gout attack peaks within one or two days, and if left alone, gradually subsides in seven to ten days.

Attacks usually recur if the disease is not managed properly (only 5 to 10 percent of patients have only one attack), and eventually damage the joints and the kidneys.

Uric acid crystals don't settle only in the joints; they can also accumulate on tendons and the cartilage of the ear, where they form lumps or nodules called *tophi*. Before modern therapy for gout, these topi would get so big they'd eventually rupture and discharge a white chalky material made up of their crystals. I haven't seen one of these in years. These crystals can also form uric acid stones in the kidney.

Treating the Acute Attack of Gout

Modern medications have essentially conquered gout. There is really no reason for anyone to suffer from it anymore.

The most effective modern therapy for acute gout is the family of *nonsteroidal anti-inflammatory drugs* (NSAIDs). Take them until the pain subsides and then go on to a different group of drugs that *prevents* the recurrence of gout. There are several effective NSAIDs against gout. You can have an intramuscular injection of ketorolac (Toradol), or oral medications such as ibuprofen (Motrin), naproxen (Naprosyn), and others. I usually prescribe 50 mg of indomethacin (Indocin) three times a day on a full stomach. The weaker NSAIDs available over-the-counter are usually not strong enough unless you take several of them. I continue the high initial dose of indomethacin for twenty-four hours after the pain has subsided, taper it during the next three days, and then discontinue it.

More important than the particular NSAID you take is how soon you start therapy. The longer you wait, the less effective it is. You may occasionally need a narcotic in addition to or instead of the NSAIDs. *Do not use aspirin in any form or combination. It makes matters worse.* When the pain is very bad and the NSAIDs and other painkillers aren't enough, you may need steroids (cortisone-like drugs).

If you're taking an anticoagulant such as warfarin (Coumadin), be very careful with any of the NSAIDs. Check your blood (prothrombin time) frequently to make sure it's not too thin. If you have some other medical problem such as peptic ulcer, gastritis, liver or kidney disease, you may not be able to tolerate an NSAID. In such cases, you may need a steroid either by mouth or injected directly into the joint.

In the 1800s *colchicine,* extracted from the autumn crocus, was the only effective agent available for treating the acute attack and preventing recurrences. It still has a place in the treatment of gout as well as its prevention in those patients who for any reason cannot tolerate the NSAIDs. Colchicine works only in gout and no other form of arthritis. Taken orally, it usually becomes effective only after it has caused nausea, vomiting, or diarrhea. That sounds awful, but believe me, the intestinal symptoms are preferable to the pain of gout. There are fewer side effects when colchicine is given intravenously, but this route has several drawbacks: It can hurt the liver; it can be very painful if any of it leaks into the tissues near the site of injection; the wrong dose can suppress the bone marrow and cause the kidneys to fail. So make sure that the doctor doing the injecting has had experience with the technique.

If you are having an acute attack of gout, remember that the sooner treatment is started, the more effective it will be. Insist on seeing your doctor as soon as possible, and no later than the next day. While you're waiting, drink five or six glasses of water, rest, and elevate the affected limb.

Long-Term Treatment of Gout

There is a drug you should take on an ongoing basis to keep the uric acid within normal limits and reduce the likelihood of recurrence of gout. Remember that repeated attacks, even if you're a stoic and able to withstand the pain, can ultimately damage your joints and your kidneys.

Allopurinal (Zyloprim) is a long-term medication that prevents the purines in your food from converting to uric acid. It is effective and very well tolerated. Start with 100 mg per day and increase it as necessary (to keep the uric acid level at 6 mgs or lower) up to 300 mg per day. Another effective medication is probenecid (Benemid) that reduces uric acid by increasing its excretion by the kidneys. If your doctor prescribes probenecid, stop any aspirin you're taking. It interferes with the action of probenecid.

It's a good idea to add one or two colchicine tablets a day for a few weeks after starting any of these drugs because they may initially increase the risk of an attack. Colchicine in these small doses does not have any significant side effects.

Remember: Do not take any agent that lowers uric acid during the acute attack. They don't work at that time and may worsen symptoms.

If you choose not to accept any maintenance or preventive therapy, avoid purine-rich foods and reduce or eliminate alcohol. But you'd better keep your fingers crossed. This strategy only works in a lucky 10 percent of patients; 60 percent have a recurrence within a year, and almost 80 percent get another attack within two years.

If your uric acid level is high, but you have never had gout, I don't recommend any treatment unless you have a strong family history of the disease. Only a very small percentage of such people ever develop gout. However, watch your diet and drink plenty of water.

Pseudogout

Pseudogout is a condition that's a dead ringer for gout. It also causes a swollen, hot painful knee, wrist, or shoulder. Pseudogout affects 3 percent of the population, mostly those in their sixties.

Gout and pseudogout are both due to the deposit of crystals in the joints. However, in gout they are uric acid crystals, while in pseudogout they're calcium. The immune system launches the same attack on both, so that the clinical presentations are almost identical.

The cause of pseudogout remains a mystery. As with gout, there appears to be a genetic connection, and sometimes the attacks occur in people with hypothyroidism and hyperparathyroidism, but that's where the similarity ends.

The treatment of the acute attack of pseudogout is the same as that for gout: anti-inflammatory drugs, steroid injections, and other painkillers. However, neither colchicine nor any of the drugs and measures to lower uric acid has any effect on pseudogout since uric acid is not the culprit.

It's difficult to distinguish gout from pseudogout on clinical grounds. However, since the incidence is almost equal in both men and women, *any female who develops "gout" should be seen by an arthritis specialist, who can make the right diagnosis by doing a needle aspiration of the joint and looking at the crystals under the microscope. Testing the uric acid level in the blood doesn't help because it may be normal in both conditions.*

WHAT TO INSIST ON IF YOU HAVE GOUT

Gout is a common form of arthritis with a specific cause—the inability of the body to deal with uric acid, a normal constituent of the blood that usually rises to abnormal levels. In persons with gout, uric acid forms crystals that are deposited in the joints. The acute pain, redness, and swelling that ensue are the result of futile attempts by the immune system to rid the joints of these intruders.

The diagnosis of gout does not usually present a problem. Although most cases are associated with elevated blood uric acid, attacks can occur when the uric acid is normal. Conversely, 90 percent of people with high uric acid never develop gout.

If you suddenly have an acutely painful joint that has all the characteristics of gout, *insist on seeing your doctor as soon as possible, because treatment is most effective when started early.* A normal uric acid level does not rule out the diagnosis. If you're having symptoms but your uric acid level is normal, *insist on a consultation with an arthritis specialist or orthopedist.* You may need to have the fluid in the affected joint removed and looked at under the microscope for the presence of the characteristic needle-like uric acid crystals.

It's very important to distinguish gout from pseudogout because their long-term management is different despite their striking similarity.

15

HAIR LOSS

Is Bald Beautiful?

Some men can parlay complete baldness into something attractive, even sexy. Yul Brynner was a case in point; so are *Star Trek*'s Captain Picard, Kareem Abdul-Jabbar, the basketball great, and my oldest son, the tai ch'i master. On them the billiard-ball head looks good. In fact, they deliberately remove every vestige of hair on their scalps, and on special occasions they even polish them to a high gloss. But hair that falls out gradually and insidiously and looks thin or straggly, with bald spots showing through wispy strands, is a cosmetic problem for many. It generates a usually fruitless search for a cause and cure; one shampoo after another is tried and discarded as the prospect of ultimately needing a hairpiece looms larger and larger. Hair loss may have cosmetic consequences, but it may also have medical implications.

There are two major kinds of hair loss. The first is "natural," so-called pattern baldness. Two of every three men develop a receding hairline by the time they're fifty, and more than a third of American women also experience significant hair loss. The second form of baldness is reversible and due to an avoidable or treatable cause.

Because cutting the hair and nails is painless, we may conclude that they are dead or inert tissues. The fact is that hair and nails are very much alive. You can't always see it, and you certainly don't hear it, but each of your scalp hairs is continually growing for anywhere from two to six years—about a half inch a month; a little less as the years go by. It then enters a resting phase for two to three months, after which it falls out. A new hair then starts growing from the same follicle, and the process then begins all over again. Normally, 90 percent of your hair is in the growing mode and 10 percent is resting. You can expect to lose up to 125 hairs per day in this way (300 on the days you shampoo). Since hair loss is balanced by new growth, the appearance of the scalp is normally unchanged.

Hereditary Thinning and Balding

When you look through the family album, you can assume that male pattern baldness is something you will ultimately develop. You father's "hairdo" is almost identical to your grandfather's, so why should familial genetics spare you?

Female pattern baldness is akin to that of the male. The hair thins a great deal, especially at the top or the sides of the head, and bald spots may also appear. As you will see below, this happens when the hormonal environment changes, mainly as a result of estrogen variations—as when women take the Pill, become pregnant, or reach menopause.

Females, as well as males, transmit the balding gene. My own family is a case in point. There has never been a bald Rosenfeld anywhere in the annals of that distinguished family. Look at my picture on the jacket. There's not a single hair missing or out of place. Yet every one of my three sons is bald—one totally. He has made peace with his genes and has even outperformed them, going so far as to remove every hair on his cranium. His two brothers are still trying to save what foliage they have, but alas, to little avail. It's my wife, not I, who's responsible for their appearance. Her father and brother were both bald; mine were not. I'm not telling you this to criticize my wife or her ancestors, for beauty is only skin-deep. Besides which, my sons inherited many fine qualities from the "other side" of the family that transcend hair in importance. I simply want to point out that either parent can transmit the baldness gene.

Hereditary baldness (androgenic alopecia) used to be considered incurable, but there are now several ways to deal with it. First, you can change your hairstyle. That's what Napoleon did. If you look at his picture, you will see how his hair is combed forward almost down to his forehead. Since Napoleon despised men who wore wigs, his hairdresser or whoever advised him at the time thought this was the most effective way to conceal his male pattern baldness. (Julius Caesar had a similar hairdo and for the same reason.)

If your bald spot isn't too large, and you've got enough hair left, you can spray some more from a can onto your scalp. It's not really hair but a powder that creates a hairy illusion. If this doesn't work, two medications, minoxidil (marketed as Rogaine) and finasteride (sold as Propecia), can sometimes improve hereditary thinning or baldness.

Rogaine has been available since 1983, and you can now buy it over-the-counter. This drug was initially developed as a blood-pressure-lowering agent. However, during its trials, doctors noted that some men and women receiving it began to sprout hair in various parts of their bodies. This observation led to its preparation in topical form for the treatment of hair loss in both men and women.

Response to Rogaine is variable and unpredictable, but often more effective in women than in men. You can often spot a Rogaine user by the peach fuzz that appears on the scalp. However, about 10 to 14 percent of those who use it do obtain visible regrowth; others just stop losing their hair, or do so more slowly. In some cases, it only maintains the status quo—things just don't get worse. This drug is most apt to be successful if you start taking it when you're young; if you've had the hair problem for less than ten years; if the bald spot on the top of your head is less than four inches across; and if the bald areas have short, little hairs, which have the potential to grow.

Rogaine comes in two strengths, 2 percent and 5 percent. I suggest that men start with the stronger dosage. Apply it to your scalp twice a day; you may not see any results for many months. Don't throw in the towel for at least a year. If there is no improvement by that time, move on to something else. But if you do see some sprouting, stay with it. If it works, you'll need to take Rogaine for the rest of your life. If you quit for whatever reason, the hair that did result from its use will disappear. Rogaine sometimes irritates the scalp, in which case don't use it.

Unlike Rogaine, which can be effective in both men and women, *Propecia* (finasteride) works only in men. It is a weaker form of Proscar, the 5-mg dose of which is prescribed to help shrink an enlarged prostate and reduce the frequency of night visits to the john. The FDA approved it for the treatment of hair loss in men at the end of 1997. The dosage is a daily 1-mg tablet. Several studies suggest that Propecia does work. In one report, after two years of therapy with this drug, hair was longer and thicker in 66 percent of cases, and the drug stopped further hair loss in five of every six men. Happily, it doesn't cause hair growth anywhere but on your head.

Propecia acts by blocking an enzyme called 5-alpha-reductase that converts the male hormone testosterone to another form called dihydrotestosterone (DHT). This DHT causes baldness. So Propecia reduces the amount of DHT in your body, without causing any decrease in masculinity. However, although it's well tolerated, some men occasionally become impotent or have less sexual desire after using it.

Propecia is available only by prescription and costs about twice as much as Rogaine (about $50 per month as compared to $20 or less). Remember that it is not meant for women or children. This medication should never under any circumstances be taken or even handled by any female who is either pregnant or potentially so, since it can cause abnormalities of the genital tract in the fetus.

Saw palmetto, an herb that's widely used in Europe (and more recently in this country as well) for the treatment of symptoms of prostatic enlargement, also blocks the 5-alpha-reductase enzyme, much as does finasteride. It, too, is said to be effective against hair loss, but the supporting evidence is still sparse.

Reversible Hair Loss

Here are some of the more common causes of *reversible* hair loss:

The cosmetics you use and how you care for your hair are the most frequent culprits of temporary hair loss. For example, teasing, perming, and coloring can make hair brittle and easily broken. Harsh hair-straightening chemicals can damage the hair follicles. Curling irons, hot rollers, hair sprays, gels, and mousses should be used as little as possible, and you're better off air-drying more and blow-drying less.

I'm not a cosmetician, but here's what my wife (who has a splendid head of hair) and her hairdressers tell me:

- Don't shampoo every day; three times a week is often enough. Use warm, not hot, water.
- Apply a gentle conditioner or hair cream to the tips of the hair after shampooing. Rubbing it into the scalp flattens the hair.
- Don't rub, comb, or brush your hair vigorously when it's wet. Frequent brushing or combing isn't good either, especially if you're beginning to find more hair than you like on your pillow.

- Your comb should have wide teeth, and your hairbrush should be soft and smooth-tipped.
- If your hair is fragile to begin with, ponytails and braids that require a lot of tight pulling can cause "traction alopecia," especially common among African Americans.

Crash diets. Hair loss is much less common in China, Italy, and Japan than it is in America. Although that's partly due to genetic differences, diet also plays a part. Populations with more hair on their head generally eat more leafy green vegetables, fish, unsaturated fats, and antioxidants such as vitamins C and E than we do. These foods nourish hair.

If you go on a "strict" diet from time to time, you should know that reducing your protein intake can put your hair into the resting phase. This is how the body conserves its protein stores. You may end up with substantial hair loss. The good news is that when you resume an adequate protein intake, your hair will begin to grow back.

Thyroid malfunction (See Chapter 38). Whether your thyroid gland is underactive or overactive, producing too much or too little of its hormone, your hair responds by falling out. Thyroid trouble is the first thing to look for when your basin is full of hair and your pillow is covered with it. Ask for a simple blood test of thyroid function. Depending on what it shows, replacing the missing hormone or cutting down its overproduction returns your body metabolism to normal and your hair will stop falling out.

Illness. If you've been pregnant, or had an infection, especially with high fever (or undergone major surgery, or been hospitalized and given a variety of drugs ranging from painkillers to antibiotics), your hair may begin to fall out—not right away, but several weeks or months later. There's nothing you can or should do about it other than maintain good nutrition. This hair loss is temporary and you can count on its growing back within 2–4 weeks. However, if you have an ongoing chronic, debilitating illness, hair loss may persist for the duration. Stress, even in the absence of surgery or chronic illness, can also affect the hair growth cycle so that the resting stage comes sooner, and is followed by hair loss. It may take several months for this to happen, but when the stress is removed, hair usually grows back.

Chemotherapy for cancer is perhaps the most devastating cause of hair loss. However, most patients who require it are so concerned with survival that baldness is of secondary importance. Most such hair loss is only temporary.

Hormonal factors. When you're pregnant, your scalp is likely to look better than ever because the hormonal changes in your body favor hair growth. However, once you have your baby, your hair starts "resting" and falls out. This can continue for about six months, after which time normal growth resumes. When you enter menopause, the change in your hormonal status can also cause temporary hair loss, which is usually reversed by hormone replacement.

Medication. If there has been any change in your hair growth pattern, review all the drugs, supplements, and herbs you're taking. Everything from vitamins (especially vitamin A) to heart medications (diuretics), blood-pressure-lowering agents, painkillers, antidepressants, blood thinners, and antibiotics can do it. Chief among the offenders are cancer treatments such as radiation and chemotherapy. Although the hair does grow back after the therapy has been completed, the therapy may have to be continued for so long that many patients buy a wig or wear a bandana for the duration.

Anemia. If you're lacking iron (because you aren't getting enough in your diet, or are losing it in your blood—a common cause is heavy menstrual flow—or aren't absorbing the iron you eat), you may begin to lose your hair. Correcting the anemia will cure the problem.

Birth control pills. Some women who have a hereditary vulnerability to do so begin to lose their hair when they take the Pill. Switching brands may solve the problem. If it doesn't, you'll have to decide which is more important to you—this method of contraception or your appearance. Sometimes the hair doesn't start falling out until two or three months after stopping the oral contraceptive. If that happens to you, don't panic. It will grow back in about six months.

Alopecia areata. This is a poorly understood disorder, probably of the autoimmune system, that causes hair loss at any age. Healthy individuals either develop discrete round, bald patches the size of a silver dollar on the scalp or, in severe cases, lose *all* their body hair. Steroid injections to the affected area can help. Some dermatologists prescribe a variety of topical agents or light therapy, but I have never been impressed with the results.

Ringworm (tinea capitis) has nothing to do with worms. It is a fungus that affects the superficial layers of the skin and no other part of the body. It's most common in children, and it's contagious. Involved areas of the scalp develop scales and lose their hair. Examine your child carefully if one of his or her classmates is diagnosed with ringworm. A cat or other pet can also transmit the disease, so take your cat to the vet to make sure it isn't the source of the infection. Remember too that ringworm has no respect for age, so you are not immune.

A variety of topical antifungal creams, as well as oral agents such as griseofulvin, Sporanox, and Lamisil will cure ringworm and restore hair growth. Some of the antifungal medications are available over-the-counter; make sure they contain miconazoles or clotrimazoles. You should also eliminate the fungal spores by shampooing with selenium sulfide.

No matter why you're bald—hereditary baldness or thinning, or your scalp has been injured or burned, or you've lost hair in some other way, if you've done all you can and you simply don't like the way you look, you should consider hair transplantation. This almost always involves taking hair from the back of the scalp and moving it to the bald spot that needs it more. There are several different kinds of procedures such as scalp reduction and flap surgery, depending on the geography of your scalp, and they're usually done by a dermatologist. I have seen the most natural results transplanting hair with "micro grafts" using 1–4 hairs per graft. Be sure to check the cost before you decide to go this route. It's expensive and not usually covered by insurance.

WHAT TO INSIST ON IF YOU'RE LOSING YOUR HAIR

Hair loss is essentially a cosmetic problem, but it can also reflect some underlying disorder. No one ever died from baldness or thinning hair. You can't expect your insurance company to reimburse you for a hair transplant. However, *if you have unexplained hair loss, you should insist on a complete physical examination because there are important diseases that can cause it.*

(16)

HEART DISEASE

When Your Ticker Isn't Tocking

Hearts don't "break," they're "attacked." Although heart disease can kill you when you're very young (usually as a result of a congenital defect), or at any age by bacteria that infect and damage the cardiac valves, or viruses that strike and weaken the muscle, the major nemesis overall is the heart attack.

One and a half million people have heart attacks every year in this country alone. It's the number one killer in the United States and in almost every developed nation except Japan (where stroke has that dubious honor). The older you are, the greater your vulnerability. Three hundred thousand of those stricken never even reach a hospital because they die suddenly wherever they happen to be—in bed, at work, watching television, or jogging in the park.

How and Why Heart Attacks Happen

You suffer a heart attack when your cardiac muscle is deprived of its blood supply. This usually happens as a result of the sudden obstruction and closure of a coronary artery in the heart that was previously affected by arteriosclerosis. Although the great majority of heart attacks occur in adult life, the process responsible for them begins in childhood, when small fatty plaques form in the arteries of the heart (and elsewhere). As we grow older, these deposits enlarge and absorb cholesterol as well as other fats and a variety of substances carried in the blood. Eventually, they also contain calcium, which is why arteriosclerosis is popularly referred to as "hardening of the arteries." The heart attack is the final event in this saga. It occurs when a plaque, regardless of its size, ruptures or a fresh clot forms on its surface.

As these coronary artery plaques gradually enlarge, reducing the amount of blood flowing through them, a protective "collateral circulation" is called into play. We're born with a network of tiny blood channels throughout the heart muscle. As the amount of oxygen to the heart muscle decreases, these vessels, heretofore only "potential," begin to widen enough to deliver a significant blood supply. Whether you live or die after a heart attack depends on several factors: The size of the blocked artery, the condition of your heart muscle (was it previously damaged or weakened by any other process such as long-standing untreated high blood pressure?), the condition of the other coronaries and how much blood they are delivering, and last but not least, the extent and efficiency of your collateral circulation. The formation of collaterals is stimulated not only by a reduced blood supply but also by regular exercise, which has the heart constantly calling for more blood to nourish it. Couch potatoes have fewer collaterals than do joggers!

Are You at Risk? Yes!

Every adult is a candidate for a heart attack, regardless of age, but some more than others, depending on the kind and number of their cardiac risk factors. The more risk factors you have, the greater the danger. So the sooner you begin to identify and correct them, the better. Here are the most important ones:

- *Elevated cholesterol.* In order to dissolve in the bloodstream, this blood fat is attached to two kinds of proteins—a "good" one called high-density lipoprotein (HDL) and a "bad" one, low-density lipoprotein (LDL). HDL is good because, together with the cholesterol it's carrying, it remains in the bloodstream away from the arterial wall. LDL and its cholesterol molecule, on the other hand, are deposited onto the lining of the coronary arteries, where they eventually form obstructive plaques. So it's not enough to know just your cholesterol level. You must *insist* on knowing the HDL and LDL breakdown. Total cholesterol should be no higher than 200; the LDL should not exceed 100; and the ratio between total cholesterol and the HDL should be less than 4 (again, the lower the better). Regardless of the cholesterol/HDL ratio, a total cholesterol reading higher than 200 accompanied by an LDL above 100 should be treated. However, the primary target is the LDL. Regardless of the other numbers, this should be lowered below 100.
- *Triglyceride,* a neutral fat made in the liver, is also a risk factor for arteriosclerosis. Unlike the blood test for cholesterol, which may be performed regardless of when you last ate or drank, you must have been fasting for at least fourteen hours when your triglyceride level is being measured. This value should not exceed 150.

- *Tobacco* accelerates the process of arteriosclerosis over the long term. However, nicotine throws all your arteries, including your coronaries, into spasm every time you inhale. If they already contain some plaques, this superimposed spasm can temporarily close them after even only one cigarette. We usually associate tobacco with cancer and birth defects. The truth is that tobacco contributes to the majority of the more than 900,000 deaths each year in the United States that are due to vascular disease and heart attacks.

- *High blood pressure* (hypertension, see Chapter 19) is a very important risk factor. Blood flowing through the arteries at an elevated pressure is constantly pounding their walls, weakening them and promoting plaque formation. So it's critical to lower the pressure as soon as possible and keep it down forever. If you're otherwise healthy, a normal blood pressure will help you stay that way; if you've already got heart trouble, it will substantially reduce the risk of a heart attack. We used to think that only the diastolic pressure (the lower of the two numbers) was important. We now know that the top figure (systolic pressure) is also critical and should not be more than 140 at any age. So forget the old myth of 100 plus your age as an acceptable reading. It's not.

- *Diabetes* is another major risk factor. A high blood sugar, especially in someone who is overweight (as many adult diabetics are) and who also has elevated cholesterol, increases vulnerability to premature arteriosclerosis. So if you're diabetic, it's extremely important to keep your sugar levels as close to normal as possible, making sure, too, that your cholesterol is below 200 and that your weight is as good as you can get it.

- *Overweight* plagues 70 percent of patients with coronary artery disease. If you weigh only 10 percent more than you should, you raise your risk of a heart attack by 30 percent.

- If your *genetics* appear to be bad—for example, several of your close blood relatives had heart attacks before age sixty—you are statistically more likely to have one too. However, even if they've passed some of their bad genes on to you (and there's no way you can be sure of that at the present time), there's more to the story. Despite their genes, these ill-fated relatives may have suffered their heart attacks prematurely because they smoked, were diabetic and paid no attention to their elevated sugar, or ignored their elevated blood pressure and cholesterol. So don't be fatalistic and nihilistic about a bad family history. Be all the more diligent in eliminating whatever controllable risk factors you can identify.

- *Lack of exercise.* Regular exercise protects the coronary arteries. Remember the collaterals! That doesn't mean running in a marathon or looking like Arnold Schwarzenegger. All you need to do is walk briskly for thirty minutes a day four or five times a week, or swim, dance, or bike. If you can't exercise outdoors often enough because you live in Alaska, where it's too cold in the winter, or in the tropics, where it's too hot, buy a small treadmill and do the walking in the comfort of your home. That's what I do every single day of my life. Aerobic exercise reduces the workload of the heart by lowering the resting heart rate and blood pressure. It also lowers cholesterol and triglyceride levels; raises the good HDL and drops the undesirable LDL; reduces blood sugar in diabetics; helps prevent osteoporosis; decreases body fat; eases stress and improves mood.

- *Certain personality types* and behavior patterns are said to increase the risk of a heart attack. The prototype is the hard-driving, aggressive, time-conscious, type A executive whose anger and hostility raise his adrenaline level. This in turn raises the heart rate and blood pressure. So if you're going through life with a chip on your shoulder, work out instead of throwing a tantrum.

- *Infections,* both viral and bacterial, are now also being implicated in the causation of heart attacks. This most surprising link was suggested after researchers found a variety of organisms inside the arterial plaques. These included *Chlamydia* (the bug that causes pneumonia, sexually transmitted disease, and other infections); cytomegalos virus, which affects the liver; and even *H. pylori* (the bacterium associated with ulcers and possibly cancer of the stomach). The *Chlamydia* story is particularly interesting. Researchers have found higher concentrations of *Chlamydia* antibodies in the blood of some persons with a history of heart attacks. When they treated them with an anti-*Chlamydia* antibiotic such as azithromycin (Zithromax) for one week, they had a lower incidence of subsequent heart attacks than did an untreated group. These observations are being tested further, but in the meantime some doctors are routinely checking all their heart attack patients for *Chlamydia* antibodies and treating with azithromycin those who are positive. I decided to do the same in my own practice, but guess what? I haven't found any *Chlamydia* antibodies in a single one of my cardiac patients. (I'm still looking, though.)

- Before *menopause,* the ovaries make lots of estrogen that protects women against heart attacks. When estrogen production declines and the periods stop, women become as vulnerable as men. Does replacing the missing hormone turn back the clock? Recent studies have not confirmed any protective effect. In fact, a woman who sustains a heart attack should not continue taking the hormone. In my own practice, I am still prescribing ERT for most menopausal women without heart disease because of this hormone's many other benefits (well-being, better skin, a more supple and moist vagina, and less osteoporosis), but not to prevent a heart attack.

- *Homocysteine,* a protein normally found in the blood in concentrations of 5 to 15 micromoles, appears to be associated with a risk of heart attack when its values exceed 20 micromoles. (But many heart attack patients have normal levels of this protein.) It remains to be seen whether lowering elevated homocysteine levels will confer any protection, but most cardiologists are now routinely screening for homocysteine and treating when it's elevated. The folic acid, vitamin B_6 and vitamin B_{12} in most multivitamins will often return these levels to normal. I routinely prescribe them for all patients with elevated homocysteine levels.

- *Excess iron* is thought by some to contribute to heart disease, presumably by enhancing plaque formation through the LDL fraction of cholesterol. This may explain the low incidence of heart disease in premenopausal women, whose monthly blood loss eliminates extra iron, as well as the observation that regular blood donors have fewer heart attacks too. Don't take extra iron unless you have an iron deficiency anemia due to any cause (menses, hemorrhoids, poor nutrition).

- The newest risk factor to be identified is a blood test called the "C Reactive Protein." When elevated this "inflammatory" marker is an independent (regardless of what all the other tests show) predictor of vulnerability to heart attack.

Sudden Cardiac Death

Of the 500,000 cardiac deaths in the United States every year, more than 300,000 are "sudden." The lowered oxygen content of the injured heart muscle triggers abnormal electrical activity that causes its ventricles (the major pump) to "fibrillate"—that is, to twitch very rapidly instead of contracting. As a result, the heart cannot expel enough blood, leaving the brain and the rest of the body deprived of the nutrients necessary to maintain life. Death follows in minutes. Ventricular fibrillation can usually be terminated by an electric shock (defibrillation) delivered by a defbrillator. This machine is carried by most emergency ambulances and is standard equipment in virtually every hospital emergency room and now also on most airliners. Every suspected heart attack patient is immediately hooked up to an ECG machine so that ventricular fibrillation can be spotted and treated as soon as it begins.

Most of those who suddenly die had some earlier warning that they didn't recognize, denied, or ignored. That's why the routine cardiac diagnostic tests described below to detect vulnerability to heart disease are so important.

Heart Symptoms *Before* the Heart Attack

Unlike a stroke, before which you may have no warning, many patients are diagnosed with coronary artery disease long before they suffer a heart attack. Such early diagnosis is especially important these days because there's so much we can do to head off the heart attack. Twenty years ago I was treating on average ten patients in the hospital at any given time for an acute heart attack. Today I still see the same number of people with heart trouble, but very few of them develop a heart attack because of the medications and procedures now available that can prevent it.

You should suspect that your coronary arteries are narrowing if you experience *pressure or pain in the chest or undue shortness of breath* while walking (especially uphill, in cold weather, carrying a heavy package, or soon after eating), during emotional duress or sexual intercourse, or even after lying down in bed at night. This symptom is called *angina pectoris.* ("Angina" is the Latin word for "pain," "pectoris" means "chest.") Angina sets in because stress or physical activity requires an increase in the blood supply to the heart that the narrowed coronary arteries can't deliver. Angina is the cry of your heart for more oxygen. Why would you get angina after just going to bed? Because when you lie down, blood held in the legs by gravity when you were standing flows back into the heart, which must then work harder to expel it.

The major characteristic of angina is that it clears up a minute or two after you stop doing whatever it is that provoked it. If it came on in bed, sitting up helps. Nitroglycerin in a tablet placed under the tongue (or sprayed there) relieves angina almost immediately. If your symptoms persist, they're either not angina or you may be having a heart attack.

Diagnosing Coronary Artery Disease

If you develop any symptom suggesting angina, think "heart," especially if you're a man over forty, a menopausal woman, or have one or more important risk factors at any age. Don't try to confirm the diagnosis yourself. That's your doctor's job. *Insist on a thorough cardiac evaluation,* which should initially include:

- A careful history
- Thorough physical examination
- Pertinent blood tests (especially for blood fat profile and sugar)
- Electrocardiogram

Although the ECG is a useful tool, it is normal in as many as 75 percent of people with angina. If your doctor suspects heart disease, you'll need a *stress test.* This extra effort makes the heart work to require more blood. If your coronaries are blocked and can't deliver what's needed, the exercise ECG usually becomes abnormal.

There are several different kinds of stress tests. Some doctors still have you walk up and down a small staircase in their office (a test devised by my late father-in-law, Arthur Master, with whom I worked for many years). However, the treadmill and the stationary bicycle are now more commonly used.

All ECG stress tests have a certain incidence of false negative results (the patient has angina but the test reads normal) and false-positives (the ECG becomes abnormal even though the subject is free of disease). Healthy women often have false positive stress tests and frequently require one of the more sophisticated procedures described below.

If your doctor suspects that your stress test is inaccurate, you'll go to the next level of testing. This may be a stress echocardiogram that provides a view of the beating heart. When the blood supply is reduced, the affected portion of the heart muscle beats less vigorously, and this "weakness" is apparent on the echocardiogram.

There are several more expensive diagnostic procedures, of which the most widely used is the nuclear stress test. It provides an image of the blood distribution to the heart muscle at rest and during exercise.

MRIs and CT scans of the heart are even newer techniques. At the moment, I believe a nuclear test is the most practical and reliable, although the others may turn out to be superior and less expensive. It's too early to tell.

If you have arthritis, or have had a stroke and find it difficult to walk or pedal, your heart can be "stressed" by injecting you with a drug such as adenosine that increases its work as much as physical exercise does.

If any of these examinations indicate angina, you will be treated with a variety of drugs, the most important of which is *nitroglycerin.* Keep it with you at all times. At the very onset of your symptoms, sit down if you can and let a nitro dissolve under your tongue. (If you remain standing, you may pass out, because nitro widens the arteries, not only in the heart, where it causes more blood to be delivered, but also everywhere else in your body, dropping the blood pressure.)

Prevention

There are many long-acting nitroglycerin derivatives that widen the arteries for a longer time. They are taken to prevent attacks—by mouth (Isordil, Ismo, Imdur, Monoket) or applied topically to the chest in a patch, cream, or ointment. These are preventives. Sublingual nitro is the only one that relieves an acute attack of angina. (Never take any of these coronary dilatory drugs along with Viagra. If you do, your blood pressure may drop too much.)

Other effective antianginal drugs include beta-blockers and calcium channel blockers. I also recommend 400 to 800 units of *vitamin E* to my patients with coronary artery disease, even though some recent studies have cast doubt as to this vitamin's effectiveness in preventing heart attacks. I usually prescribe a *"statin" drug* as well to reduce even slightly elevated cholesterol levels. As far as I am concerned, the lower the cholesterol, the better, especially in someone with angina.

A daily low dose of *aspirin* (81 mg) has been shown to reduce heart attacks by almost 50 percent. Aspirin works by preventing platelets in the blood from clumping together to form clots.

If your coronary artery disease is mild, then the regimen I've described will usually allow you to lead a normal life. However, because severity of symptoms does not always correlate well with the extent of disease, many cardiologists encourage their angina patients to have an angiogram, especially if their symptoms are worsening, however subtly. This procedure consists of injecting dye into the coronary arteries through a catheter placed in an artery (usually in the groin, but sometimes in the forearm). You remain awake while it's done, and it's painless. An angiogram allows the doctor to view the entire circulation in the heart and to see which vessels are diseased and how badly. (You come to the hospital in the morning without breakfast and can usually go home that evening.)

Balloon Angioplasty

If the angiogram reveals one or more critically narrowed arteries in danger of closing completely and causing a heart attack, you may be advised to have angioplasty to unclog them. This is often done while you're still on the table. A catheter with a tiny collapsed balloon at its tip is threaded to the obstructing plaque, positioned alongside it, and then inflated. This compresses the plaque against the vessel wall and removes the blockage. To ensure that the artery remains open, a stent (like a sleeve) is usually placed in the ballooned artery.

Instead of ballooning open the diseased artery, the plaque can be scraped away (atherectomy) or, less frequently, vaporized by a laser beam, or if there is a great deal of calcium, roto-rootered with a tiny burr. You can usually go home the morning after any one of these procedures, armed with prescriptions for aspirin and some other super-aspirin such as clopidogrel (Plavix) to help prevent clots from forming in the treated vessel.

If the blocked arteries cannot be angioplastied, and something needs to be done, your next option is bypass surgery.

The Bypass Operation

An experienced surgeon (the only kind to have) can bypass several arteries in three or four hours. In this operation the obstruction in the coronary artery is circumvented by a vein graft from the legs or with an internal mammary artery from the chest wall. One end of the graft is connected to the aorta, from which it receives its blood; the other end is inserted into the diseased artery below the location of the plaque. Hence the term "bypass." This operation is only feasible if the portion of the artery below the obstruction is free of disease and wide enough to accept the graft. Sometimes the affected vessel is so small and so diffusely narrowed that there's nowhere to insert the graft.

The traditional bypass operation requires opening the chest through the middle of the breastbone. However, newer techniques such as the Minimally Invasive Direct Coronary Artery Bypass (MIDCAB) procedure do not require the chest to be opened. Instead, the surgeon inserts the instruments through a small hole in the front of the chest. Several of my patients have had successful bypasses, and even valve replacements, done this way. They've left the hospital in a day or two instead of the usual five to seven days after the open procedure. This procedure is less traumatic than the open operation and accompanied by fewer neurological complications. You should ask about it. If you're told you need the more extensive surgery, make sure it's not because your heart surgeon isn't trained to do the newer operation. Unfortunately, that's too often the case. *Insist on speaking with a doctor in your area who knows about the MIDCAB, so you can make an educated decision on how you'd like to proceed.*

When a bypass cannot be done for any reason, usually because the vessels are too diffusely diseased to accept a graft, three new approaches, still in the experimental stage but that might soon be available—laser revascularization, in which laser beams are directed into the heart muscle to form new arteries several weeks later; the injection of genes containing vascular growth factor (that makes new blood vessels), also directly into the heart muscle; and the introduction of stem cells into the diseased area of the heart to create new tissue.

Is It a Heart Attack?

Remember this cardinal rule about heart attacks: Better safe than sorry. Don't worry whether your spouse, doctor, boss, friends, or emergency room personnel think you're a hypochondriac because you're worried that your symptoms are cardiac. A mistake in judgment can be fatal; a correct call can save your life. *Don't hesitate to cry wolf!*

The typical symptoms of a heart attack are a pressure, fullness, squeezing, ache, or pain in the chest, usually behind the breastbone. I deliberately put "pain" last on the list. More commonly, it's pressure, like "an elephant sitting on my chest." So many patients ignore the classic symptoms just because they're not "painful." Doctors tend to compound this dangerous misapprehension by asking patients, "Do you have any chest pain?" The symptom, however you describe it, may spread to both arms but more commonly the left one, the shoulders, the back, up to the jaw, and even into the ears. If you've had angina before (see above), these heart attack symptoms will be familiar to you, but they're more severe than angina, and they occur at rest, not after exertion. A nitroglycerin tablet under the tongue may ease the discomfort for a few moments, but then it returns. You may also feel short of breath, lightheaded, nauseated, faint, and have palpitations.

I can't emphasize strongly enough that the symptoms of a heart attack vary from person to person. *If you have the slightest suspicion that your pain is coming from the heart, take an aspirin (any strength will do) and get to the nearest hospital as soon as you can.* Either call for an ambulance or have someone drive you. Don't wait for your doctor to return your call and don't drive yourself.

Once you get to the ER, the doctor will first make sure you're not merely having an attack of indigestion, gastric reflux, some lung problem such as pleurisy or pneumonia, or referred pain from a disk in your neck. The ER team will immediately record an ECG, but you can't depend on that alone. The annals of tragedy are filled with stories of patients who came to an ER with chest symptoms, were reassured because their electrocardiogram was "normal," and sent home, where they died of a heart attack. Blood will be drawn to see whether your cardiac enzymes are high (damaged heart muscle leaks these enzymes, and they are diagnostic of a heart attack); your blood pressure will be taken (it can drop perilously during a heart attack); your lungs will be examined; and a final diagnosis will be made.

If the ER team concludes that this is a heart attack, there are several treatment options. You may be managed conservatively: Given oxygen, intravenous nitroglycerin, and anticoagulants along with aspirin to thin your blood, other medications such as ACE inhibitors and beta-blockers to ease the strain on your cardiac muscle—and then carefully observed. If you arrived in the hospital within three or four hours of the onset of your symptoms, you will also be given thrombolytic therapy, a "clot buster" medication such as tPA, which dissolves the fresh clot and restores blood flow to the heart muscle.

However, many heart attacks are treated more aggressively, especially in larger centers. If you're lucky, the fresh obstruction in the artery can be opened by a balloon (angioplasty) and flow restored before there has been permanent damage to the heart. This is done by means of a cardiac catheterization (a tube is threaded from the artery in your groin into your heart arteries). You remain awake throughout this essentially painless procedure.

Should these measurers fail and the chest pain persists, along with worsening ECG abnormalities and rising cardiac enzymes, you may need emergency bypass surgery, especially if the blood pressure remains too low.

Life After a Heart Attack

There was a time when, if you survived a heart attack, you were expected, indeed obliged, to retire—not only from work but from life itself. How that's changed! The world is full of heads of state, CEOs, doctors, lawyers, and blue-collar workers who returned to their jobs after a heart attack and lead active, normal lives. However, you can't be cavalier about your health. Remember that bypass surgery, angioplasty, and all the other miracle interventions that have saved your life are only holding measures. Take advantage of the time they've bought to reduce the risk factors that caused your coronary disease in the first place.

WHAT TO INSIST ON IF YOU HAVE CORONARY ARTERY HEART DISEASE

Coronary artery disease and its ultimate culmination, the heart attack, is the number one killer in most of the developed world. There are several risk factors, the most important being a high cholesterol, particularly the LDL. Others include blood pressure, diabetes, and tobacco. Any and all of these accelerate closure of the coronary arteries in the heart. Most of them are under our control. Everyone begins to develop plaques in the coronary arteries early in life. The rate at which they enlarge, as we grow older, varies from person to person. When they interfere with blood flow significantly, angina (chest pain or pressure on effort) may develop. Such blockages can be treated with medication, angioplasty, or bypass.

A heart attack occurs when a coronary artery, regardless of its size, is suddenly completely blocked. The chest symptoms you then experience are not related to effort and are often accompanied by sweating, weakness, and shortness of breath. It's critical to take an aspirin immediately and be taken to the nearest emergency room. Depending on the findings there, you may be treated with medication alone, or be sent for emergency cardiac catheterization to decide whether you need angioplasty or surgery.

Preventing heart disease is largely up to you. But there are certain aspects of your medical care that you should insist on. For example, early detection is critical. A normal ECG does not necessarily mean that you are free of significant coronary artery narrowing. *Men over forty and postmenopausal women who have any of the risk factors for coronary artery disease should insist on a stress test.* Everyone should have a cholesterol profile done, including HDL, LDL, homocysteine, and CRP levels. *Insist on it.* If they're abnormal, follow a low-fat, low-cholesterol diet as best you can. If you cannot normalize the numbers, *insist on one of the several available drugs, preferably a "statin" or niacin.*

If you do develop angina pectoris, you should be considered for angiography and possibly angioplasty. Insist on a second opinion from a cardiologist as to whether you are a candidate for this procedure.

If bypass surgery is recommended, ask about the minimally invasive operation that is now available. If it is not offered to you, insist on a second opinion.

17

HEMORRHOIDS

No Thanks, I'd Rather Stand

Everyone has hemorrhoids. They don't always cause symptoms, but they do act up from time to time in one of every two Americans of both genders, usually between the ages of twenty and fifty. When they do, they cause pain, itching, or bleeding. If you need proof about the prevalence and importance of hemorrhoids in our country, ponder on this statistic: The second most commonly shoplifted item from our nation's pharmacies is Preparation H, arguably the best-known and most widely used hemorrhoidal cream in the United States! (I wonder what number one is.)

Like every other organ, the rectum has a network of veins. When they become engorged, enlarged, and often inflamed, they are called hemorrhoids (affectionately known as "piles"). They can be external (at the anal opening), where they are visible to anyone who's looking, or internal (at the beginning of the anal canal inside the rectum), where they can be felt but not seen. Hemorrhoids are not contagious and never become cancerous.

What is it that turns these harmless little rectal veins into nasty, big, painful, bleeding piles? The major offenders are constipation and diarrhea, repeated heavy lifting, coughing, standing or sitting for long periods of time, overweight, and pregnancy. And then there's anal intercourse. Here's how hemorrhoids form:

- Sitting or standing for long periods of time (bus drivers, pilots, flight attendants, and elevator operators are especially vulnerable) causes the force of gravity to pull the blood down into the rectal veins where it stagnates, enlarging and ultimately inflaming them.
- When you're constipated, the stool is hard and dry because the bowel has absorbed much of its water as it sat there waiting to be excreted. So you have to strain to eliminate it, increasing the pressure on the rectal veins.
- Hemorrhoids tend to develop in overweight people whose extra pounds cause more pressure on their rectal veins. However, they can occur in thin people as well, or flare up after any major dietary change.
- Most pregnant women become constipated because the pressure of the enlarged uterus on the bowel is transmitted to the rectal veins. But that's not all. During those nine months, the woman's blood supply increases in order to nourish the fetus, and her hormone profile changes too. The pelvic muscles relax in order to make the delivery easier, and this allows the fetus to press on the rectal veins. Other reasons for the constipation are not drinking the extra water needed and the failure to take stool softeners to counteract the effect of the supplemental iron prescribed. Happily, the hemorrhoids of pregnancy usually clear up.

External hemorrhoids are not apt to cause symptoms until the blood within them clots. When that happens, they enlarge, hurt, and itch. If you rub, wipe hard, or strain, they bleed. The moist and irritated skin around them adds to the discomfort.

Internal hemorrhoids can remain dormant for a long time too. However, they can slip out from the rectum at any time (doctors call it prolapse). They bleed unpredictably, usually after a bowel movement. The blood appears in streaks on the surface of the stool or on the toilet paper, or it trickles slowly into the bowl. It's hard to estimate how much blood you've lost by looking at the color of the water, because even a couple of drops turn it frighteningly red.

Anything in the rectum whether it's stool or a big vein, may give you the urge to "go." If your hemorrhoids are large enough and become irritated and inflamed, they leave you with this feeling too. When you strain to eliminate a stool that isn't there, the bleeding becomes worse, and so does the pain.

Let your doctor know if your hemorrhoids are painful. A blood clot (thrombus) has probably formed within one of them. Iced compresses often relieve the pain and reduce the swelling, but a small incision may have to be made to reduce the pressure. Hemorrhoidal pain can also result from infection or ulceration of the enlarged veins.

Believe it or not, hemorrhoids can save your life! If they bleed, a competent doctor will examine the lower bowel with a sigmoidoscope or colonoscope just to make sure that something else isn't responsible for the blood. *Insist that this be done.* A colonoscopy may reveal a coexisting previously undetected cancer that can be cured. Persistent rectal bleeding should be clearly diagnosed as coming from your hemorrhoids or due to something else.

It's not always possible to prevent hemorrhoids, but give it a try. Here's what to do:

- Since constipation is the handmaiden of hemorrhoids, it's very important to keep "moving." Respond as soon as possible to nature's signal.
- Eat the right diet: Lots of fiber (whole-grain breads, three to four tablespoons of bran per day), cereals, bran muffins, beans, fresh fruit (especially plums, apricots, and apples), stewed or canned fruit (prunes, figs), fruit juices (orange, prune, fig), vegetables (celery, lettuce,

spinach, turnips, carrots, cabbage), brown rice, nuts, and lots and lots of water (two quarts or more per day).
- Cut down on caffeine and alcohol, both of which tend to make the stool dry and hard.
- Laxatives are irritating; avoid them if you can.
- Exercise helps prevent constipation and also improves the tone of the muscles supporting the rectal area.
- Lose weight.
- Don't strain at stool. Do your reading somewhere other than on the toilet.

When hemorrhoids become troublesome, here's what you can do:

- Rest your feet on a low stool when you're sitting on the toilet. This makes it less painful to move your bowels.
- Apply ice to the rectal area. Some patients prefer a wet, warm tea bag or a witch hazel compress. Apply any of these for about ten minutes three or four times a day. Unfortunately, that's not easy to do on the job. When you get home, sit in eight to ten inches of water for fifteen to twenty minutes at least a couple of times before you go to bed.
- Sleep on your stomach rather than on your back. You can see why, given the location of your problem.
- Use moistened toilet paper, and pat, don't wipe vigorously.
- It's easier said than done, but try not to scratch the area.
- Be very careful about the painkillers you take. Avoid narcotics such as codeine, which, though effective, can cause constipation. Stay with a nonprescription medication such as a nosteroidal anti-inflammatory drug (Advil, Aleve) two or three times a day.
- Several over-the-counter topical agents—ointments, creams, and suppositories—can provide relief from the pain and itching of hemorrhoids. The best known

are zinc oxide ointments such as Preparation H, and Anusol-HC cream with 1 percent hydrocortisone to reduce the swelling, burning, and itching of external hemorrhoids. The same formulation comes in suppository form for internal swelling and discomfort.

- Straining increases pressure on the rectal veins. A stool softener such as docusate, a stimulant to bowel contraction such as senna (Senokot), or a bulking agent containing psyllium seed, such as Metamucil, Konsyl, and Citrucel, all of which you can buy without a prescription, will help keep the movements soft and easily passed.
- Indulge yourself with a doughnut-shaped cushion on which to sit for long hours at your desk or in your car.

Chronic hemorrhoids can result in the continuous loss of small amounts of blood with virtually every bowel movement. That doesn't seem like much to worry about because it's not dramatic like a hemorrhage. However, it can cause anemia, and that can be dangerous, especially in the elderly and chronically ill.

Treatment of Hemorrhoids

If the symptoms become more severe despite all the palliative measures described above; if the bleeding is more than just a streak on the bowel or the toilet paper; or if you find a hard lump where there used to be a hemorrhoid; or if you clotted one of your hemorrhoids and it hurts real bad, more aggressive management may be necessary. There are several options:

- Internal hemorrhoids that are troublesome, that is, bleed or protrude after bowel movement, can be tied off at their base with a small rubber band that cuts off their blood supply. The rubber band and the hemorrhoids both fall off in about seven days.

- Bleeding hemorrhoids that do not protrude can also be injected with a chemical that scars them (sclerotherapy).
- Cryosurgery using liquid nitrogen freezes the hemorrhoids. I don't recommend this procedure because it's no better than the others and is very painful.
- Hemorrhoids can be coagulated (clotted) by infared photocoagulation. (Unlike the other techniques, this one may require more than one treatment, but it is relatively painless.)
- Lasers direct a high-intensity light beam at the hemorrhoid, cauterizing or coagulating it. Laser therapy is expensive, and it can hurt just as much as surgery to remove the hemorrhoids.
- You may have no choice but an operation if clots keep forming in your external hemorrhoids, or if the rubber band ligation and other methods fail to prevent the internal hemorrhoids from slipping out of the rectum (prolapsing).

My first choice among all of these is the rubber band ligation, which is easily, quickly, and painlessly done. But any intervention is not something your primary doctor should do. It's the field of the colon-rectal specialist. *Insist on such a consultation.*

WHAT TO INSIST ON IF YOU HAVE HEMORRHOIDS

A soft seat!

Hemorrhoids are the consequence of increased pressure on the veins in the rectal area and usually result from chronic constipation, prolonged sitting or standing, pregnancy, obesity, laxative abuse, and poor bowel habits. There are several topical medications and suppositories that alleviate the pain, itching, and bleeding. Make sure that the bleeding is not masking a tumor in the bowel. *Blood in the stool, regardless of whether or not you have hemorrhoids, should always be investigated further. Insist on it.*

When home remedies fail to control the pain or stop the bleeding, several measures are available. These include tying off the vein with a rubber band; injecting chemicals into the hemorrhoid in order to close it by scarring; photocoagulation; laser therapy; cryosurgery; and surgical removal. Try ligation with the rubber band first. However, hemorrhoidectomy is the most predictable way to solve a recurring problem. *A colon-rectal specialist, not a primary doctor, should perform these procedures. Insist on it.*

18

HEPATITIS

Better Never Than Late

It was my fourth-grade teacher who whetted my appetite to be a doctor. She did it with her biology course to our class of nine-year-olds. She had an unusual gift of being able to explain even the most complicated facts so clearly that we all felt like health professionals at the end of each session. She communicated the miracle that is the human body with contagious passion that has remained with me ever since. (I later learned that teaching in elementary school was but a way station in her career and that she later became a physician herself.)

I would go home after each of her classes and think back about what she had taught us. One of my favorite pastimes was to speculate about the relative importance of each of the organs we had learned about. I wondered how the body could function without one or another, and always concluded that we could manage as long as our brain, heart, and kidneys were intact. I knew about the liver, but it never really struck me as being critical, or that its malfunction could cause death. I was wrong. (Ask any Frenchman what our most common ailment is and he'll surely tell you that it's *mal de foie*—a bad liver.)

The liver (of which, unlike the kidneys, there is only one) is situated in the right side of the abdomen behind the lower ribs.

The right kidney lies behind it, the gallbladder is on its under-surface, the pancreas is to the left, and the intestines are in front. A doctor normally cannot feel the liver when he examines your belly, although when you take a deep breath, it descends, so he can make out its lower edge. The adult liver weighs three pounds and is the largest *internal* organ of the body (the skin, which few of us think of as an organ, is the biggest one overall).

What the Liver Does for a (Your) "Living"

It's amazing that despite all the liver's myriad critical and complex functions that are necessary to maintain life, it's really quite an unobtrusive organ. Most people don't even know it's there until something goes wrong. It doesn't breathe like the lungs, beat like the heart, think like the brain, move like the bowels, or pee like the kidney. But just look at all the things it does every moment of our lives:

- It's the body's refinery. How do you think that the huge steak, two-pound lobster, chicken, or carrots you eat end up as protein, calcium, iron, fat, or vitamins in your body tissues? You can thank your liver for that. Food absorbed from the intestinal tract enters the bloodstream, which, before it goes anywhere else, must first pass through the liver where it is processed and converted into the chemicals necessary for life and growth.
- The same is true for most medications. The liver converts them into their biologically active form.
- The liver cleanses the blood of toxic substances that we consume or that our body produces during its many energy processes.
- The food, vitamins, and minerals we eat are not always needed right away, so the liver stores them for a rainy

day. For example, when you suddenly need more "fuel," the liver releases whatever glucose is required. It also stores iron.

- Guess where many of those immune factors that fight infection and cancer are made? You're right—in the liver. And just for extra measure, it also removes bacteria floating in the bloodstream.

- Cholesterol is a dirty word in today's health lexicon, but we need some to sustain life. The liver manufactures cholesterol; it also eliminates and transports it along with all its component fractions. So an elevated cholesterol level may be due not only to what you eat but also how the liver is behaving. The life-prolonging "statin" drugs that reduce high cholesterol levels do so by interfering with some of these liver processes.

- The liver makes and delivers bile, a greenish-brown fluid, to the small intestine to help digest the fat we eat.

- The liver produces chemicals that allow the blood to clot so that we don't hemorrhage when we're cut accidentally or during surgery.

- The liver metabolizes alcohol. That means that the booze you drink is "digested" by the liver and doesn't accumulate in your body.

- We think of our "hormone centers" as being mainly in our testicles, ovaries, and adrenal glands atop the kidneys. But the liver is also important in maintaining hormone balance. Just look at a man with severe liver disease such as cirrhosis—big breasts, small testicles, no hair on his face, and no sex drive—a classic example of hormone balance gone awry because the liver can no longer break down the normally small amounts of estrogen constantly being produced in all males.

- The bone marrow makes most of our blood cells after we're born, but the liver is responsible for making the blood of the fetus.

These are just the highlights of liver function. No wonder the French are in awe of it—and its potential to make you sick.

Liver Diseases

The liver is vulnerable to many of the same problems that can affect any organ: trauma, infection, cancer, and chemical injury, mainly due to drugs. For example, a vigorous blow during a contact sport such as football can hurt the liver, as can an accident that involves the abdomen. Many drugs can cause liver problems too, the most common and notorious of which are antibiotics, cholesterol-lowering agents, chemotherapy, even something as benign as acetaminophen (Tylenol) in large doses, and a wide range of industrial toxins.

The most important cause of chemical damage is alcohol, which, if taken for long enough and in large quantities, can cause permanent scarring (cirrhosis). The most common circumstance in which a cancer *originates* in the liver (primary cancer) is the presence of underlying cirrhosis due to alcoholism and the long-standing viral infections discussed below. However, the vast majority of liver cancers are *metastases,* tumors that have spread to the liver from elsewhere in the body. This is understandable, because so much blood flows through the liver for processing that cancer cells floating within it are trapped and take up residence there. Most of these cells originate in the bowel and the pancreas. When a gallstone obstructs a duct that carries bile from the liver, the bile backs up into the liver, and eventually into the bloodstream, making your skin and eyes yellow. (See Chapter 13 on gallbladder disease.)

Although any bug or parasite (amoebas are notorious) can infect the liver, the most important ones in our part of the world are viruses. There are several different kinds of viral hepatitis, each one of which is labeled with a letter of the alphabet. As we learn more and more about the liver, new forms of viral hepatitis are identified. At the moment, the list ranges from A to G. However, I will only tell you about the three most important and common ones, which account for 90 percent of the seven types of viral hepatitis—hepatitis A, B, and C. (If you want to know more about all of them, read Dr. Alan Berkman's book *Hepatitis A to G* [Warner Books, 2000].)

Symptoms of Liver Trouble

The liver reacts to most "insults"—traumatic, infectious, or cancerous—with symptoms that immediately suggest the site of the problem.

- *Jaundice,* an abnormal yellow discoloration of the skin and eyes, is the hallmark symptom indicating that some disease process has involved the liver. (Don't confuse it with the carotenemia you get from eating too many carrots, which turns the palms, soles, and skin yellow but never the eyes.)
- *Dark urine.* When the same bile that makes your skin yellow reaches the kidneys through the bloodstream it turns the urine brown.
- *Gray, light, or clay-colored stools.* Bile is what gives the stool its brown color. When the bile is prevented from reaching the intestine because the ducts that carry it are obstructed by swelling of the liver, gallstones, or a cancer pressing on them, the stools become "pale."
- *Nausea, vomiting, and loss of appetite.* This, of course, can result from any number of causes, ranging from drug toxicity to depression, but you can blame it on the liver when the other classical symptoms of liver disease are present.
- *Abdominal swelling.* If the liver is badly scarred (usually by cirrhosis), blood can't flow freely through it, and backs

up so that its plasma leaks out of the vessels into the surrounding tissues. That happens first in the belly and later
in the legs. When your abdomen becomes distended and
there's no chance you could be pregnant (because you're
a man, a menopausal woman, or a nun), suspect fluid. If
you've recently gained a lot of weight (more than 5 percent) despite a poor appetite, and you can't get into your
clothes because your belly is too big, it contains water
(doctors call it ascites).

- *Abdominal pain,* most marked in the right upper portion
  of the belly, is due to swelling of the liver and distension
  of the lining that covers it.

- *Generalized itching of the skin.* If you itch all over without any rash and it continues after you've excluded the
  possibility of an allergic reaction, suspect the liver. Bile
  salts made by the liver and present in bile make the skin
  itch, and the itching is often accompanied by jaundice.

- *Feminization of men.* Each gender has some of the
  other's hormones, albeit in very small quantities. Although men have a great preponderance of testosterone,
  they do also have a little estrogen. The liver normally
  keeps breaking down this estrogen so that it doesn't accumulate. When this estrogen-regulating function is impaired due to chronic liver disease, estrogen levels rise,
  men lose their libido as well as the secondary sex characteristics such as facial hair (so that they don't need to
  shave every day). They also develop breasts that make
  them the envy of women.

- *Insomnia, mental changes, and coma* are late symptoms
  of chronic liver disease and result from the accumulation
  of many of the toxic substances that the healthy liver
  breaks down and excretes from the body. They eventually affect brain function, and the last stage of liver failure
  is coma. Fatigue and loss of energy, of course, precede
  these terminal symptoms.

Regardless of the cause of your liver disease and whether it is transient or ongoing, here are three important suggestions for dealing with it:

- Avoid all alcohol for the duration—that is, until your doctor tells you that liver function tests are stable or have returned to normal.
- Take only those medications that are absolutely necessary. That includes nonprescription items as well as herbal preparations. Since the liver processes so many drugs, the fewer you consume while your liver is sick, the smaller the burden you place on it.
- Eat nutritiously and reduce your fat intake to a minimum. If you're retaining fluid, cut down on your salt intake.

Hepatitis A

Hepatitis A is almost always a "benign" infection; it makes you sick for a while, but unlike its sister infections, B and C, it clears up completely and does not affect your liver permanently.

How It's Transmitted

The hepatitis A virus (HAV) is ingested in both cooked and uncooked food as well as in drinking water contaminated with the feces of an infected person. That's one of the reasons you often see signs in restaurants exhorting their employees to wash their hands with soap and water after using the bathroom. The HAV is a hearty little scoundrel. It can survive for as long as three to ten months in sewage-contaminated waters. So the raw shellfish you eat from those waters even after they have been cleaned up may still harbor the virus. You can, of course, also contract HAV from drinking that water or swimming in it. HAV is not transmitted in the saliva. In the United States, some 150,000 people come down with HAV every year, often after traveling out of the country. Substance abusers who have used infected needles can also contract this form of hepatitis. You can "catch" it from close personal contact with someone who's already infected—such as sexual contact, especially among male homosexuals, and contact with others in day-care centers as well as in other crowded facilities. Health-care providers working in institutions are especially at risk.

Symptoms of Hepatitis A

After you've been exposed to HAV, the incubation period is about thirty days. When you're infected, you'll feel out of sorts for a while and your appetite won't be anything to write home about. The older you are, the more severe the symptoms. In fact, most kids infected before age five are rarely diagnosed because they have no symptoms unless they are among the 10 percent who do become jaundiced. That number increases to 50 percent in older children and to 80 percent in adults. Now and then the infection is severe. Only one in every fifteen hundred patients with HAV dies from it, and it's usually someone older than fifty. Also, the illness may be more severe if there is pre-existing liver disease. The important thing to remember is that HAV never becomes chronic. In other words, no matter how sick it makes you (and it doesn't usually), it will clear up completely.

If you've been recently exposed, say in the past fourteen days, *insist on receiving a shot of gamma globulin*. It may prevent the disease from striking you, or reduce its severity. Maybe it's just the way my nurse gives these shots, but my patients tell me they're painful.

Treatment of Hepatitis A

Don't expect more than tender, loving care from your doctor, because there is no specific treatment. Your symptoms will gradually disappear over a six-week period. During that time most people who like their work can continue to do so. If you don't, or if your job is physically demanding, you can recover at home.

Hepatitis A Vaccine

The good news about HAV is that there is now a vaccine that will prevent it. If you've already had the infection, it confers lifelong immunity, so you don't need to be vaccinated. But if you're a health-care worker and vulnerable, or if you're a man who has sex with men, or you're a substance abuser and in the habit of sharing needles, or if you're traveling to some place where the hygiene isn't great, you should have the shot. (Formerly, going abroad meant getting a gamma globulin shot every time. Now just one vaccination will protect you for much longer.) I also recommend an HAV vaccination to all my patients with other forms of liver disease that would be worsened if they were to become infected with HAV. It's also a good idea for Alaskan and other Native Americans, whose incidence of HAV infection is high, to have their children vaccinated at two years of age.

The HAV vaccine is not a live virus and so can't infect you. Usually given in the arm muscle, it's at least 90 percent effective. Adults over the age of eighteen need two shots, six to twelve months apart. Children and adolescents should receive it in three doses; the second one about one month after the first, and the third shot six to twelve months later.

Hepatitis B

This form of hepatitis is a different kettle of fish. Unlike HAV, the hepatitis B virus (HBV) causes a serious disease that can make you very sick, and may eventually kill you. It strikes about 200,000 Americans every year. Although most patients recover completely, the virus persists in the blood of 5 to 10 percent of them for longer than six months.

Carriers of HBV

Carriers, of whom there are 280 million worldwide and more than 1 million in the United States, usually feel well themselves but can infect others. The virus stays with them for years, often for the rest of their lives. Some do become sick and are at higher risk for liver failure or cancer. If you're a carrier, you should have your liver function tested every year, be careful with any drug you're taking, because so many of them can hurt the liver, and take little or no alcohol.

After being treated by a wonderful dentist for several decades, I discovered after he died that he was an HBV carrier! He was "old-fashioned," and didn't use gloves. It's a wonder that I didn't contract the disease what with his fingers pressing on my bleeding gums! But HBV can also be transmitted from patient to doctor. You owe it to your doctor, dentist, and sex partner to tell them if you are a carrier. Ninety percent of pregnant women who are carriers infect their babies, so being tested for HBV is a must if you're expecting.

The major problem with HBV is the chronic liver disease it causes in anywhere from 30 to 90 percent of young children and 5 to 10 percent of adults who are infected. One in four patients dies from either cirrhosis (scarring and destruction of liver cells) or liver cancer.

It's easier to "catch" HBV than AIDS. The virus is transmitted not only through blood but also through a variety of other body fluids—open sores, semen, vaginal discharge, tears, saliva, and breast milk. There are so many possible ways that more than a third of patients with HBV don't know how they got it!

Given the myriad infection possibilities, you should be especially careful if you:

- Are in contact with blood
- Use intravenous drugs
- Are a health-care provider—from dental worker to policeman—particularly if you're called on to render first aid
- Live with or have (heterosexual or homosexual) sex with a carrier or an infected individual
- Travel to underdeveloped areas of the world where the incidence of HBV is high
- If you received blood before 1975, when we were unable to detect HBV in blood for transfusion, you may have acquired the disease at that time and now be a carrier
- Have been contaminated with a needle. Make sure that a new one is being used if you are having your ears pierced, or receiving acupuncture, or if you're foolish enough to be tattooed. (Improperly sterilized needles used to be a problem in hospitals and doctors' offices, but virtually every health-care provider now uses disposable needles and syringes.)
- Share razors. I may be overreacting, but I include electric shavers in this warning. Toothbrushes can spread the disease and so can pierced earrings.
- Are an infected mother. You can transmit the disease to your infant should it come in contact with your virus-laden blood.

Always use condoms during sex. Wear gloves when handling blood or other secretions. If you come across blood on any object, clean it with a mixture of household bleach and water, in a ratio of 1 to 10. The best protection, however, is to get yourself vaccinated with all three shots of the HBV vaccine (see below). Everyone should have it, including newborns everywhere.

Symptoms of Hepatitis B

Most people don't know they've been infected with HBV until they become jaundiced. Before that happens, however, you may lose interest in food and experience nausea and vomiting; you may feel weak and tired and have a low-grade fever along with some "nonspecific" (by which I mean it could be due to anything) abdominal pain. Your skin may itch. Some patients develop swollen, painful joints. Within a few weeks the telltale jaundice and dark urine (dark because it contains liver bile) become apparent. These symptoms may last for a few days.

The good news about HBV is that once you get it, you're immune to reinfection for the rest of your life. (But only to the HBV. You're still fair game for any other form of hepatitis to which you were never previously exposed.) You can now do all the things I warned about above—take a job as a health-care worker, drink the water in Mexico, and even share chewing gum. You'll never get HBV again. But before you go overboard, remember all the other forms of hepatitis to which you're still vulnerable.

You're immune, but your blood will always have the HBV antibodies. So quash the humanitarian impulse to donate your blood. Forget also about offering body organs, sperm, eggs, or other tissue. Incidentally, vaccination also leaves you testing positive forever. I've had patients who either forgot or didn't realize that they'd had the HBV vaccine and who called me puzzled and panic-stricken because their blood had been rejected by the blood bank.

Someone who's had HBV and recovered no longer carries the virus (although the antibodies that make their test positive for HBV remain). By contrast, a carrier does have the virus, although it is no longer causing any symptoms.

When You Remain Chronically Infected

If the virus remains in your blood after six months, but your liver function (blood) tests are normal, you're a carrier. If they're abnormal after that period of time (even though you have no symptoms), you are designated as having a chronic disease. The abnormal blood tests indicate that HBV is hurting your liver cells, which may someday be replaced by scar tissue—in other words, that you could develop cirrhosis. The liver shrinks and becomes hard, and its lower edge feels irregular on examination; blood has a difficult time flowing through it. As a result, veins carrying blood to and through the liver from the lower extremities, abdomen, and stomach back up and become distended, forming *varices*. When these become large enough, they can rupture and cause a hemorrhage. When varices in the food pipe (esophagus) burst, the patient can bleed to death. The other major consequence of chronic hepatitis is liver cancer, which kills more than a thousand Americans every year.

Treatment of Hepatitis B

There is no specific treatment for hepatitis B; 90 percent of those infected recover completely. Of course, you should get plenty of rest in the critical weeks during which the course of the illness will be determined—spontaneous cure, the carrier state, or chronic hepatitis. Eat a nutritious low-fat diet with lots of fruits and vegetables. *Avoid all forms of alcohol* and any unnecessary drugs with the potential to harm the liver.

If you develop chronic hepatitis B, ask your doctor about interferon alfa-2b and lamivudine, the two drugs that have been approved for this disease. These drugs can result in prolonged normalization of liver status in about one-fourth of the cases. (I'm hedging on using the word "cure" because so many treated patients respond for a while, then relapse.) Several other medications are currently being evaluated as well.

Hepatitis B Vaccine

If there is any possibility of your becoming infected, you should be vaccinated. Infants of infected mothers must be vaccinated at birth. So many of us are vulnerable these days that I recommend it to all my patients, including all newborns, regardless of whether the mother has hepatitis B. The vaccine is safe and effective (it's genetically engineered so there's no risk of it infecting you) but not cheap. You need three shots over a six-month period. They're injected under the skin and are 90 to 95 percent effective. You should have a blood test after the last dose to see whether it has "taken." If you do not respond the first time—that is, if your blood doesn't show the protective antibodies have another go at it.

Children under eighteen can get the HBV vaccine free of charge if they're not covered by their parents' health insurance. It costs less at a public health station than what a private doctor usually charges. Don't bother asking for the vaccine if you think you're already infected. It won't do you any good now. However, if you've recently been exposed or have been accidentally stuck with an infected or questionable needle, *insist on the hepatitis B immune globulin.* And the sooner the better— preferably within twenty-four hours, but no later than seven days. Then get a repeat dose thirty days later. You should have the vaccine as well as the immune globulin because the vaccine adds long-term protection to the short-term benefit of the immune globulin.

Hepatitis C

For years, HAV and HBV were the only two hepatitis viruses identified. The existence of a third one was recognized in the late 1960s in patients who had received blood transfusions. For years this newcomer defied identification, and so was called non-A, non-B hepatitis. In 1989 it was finally isolated and named hepatitis C virus (HCV). Today it's recognized as a serious and common blood-borne infection in the United States. Though no longer caused by infected blood transfusions, since we can screen for HCV, the disease is still being spread by carriers (who contracted it years ago and are unaware that they have it) to health-care workers and others vulnerable to needle pricks from infected blood; to those with whom the carriers share contaminated needles, razors, toothbrushes, and other personal items and their sex partners; by pregnant women; and by drug users who share needles.

We were unable to screen blood for the presence of this virus before 1990, and blood banks began testing for it in 1992. Since then, the risk of contracting hepatitis C from transfusions has been very small. Still, there are currently 4 million people (almost 2 percent of the population) infected with the virus in this country. Ten thousand of them die every year from the complications of liver disease. (By comparison, there are fewer than 1 million cases of AIDS.) Seventy percent of those infected with HCV have no symptoms whatsoever; most don't know they have it.

Screening for Hepatitis C

For years, doctors couldn't decide what to do about all those people who'd received transfusions with possibly tainted blood before 1992. Should they be tracked down and tested? Those opposed to doing so argued that this would be a monumental and costly task, and to no avail, since there is no cure for the disease. However, the proponents of testing won out, and blood banks across the country sent letters to all known recipients of blood prior to 1992 advising them to be tested for hepatitis C.

Unfortunately, this search will only identify a fraction of the cases of hepatitis C, since there are so many others who contracted the disease after coming into contact with an infected person's blood. This includes millions of drug users who have ever shared needles and syringes, even only once (among six hundred IV drug users being studied for a needle-exchange program in Canada, 90 percent were found to harbor the virus); anyone who was tattooed or underwent any other surgical or dental procedure in which the equipment used was not properly sterilized; persons who had intercourse with a carrier, whose semen, urine, or other body fluids can contain the hepatitis C virus (a low-risk route of transmission); anyone who has ever shared a toothbrush, razor, or other contaminated household utensil with a carrier; health workers exposed to infected blood from their patients' minor cuts or abrasions. Frustratingly, even the most detailed history looking for possible exposure fails to reveal the source of the infection in some cases! That's why I advise such screening for all these individuals, as well as for all kidney dialysis patients who are exposed to equipment through which large amounts of other people's blood courses.

There is one major difference between HCV and the other two, A and B. If you contract hepatitis A, you're almost certain to make a complete recovery. Most patients with hepatitis B also get better on their own, although a small number do develop serious chronic liver trouble. HCV, on the other hand, causes potentially serious chronic infection of the liver in 85 percent of those whom it infects. Also, unlike hepatitis A and B, which usually make you sick shortly after they infect you, hepatitis C enters your body and usually remains silent or dormant for ten or twenty or more years. But it's not hibernating all that time, for, although you may feel perfectly well, the virus is working on your liver.

Symptoms of Hepatitis C

The most common symptoms, when they finally appear, are fatigue, loss of appetite, and vague abdominal pain. About 20 percent of cases of chronic hepatitis C go on to develop cirrhosis. Some patients with cirrhosis from chronic hepatitis C develop cancer of the liver. To give you some idea of the magnitude of the problem, *hepatitis C and its complications account for more liver transplants done in this country than any other disease.*

The only way to diagnose hepatitis C is with a blood test for its antibodies. You can't depend on liver function tests that may not become abnormal until much later. If you think or know you have been exposed to HCV, *insist on a blood test.*

Treatment of Hepatitis C

What should you do if you're found to be harboring the virus? Although we can treat the symptoms of hepatitis C once they appear, there is no predictable way to prevent the disease from becoming chronic. Still, I believe that even if you have no symptoms, you should *consider current antiviral therapy.* You may be one of the lucky few who respond.

Treatment regimens vary somewhat. My consultants advise Pegylated interferon once a week, as well as two capsules a day of the antiviral drug ribavirin, continued for six to twelve months. This program has resulted in a sustained response in more than half the patients.

No Hepatitis C Vaccine

Unlike hepatitis A and B, there is no vaccine as yet for hepatitis C. If you have the virus, do everything in your power not to infect others; avoid alcohol, which may accelerate viral damage to the liver; and get yourself vaccinated against hepatitis A and B. I have no data confirming this impression, but it seems to me that a superimposed viral infection on one that you already have can only make matters worse.

WHAT TO INSIST ON IF YOU HAVE VIRAL HEPATITIS

Hepatitis A

HAV is almost always a benign disease that does not hurt the liver over the long term. However, you may feel lousy for weeks. So if you've been in close contact with someone who has HAV during its early communicable phase, *insist on a gamma globulin shot to prevent becoming sick yourself.*

There is a vaccine against hepatitis A that you should *insist on if you fall into any of the following categories:*

- Health-care worker or someone in close contact on an ongoing basis with infected persons
- Male homosexual
- Substance abuser who may share needles
- If you have any other underlying liver disease that would be worsened if you were to "catch" hepatitis A

Don't take no for an answer. *Insist.*

Hepatitis B

Unlike hepatitis A, hepatitis B is potentially serious. Although the great majority of those who develop it do recover, some do not. Either they can become carriers who, though free of the symptoms themselves, can transmit it throughout their environment, or they can develop chronic liver disease that can in turn progress to life-threatening scarring (cirrhosis) or liver cancer. So it's critical that you be protected whenever possible. That means:

- If you are diagnosed with chronic hepatitis before it has progressed to its late stages, *ask about treatment with interferon alfa-2b or lamivudine.* They're not a cure, and only a minority of patients respond, but they're your best chance.
- If you're an infected mother, *your infant should be vaccinated at birth.* No one is apt to argue about that, but if they do, *insist.* In fact, *all newborns should be so vaccinated.*
- If you're at high risk for the disease because of exposure at work (or from a friend), *insist on being vaccinated.* A small number of vaccinations do not take. *You should have a blood test after the last of the three shots to see if they were successful. If not, insist on another round.*
- If you were never vaccinated and were exposed to someone with hepatitis B within twenty-four hours and before seven days, *insist on hepatitis immune globulin* and get a second shot in thirty days. It can protect you against a bad disease.

Hepatitis C

This viral infection is a silent killer. Unlike A and B, it quietly destroys your liver over the years. If you fall into a high-risk group—that is, if you received any blood transfusions before 1992 (when the virus was not detectable in routine screening), ever used intravenous drugs, have been receiving kidney dialysis, or fall into any of the other high-risk categories described above—you should be screened for hepatitis C.

If you test positive, even if you still feel well, you should be treated to arrest the progression of the liver damage. It's not a sure thing, but many patients do respond for years. *The treatment of choice is a combination of alfa interferon and ribavirin.* It's expensive. Don't be deterred. *Insist.*

(19)

HIGH BLOOD PRESSURE (HYPERTENSION)

When Ignorance Isn't Bliss

You either have high blood pressure yourself or know someone who does. Yet how many of these critical questions about this almost universal condition can you answer correctly:

- What is blood pressure?
- What percentage of Americans have high blood pressure?
- What percentage of persons who know that their pressure is high are being adequately treated?
- Are men more likely to have high blood pressure than women?
- Is high blood pressure curable?
- How many readings should be taken before the diagnosis of hypertension is made?
- What is white-coat hypertension?
- Is there a form of high blood pressure that is not harmful?
- Which of the two blood pressure readings is more important, the top figure (systolic) or the bottom (diastolic)?

- How often should someone without known high blood pressure be tested?
- Does chronic alcohol excess increase blood pressure?
- Does cigarette smoking raise blood pressure?
- Is excessive salt intake an important cause of high blood pressure?
- What is secondary hypertension?
- What blood pressure reading is optimal?

Write your answers down before you read this chapter. If I were a betting man, I'd give you odds that you'll get no more than ten correct answers. Go ahead. Prove me wrong!

The Statistics

Fifty million Americans have high blood pressure (that's nearly 25 percent of the population). Only 70 percent of them are aware of it. Among those who are, fewer than 30 percent are controlling it successfully.

Patients ask me every day about this very common and important disorder. Here's what I tell them:

Blood pressure is not a numbers game. It's a measurement of an important biological phenomenon. Your heart beats more than 100,000 times a day, sending a surge of blood into every artery of the body with each contraction. The force with which it flows through them is the "blood pressure." If the artery walls are compliant and free of disease, the pressure of the blood circulating through them is normal. However, if they are rigid, hard, in spasm, and constricted, the blood flows under high pressure. As it does so, it pounds the walls of these vessels with every beat, causing them eventually to thicken and "harden." This process, called *arteriosclerosis*, eventually narrows and blocks arteries in the heart, brain, eyes, legs, kidneys—indeed, everywhere—cutting off their blood supply. In the heart, such blockage causes exertional chest pain called *angina pectoris* and finally a *heart attack;* in the brain, rupture of the artery or its occlusion causes a *stroke;* in the legs, the vessels narrow so that your muscles don't get enough blood and *walking becomes painful;* in the eyes, arterial rupture and hemorrhage lead to *blindness;* in the kidneys, the diseased vessels damage the renal cells so that they fail and retain toxic substances that the kidneys would normally excrete, and the end result is often *dialysis.*

The pressure within the arteries immediately after the blood is ejected into them from the heart is called the *systolic blood pressure.* That's the top figure in the reading. Between beats, when the heart is resting and not pumping any blood, the pressure falls. That's the *diastolic pressure.*

Ninety-five percent of the time, the doctor can't find an obvious cause of the elevated blood pressure and calls it *essential hypertension,* although some of the mechanisms involved are understood. For example, we know what it is that constricts the arterial wall, raising the pressure, but we don't know *why* it happens. (It's too bad we're stuck with the term "hypertension," because in so many people's minds that means "too much tension." If that were true, given the many stresses of normal living, we'd all be hypertensive. Although stress can elevate blood pressure temporarily, it is not a cause of high blood pressure.)

Essential hypertension can be controlled; the numbers can be normalized and that's what counts, even though *the underlying disorder cannot be cured.* This means that therapy must be continued "for the duration."

The cause can be determined in five percent of cases of high blood pressure: a blocked artery going to one of the kidneys; some form of kidney disease; a medication (for example, steroids); or a hormone-producing tumor of the adrenal gland. Such cases are referred to as *secondary hypertension.* By contrast with essential hypertension, secondary hypertension can often be cured.

What's High?

Generally speaking, the lower the pressure, the better (except, of course, when there is a major drop after a heart attack or hemorrhage, or readings are so low because of too much medication that you are tired and dizzy). Forget about such myths as 100 plus your age is normal for the systolic reading or that as long as the diastolic number is not high, the systolic figure doesn't matter. We now know that *isolated systolic hypertension*—that is, an elevated top figure and a normal lower number—is associated with a significantly higher risk of stroke, especially in the elderly.

Generally speaking, your target pressure should be 120/80, no matter how old you are (it can normally be as low as 80/60 in children), but anything less than 130/85 is acceptable. *If your pressure is always above 140/90, it should be lowered one way or another. Insist on treatment even if you feel perfectly well.*

There's only one way to determine whether or not your pressure is elevated, and that's to have it measured. Hypertension rarely produces recognizable symptoms before it has done its damage. That's why it's called the silent killer. So don't look or wait for symptoms. Headache, nosebleeds, and a feeling of fullness in the head aren't common, and when they do develop, they may be due to something other than high blood pressure.

Insist that your doctor measure your pressure at every visit, no matter why you're there or what his or her specialty happens to be. It only takes a minute. Some of us are more vulnerable than others and should be checked regularly. As, for example:

- Every man and woman over thirty-five
- Anyone with a family history of high blood pressure. Fifty percent of hypertensives have at least one family

member with the disease. The gene responsible for it has not yet been found.

- Pregnant women
- African Americans. More than half the men and slightly less than half the women suffer from it, and the disease accounts for 30 and 20 percent of all deaths in males and females respectively.
- Women taking oral contraceptives
- Couch potatoes
- Anyone who's overweight. One-third of patients with hypertension weigh too much.
- Those who drink too much alcohol

Even if your blood pressure is found to be normal, and less than 130/85, recheck it every two years for the rest of your life. It may become elevated later on. If it's 130/85–89, come back in one year. If it's 140/90 or higher, consider the circumstances under which it was taken. For example, was it done when you'd just arrived at the doctor's office after running a couple of blocks because you were late? Sit for at least five minutes before you allow the cuff to be put on your arm. Did you smoke (shame!) or have any caffeine prior to the reading? Both can raise pressure temporarily (tobacco use does not cause *chronic* high blood pressure). If you're "heavy," make sure the doctor uses an extra large cuff on your arm in order to get an accurate reading.

If the blood pressure is high, insist on at least two more measurements a couple of minutes apart, lying, sitting, and standing—and in both arms. In today's "in and out" doctors' visits, such extra time is not always granted, but you must have it because once you're labeled "hypertensive," it's usually forever.

Even if the pressure is recorded properly during that first visit, don't buy the diagnosis of high blood pressure just yet. Unless the readings are dangerously high and call for immediate treatment (200/110 or higher), make two or three more appointments a few days or weeks apart—just to be sure. You may be one of the 20 percent of people with *white-coat hypertension* (I am) whose pressure is higher in the doctor's office than it is at home. White-coat hypertension is not innocent. There are studies suggesting that people who react in this way eventually end up with "real" hypertension. They are more apt to be overweight or diabetic than those whose pressures don't fluctuate in this manner. So consider your white-coat reaction a reason to be closely monitored in the future.

If the high blood pressure isn't giving you any symptoms, should you leave well enough alone? Believe it or not, when I was a medical student, that was what we were taught to do! But over the years it has become clear that men and women with untreated hypertension are at greater risk for dying from heart disease, strokes, kidney trouble, and vascular disease.

It's especially important for diabetics to keep their blood pressure as close to normal as possible because they are more prone to vascular disease. Adding the burden of high blood pressure further aggravates the situation.

In addition to harming blood vessels, long-standing untreated high blood pressure creates a burden for the heart, which must work harder to eject its blood against the increased resistance in the vessels that receive it. It enlarges as it tries harder and harder to pump its blood. Eventually, it can thicken no more, it gives up, and it "fails." When that happens, its contractions weaken; the heart dilates with the blood that it can't squeeze out; the blood backs up into the lungs; breathing becomes more difficult; physical activity is reduced; the feet swell. It's a mess. It's much easier to prevent all of this and treat the pressure in time.

What should you do when you're told your blood pressure is too high? Although 95 percent of cases are of the "essential" type, for which there is effective treatment but no cure, make sure that you don't fall into that curable category, uncommon as it is. The following should raise your suspicion that such may be the case:

- You're younger than fifteen and your hypertension is recent
- You're older than sixty-five and *suddenly* found to have very high blood pressure
- You have suddenly developed severe headaches
- The onset of heart palpitations associated with the elevated pressure
- Excessive sweating
- Muscle cramps or weakness
- Excessive urination

The search for secondary, curable hypertension can be expensive, and the chances of a "hit" are low. But if you are so diagnosed, the testing can save your life. So *insist on a full workup, no matter what it costs.*

Managing Hypertension

Let's assume that the curable causes of hypertension have been ruled out and that you have essential hypertension. What now? Don't be tempted to opt straightaway for the quick fix of medication even though that's probably what you'll end up with in the long run. In every medicine there's a little poison. Pressure no higher than 150/100 is not an immediate threat, although it is dangerous in the long run. *Insist on three to six months to normalize it without drugs.* First try to modify your lifestyle. Here are some of the more effective measures you (and you alone) can take. They are successful in as many as 50 percent of people with early and mild hypertension. But be forewarned. You're on your own. Your doctor can't lose weight for you, or stop smoking, or do the necessary exercise.

- Weight loss. Overweight is the single most important risk factor for hypertension. Losing as little as ten pounds can have a significant impact on your pressure. The only way to lose weight over the long term is to cut calories and exercise. You may be tempted to try some weight-reduction pills. Don't! Most of them *raise* blood pressure! And don't be in a hurry: Weight that's lost quickly is regained quickly. Start a program with which you can live, stay with it and lose the excess pounds slowly but surely.

- Alcohol. Booze in all its forms—hard liquor, beer, and wine—raises blood pressure over the short and long term. A couple of drinks will increase the pressure temporarily, and chronic excess intake (more than two drinks a day) can result in ongoing hypertension.

- Exercise reduces blood pressure, especially if you're overweight. And it doesn't have to wear you out either. Walk briskly for thirty minutes to an hour three or four times a week and your pressure will fall. But you've got to do it regularly on an ongoing basis. Get into the habit of taking your pressure before, during, and after exercise as well as later in the day to assess its impact.

- Biofeedback and other stress-reducing techniques such as meditation can help lower blood pressure, especially in conjunction with weight loss and exercise.

- A diet rich in fruits and vegetables and low in saturated fat also helps you lose weight and so eventually lower blood pressure too.

- Salt reduction is controversial. We Americans eat much more salt than we need or than is good for us. Hypertension aside, reducing your salt intake makes you less vulnerable to osteoporosis and kidney stones. If you already have some heart trouble, the less salt you consume, the better. There is no question that many hypertensive individuals are salt-sensitive—that is, their elevated pressure is related to their salt intake. This is especially true for African Americans, women, and the elderly, but not for everyone. I advise my newly diagnosed patients with high blood pressure to reduce their salt intake to no more than 2,400 mg a day (about a teaspoon) for several weeks to see whether it makes a difference. The best way to do that is to avoid frankly salted foods such as herring and to remove the salt shaker from the table. You may add a little salt to taste in the cooking. Many packaged foods contain sodium that you may be consuming unknowingly. Check the label of all packaged foods for their salt (sodium) content. If you need to spice up the taste of your food, try an herb or salt substitute. Those that contain potassium are especially tasty.

You should also reduce the other risks of vascular disease to which you are more vulnerable because of your hypertension. If you haven't already quit smoking, do so now. Have your sugar checked *again* to make sure you're not diabetic. The combination of diabetes and high blood pressure favors early arteriosclerosis. Check the level of your blood fats and start the necessary dietary and/or drug therapy to normalize all the fractions of your cholesterol.

If you've tried your best for three to six months to control everything that can contribute to your high blood pressure, and you just don't have the discipline to stick with the regimen (believe me, you're not alone), or you really have been very "good" but your pressure stayed high anyway, you'll have to start medication. But that doesn't mean that you should abandon these healthful lifestyle changes. If you continue to follow them, you will be able to control your pressure *with less medication and therefore have fewer side effects.*

Once you've been found to have high blood pressure, arrange for a complete physical and some other special tests. They should include a complete blood count, urinalysis (looking for the presence of albumin, an indicator of kidney malfunction), potassium level, urea nitrogen (again to determine kidney function), fasting blood sugar (to see whether you're diabetic), and an electrocardiogram. If you're under forty, ask for a renin level be done too. (Renin is a hormone that stimulates the kidney to make angiotensin, another hormone that constricts the blood vessels and raises pressure (discussed below). If you're male and over forty, you should also have a stress test. After all, you don't know how long your pressure has been high and your heart may already have been affected. A stress test will detect cardiac abnormalities before the resting ECG becomes abnormal. *Insist on all of them.*

High Blood Pressure Medications

Here are the cardinal rules about drug therapy for hypertension:

- Never throw in the treatment towel because the side effects "are worse than the disease." There *is* a combination of medications that will eventually work *for you*. It takes time and patience on your part and your doctor's, but the right mix of drugs can always be found. Stick with it. No side effects are nearly as bad as the paralysis that follows a stroke—which is just one of the possible outcomes of untreated hypertension.
- By the same token, do not accept troublesome side effects of the medication as inevitable and the price you have to pay to control your blood pressure. That was true years ago, but today there are scores of drugs that you can try. If your doctor can't find an effective one with which you're comfortable, *insist on a second opinion from a specialist in hypertension.* Side effects are not only unpleasant; they are nature's way of telling you that the medicine causing them is not good for you.
- Until fairly recently, doctors believed that as long as the blood pressure was normalized, it didn't matter how it was done. There is a growing suspicion that some agents more effectively prevent long-term complications of hy-

pertension than do others, even though they lower pressure to the same extent. These differences are discussed later in this chapter.

- Start with *one* drug and only change it or add another after you've given it a chance. Be patient. Work with your doctor to keep the treatment as simple as possible. If your blood pressure is not responding to a given agent, it's better to add another rather than increase the dose of the first one. You're less likely to experience side effects from small doses of several medications than larger doses of fewer ones.

- Learn all you can about every single medication you're given. If your doctor is too busy, ask your pharmacist and read the package insert carefully. It was written for you. Pay particular attention to possible drug interactions. Make note of any precautions to take if you're on any other medication too. For example, the mainstays of therapy for hypertension are diuretics (water pills), which sometimes cause a loss of too much potassium along with the salt and water they eliminate. If you're also taking digitalis, low potassium can result in toxic side effects. Also, some diuretics increase blood sugar in diabetics. These are just two examples of how careful (and knowledgeable) you must be when taking any medication, including herbs. As far as the latter are concerned, always tell your doctor which ones you are taking if he or she didn't recommend them.

- The price range for blood pressure drugs varies considerably. As many as 25 percent of Americans, many of them senior citizens, can't afford to fill their prescriptions. I see this every day in my own practice. Ask your doctor to prescribe generic preparations rather than brand names when possible. I always do so because I don't believe there is any real difference between them, and the generics are a lot cheaper. And don't be shy about asking for samples. Drug houses give them to doctors. I save mine for patients with economic problems. Finally, there is almost always a reasonably priced pill that you can take instead of the one you can't afford. It may not be quite as effective, but it's far better than no pill at all. And if there is really no alternative to something you just can't buy, ask your doctor to contact the manufacturer on your behalf. Every pharmaceutical company has some type of plan that makes its product available to someone who simply doesn't have the means to buy it.

- The goal of treatment should be to lower blood pressure to below 130 systolic and less than 85 diastolic, no matter how high it was before therapy.

When I started practice in the 1950s, there were only a few drugs with which to treat hypertension. Today there are scores of effective medications. They fall into seven main categories:

- Diuretics
- Beta-blockers
- Angiotensin-converting enzyme (ACE) inhibitors
- Calcium channel blockers
- Alpha-blockers
- Angiotensin II receptor blockers (ARBs)
- Vasodilators

Drugs in every one of these categories have advantages and disadvantages. The one(s) your doctor selects will depend on your age and whatever other diseases you happen to have or to which you are vulnerable. For example, if you're both hypertensive and asthmatic, you probably won't be given beta-blockers as the first choice. On the other hand, if you have a cardiac rhythm problem, a beta-blocker might be ideal. If you have kidney trouble, a diuretic, often the agent most doctors prescribe first, may not be safe. So bear all these caveats in mind as you read about the various treatment options.

Diuretics are the first choice of most doctors, especially for older patients and African Americans. They should first be used alone, but if the pressure does not fall sufficiently, other agents are added. Their long-term results are impressive. They substantially reduce the incidence of strokes and heart attacks. Unless you don't mind getting up at night, take them in the morning—assuming, of course, that you have access to a john during the day. If you don't, or have errands to do all over town, or are going on a long car trip, then wait until you're back home or in your office before you take this medication.

There are three main types of diuretics: thiazides, such as chlorothiazide (Diuril), chlorthalidone (Hygroton), and hydrochlorothiazide (Hydrodiuril); loop diuretics such as furosemide (Lasix), bumetanide (Bumex), and ethacrynic acid (Edecrin); and spironolactone (Aldactone), and triamterene (Dyrenium). In addition to promoting loss of salt and water, the thiazides and loop diuretics (but not Aldactone and Dyrenium) also result in the excretion of other substances such as potassium. Too little potassium can cause potentially serious disturbances of heart rhythm and may also interact adversely with digitalis, other heart drugs, and some antidepressants. That's why many doctors give potassium supplements to patients who are taking diuretics. In fact, many of these diuretics come with built-in potassium supplements.

Don't take supplemental potassium just because you're on a diuretic if your kidneys are damaged and are not eliminating potassium efficiently. You also probably don't need the extra potassium if your diet contains enough of it in all the bananas you eat and orange juice you drink. Too much potassium can cause heart rhythm disorders.

Diuretics do more than just lower blood pressure. They also prevent the formation of calcium-containing kidney stones and reduce the severity of osteoporosis.

Although these drugs are usually well tolerated, they can cause some problems. For example, they can leave you tired (especially if you're losing too much potassium), reduce your

sex drive, raise the level of uric acid in the body (and precipitate an attack of gout), increase the cholesterol level, cause
one or both breasts to swell and become tender in men, and
render incontinent those elderly people who already have a
problem holding their urine. But don't let these potential problem deter you from using these drugs. On the whole, they are
easy to take.

Beta-blockers lower blood pressure by reducing the force
with which the heart contracts and slowing the heart rate.
They also counteract the effect of adrenaline-like chemicals
that raise blood pressure. They are among the most useful and
versatile agents in medicine. Doctors prescribe them for everything from preventing panic when you're making a public
speech to slowing a rapid heart rate, controlling dangerous
abnormalities of cardiac rhythm, reducing the frequency of
angina pectoris, improving tremors, preventing migraine
headaches—and lowering blood pressure.

Because beta-blockers have so many uses, drug companies
make a host of them. Although there are some differences
among them, many are me-too preparations, especially with
respect to blood pressure therapy. The best-known beta-
blockers are popranolol (Inderal), atenolol (Tenormin), metoprolol (Toprol), acebutolol (Sectral), and nadolol (Corgard).
One of them in particular, carvedilol (Coreg), is especially useful for treating severe heart failure. It also works better than
the others for diabetics.

Beta-blockers generally go very well with diuretics. In fact,
combining them is more effective in reducing the incidence of
heart attacks than either drug alone, regardless of the extent to
which each lowers blood pressure.

Beta-blockers also have their downside. They can cause the
airways to go into spasm, so avoid them if you have any kind
of chronic lung condition such as asthma, bronchitis, or emphysema. These drugs can increase arterial spasm and further
constrict them, so avoid them if you have pain in your legs
when you walk because your blood vessels are narrowed.

Check your cholesterol level if you're on a beta-blocker. These drugs can reduce the level of the good cholesterol (HDL) by as much as 10 percent.

Beta-blockers can also mask the symptoms of a low blood sugar (hypoglycemia) in diabetics. That's why I don't usually prescribe them as the first choice for such patients. Finally, beta-blockers can result in an array of unpleasant side effects that include impotence, fatigue, bad dreams, depression, memory loss, and cold extremities.

If you've been taking a beta-blocker for any length of time to treat angina and have to stop it because of an adverse side effect, do not do so suddenly. Reduce the dosage gradually before discontinuing it, otherwise your angina may worsen and even leave you vulnerable to sudden death.

Despite this long list of precautions, beta-blockers in the right dose have myriad beneficial effects, not the least of which is that they safely and effectively lower elevated blood pressure. They are for the most part very well tolerated. However, you should be aware of their potential side effects and tell your doctor if you're experiencing any of them.

ACE inhibitors are blood-pressure-lowering agents. Their mechanism of action is very different from those of diuretics and beta-blockers. There are three proteins that interact to cause most cases of essential hypertension—renin, aldosterone, and angiotensin. The ACE (angiotensin-converting enzyme) inhibitors prevent the formation of one of them, angiotensin, by blocking the enzyme that converts it into its active form. Without angiotensin, the other two proteins are less potent and do not raise blood pressure nearly as much.

Whenever a good medication appears on the market, many others follow. So there are several ACE inhibitors, including some generics. The best known are captopril (Capoten), enalapril (Vasotec), quinapril (Accupril), ramipril (Altace), and lisinopril (Zestril, Prinivil). *Insist on an ACE inhibitor or one of the ARBs discussed below for your high blood pressure if you are a diabetic, especially if you already have some kidney trou-*

ble or heart disease. There is mounting evidence that these agents are actually the best for preventing many vascular and kidney complications even in the absence of hypertension. More and more doctors are prescribing them, especially in combination with diuretics.

Like any medication, ACE inhibitors have potential side effects of which you should be aware. The most common one is a dry, irritating cough. You'll save lots of time and money if you remember this particular complication. I can't tell you how many patients go from doctor to doctor, from nose and throat specialists to lung experts, trying to find out why they're coughing. If you're taking an ACE inhibitor, chances are that's what's doing it. Switch to some other drug (but not a different ACE inhibitor) and the cough will go away. If you must continue with an ACE inhibitor, try taking iron supplements. They were recently reported to lessen the cough.

A more serious complication of ACE inhibitors is their ability to cause kidney damage in some patients. Although they are usually good for that organ, their use can result in retention of potassium, too much of which can cause fatal cardiac rhythm disturbances. So if you're taking a diuretic along with an ACE inhibitor (an otherwise excellent combination), *you may not need supplemental potassium or a potassium-sparing diuretic.* Also, *don't use an ACE inhibitor when pregnant.* If one was prescribed for you before you became pregnant, stop it as soon as you hear the good news.

What a great advance the angiotensin II receptor blockers (ARBs) have been! This latest group of drugs acts in the same general way as the ACE inhibitors and they're just as effective, but they have fewer side effects and they rarely if ever result in a chronic cough. So if you are taking an ACE inhibitor and are coughing, consider switching to an ARB. These agents may also have an additional protective effect on the arteries and can also be combined with a diuretic. Indeed, some of them are marketed in such combinations. Among the most widely used ARBs are losartan (Cozaar), which when combined with the diuretic hydrochlorothiazide is sold as Hyzaar, irbesartan (Avapro), candesartan (Atacand), and valsartan (Diovan). I don't think there's much difference among them, although some are said to be longer-acting and therefore better suited for one-a-day dosage. ARBs and ACE inhibitors can also be used together to lower the blood pressure when necessary.

Alpha-blockers lower blood pressure by blocking nerve impulses that constrict the blood vessels. Drugs in this category include doxazosin (Cardura), terazosin (Hytrin), and prazosin (Minipress). I have not found them very effective against hypertension, although they do reduce the frequency of urination at night in men with prostate enlargement. They have the troublesome propensity to increase heart rate, retain fluid, and drop blood pressure too much and too quickly, especially when you suddenly stand up from the lying or sitting position. There have been some reports that these drugs may actually increase the risk of heart attack. If you need an alpha-blocker to help control your urinary symptoms and you find it's causing too much of a blood pressure drop, especially if you have normal blood pressure to begin with, there's a newer one called tamsulosin (Flomax), which is just as effective for the prostate but doesn't lower pressure nearly as much.

Vasodilator drugs reduce blood pressure by widening the arteries. They are not used nearly as often as they used to be since the advent of more effective newer drugs. The best known are hydralazine (Apresoline) and minoxidil (Loniten, which actually grows hair when applied to the scalp; you're more likely to recognize it by its other name, Rogaine). I don't advise any of these agents if you have angina pectoris or have had a heart attack.

Calcium channel blockers are very effective blood-pressure-lowering agents. Because of some reports that although they normalize pressure, they do not protect against the cardiac complications of hypertension (such as heart attack and heart failure) as well as do diuretics, ACE inhibitors, and beta-blockers—some doctors hesitate to use them as a first-line drug.

They do, however, protect against stroke, particularly in the elderly. I still prescribe them together with other medications that I know are protective just to get that extra blood-pressure-lowering effect.

There are three main categories of calcium channel blockers: the phenylalkylamine group (verapamil [Calan], Isoptin, Verelan); the benzothiazepines (diltiazem—Cardizem, Dilacor); and dihydropyridines, such as nifedipine (Procardia, Adalat), amlodipine (Norvasc), and felodipine (Plendil). They differ from one another in the mechanism by which they lower blood pressure. Incidentally, if you have Raynaud's phenomenon (your fingers or toes turn blue when exposed to cold), these drugs can help. They also prevent migraine. Grapefruit juice enhances their effect. You'll get more of the drug than you bargained for, so take them with water or orange juice instead.

The main side effects of calcium channel blockers are swelling of the feet, inflammation of the gums, constipation (especially with the phenylalkylamine group), impotence, and fatigue.

Other Treatment Options

Many doctors believe that *calcium supplements* lower blood pressure. I consider the data to be inconclusive. So I limit this recommendation to women of all ages to prevent osteoporosis, not to lower blood pressure.

What about *potassium?* There's no question in my mind that a high intake of potassium from natural sources (fruits and vegetables) is good for you and may have a beneficial effect on blood pressure. There have even been some studies indicating that potassium supplements lower blood pressure. However, the doses required to do so often produce intestinal side effects, so I don't prescribe them except for patients taking diuretics. The same is true for *magnesium.*

I love *garlic*, but despite the rumors, I'm not convinced that it lowers blood pressure.

When You're Being Treated for High Blood Pressure

If there is any question about whether or not you have the kind of blood pressure numbers that require therapy, there is one further step you can take. It's called *ambulatory monitoring*. A blood pressure cuff is placed on your arm and you wear it for the next twenty-four hours—eating, arguing, working, making love, sleeping (but don't take a bath or shower—that's an expensive piece of equipment and you'll ruin it if you do). You keep a diary of everything that's happening and when. All this time, the cuff keeps inflating and deflating every thirty minutes, and the unit records all the pressures it takes. No chance of a white-coat syndrome here! The next morning you return the instrument, and the record of the past day is printed out.

I don't obtain ambulatory monitoring very often. In my experience a careful doctor and an intelligent patient working together can usually tell whether the blood pressure is high.

More important and much more practical than ambulatory blood pressure recording is *home blood pressure monitoring*. This is something I insist on for every patient with hypertension. The machines are not expensive or unwieldy, and their digital readout is as accurate as what your doctor obtains with the cuff and stethoscope. Make sure when you buy the unit that the cuff is the right size for your arm, especially if you are overweight.

Home pressure monitoring is, in my view, as much an advance in the management of hypertension as the home glucose machine is for diabetics. It frees you from the need (and expense) of coming to the doctor's office for a routine reading; it allows you to check your pressure several times a day under different circumstances and after you take your medication. It reveals the effectiveness of your treatment. All this is useful information for you and your doctor in determining the timing and dosage of your drugs. You can buy one of these machines at most drugstores for less than $100. But remember this: Some of these units are inaccurate. *Bring it to your doctor's office to have it checked out against the blood pressure machine in the office.* Do this every few months just to make sure that the unit is maintaining its accuracy.

Reviewing Your Answers to the Questions

It's now time to see how you made out on the questionnaire at the very beginning of this chapter. Was I right, or did you get more than ten correct answers?

- What is blood pressure? It's the measurement of pressure under which blood flows inside your arteries.
- What percentage of Americans have high blood pressure? Twenty-five percent, or fifty million people.
- What percentage of persons who know that their pressure is high are being adequately treated? Fewer than 30 percent.
- Are men more likely to have high blood pressure than women? Only until age 55, when the ratio reverses.
- Is high blood pressure curable? In only 5 percent of cases, but it can always be successfully treated.
- How many readings should be taken before the diagnosis of hypertension is made? In at least two or three follow-up visits.
- What is white-coat hypertension? When the readings are higher in the doctor's office than at home. It is not always a benign phenomenon, since many patients who attrib-

ute their pressure elevation to "nervousness" later do, in fact, develop high blood pressure.

- Is there a form of high blood pressure that is not harmful? No, every case of hypertension is a potential vascular threat down the road.
- Which of the two blood pressure readings is more important, the systolic or the diastolic? They are both important.
- How often should you be checked if you have high blood pressure? Buy a home blood pressure cuff and do it routinely once or twice a week.
- Does chronic alcohol excess raise blood pressure? Yes.
- Does cigarette smoking raise blood pressure? Only within half an hour of smoking. It does not cause chronic hypertension.
- Is excessive salt intake an important cause of hypertension? In many but not all cases, especially in African Americans.
- What is secondary hypertension? The blood pressure elevations that occur in 5 percent of cases and are due to some known cause that can usually be cured.
- What blood pressure reading is optimal? Any number below 130/85.

WHAT TO INSIST ON IF YOU HAVE HIGH BLOOD PRESSURE

Hypertension is a major cause of life-threatening vascular disease, especially affecting the brain, heart, eyes, kidneys, and the circulation in the legs. It does not usually result in symptoms until it has already damaged these vital organs. So it is extremely important to be checked regularly throughout life for the presence of this disease.

Do not accept the diagnosis of hypertension on the basis of one or two "borderline" readings. However, *if your pressure is consistently 140/90 or higher, insist on treatment.*

Although eminently manageable, 95 percent of cases of hypertension are not curable. However, the other 5 percent may be. *You must insist on a full diagnostic evaluation to make sure that you are not among that 5 percent.* You are most likely to be if you are younger than fifteen or over sixty-five and have suddenly developed very high pressure. Other telltale symptoms include excessive sweating, palpitations, increased urination, and hormonal or kidney problems.

If you're male and over 40 or female, postmenopausal, and have high blood pressure, insist on a cardiac and neurological evaluation. This should include the pertinent blood tests, and a cardiac stress test to identify silent heart disease.

Unless your pressure is very high, *insist on being observed for up to six months while you make the necessary changes in your lifestyle that can normalize blood pressure without drugs.*

There are several categories of drugs to treat high blood pressure. Do not accept a combination that leaves you with miserable side effects. Everyone with high blood pressure can be successfully treated with little or no toxicity. *Insist on a consultation with a hypertension specialist if the quality of your life is unacceptable because of these side effects.*

20

INFERTILITY

When Your Stork Won't Fly

"Barren" marriages are the stuff history, drama, and political intrigue—all wound up in love, passion, and frustration. Thrones and dynasties have risen and fallen on the ability to produce an heir. The seeming inability to have a baby continues to disappoint and frustrate couples throughout the world. Their ongoing attempts to overcome the problem have changed lovemaking from what should be a normal, spontaneous outpouring of passion to "performance on demand." Sex often becomes a calculated clinical act fraught with anxiety, performed under the supervision of caregivers and enveloped in the trappings of medicine—record-keeping thermometers, medications, calendars, and hospital clinics. Millions of women go to bed at night hoping and praying to wake up nauseated in the morning!

Despite all the playgrounds teeming with children, the crowded schools, and the fact that every one of your friends who wants to be pregnant either is or has been, more than 5 million couples of childbearing age in the United States want to have a baby and can't. If you're among them, at what point should you conclude that you are infertile and seek help? The following numbers may guide you. In this country, normal couples in which the woman is under the age of thirty and who engage in regular intercourse, pregnancy will result within six months; 90 percent of these women will give birth within a year; it will take two years for the rest. The statistics become less favorable as you grow older. So if your gynecologist and internist are stumped, *insist on a consultation with a fertility specialist* if you're younger than thirty-five and have been trying for two years; or are between thirty-five and forty and have been unsuccessful for six months; or are over forty and have had no luck for three months. But get such expert help *now* if you're infertile and have ever had pelvic infections, a sexually transmitted disease, endometriosis, gynecological surgery, or your periods have changed, are irregular, painful, very heavy, or sparse.

After one year of infertility, there is a 50 percent chance that you can be helped by a specialist. On the other hand, if you keep trying on your own in the hope that nature will "take its course," the likelihood of having a baby is only 5 percent.

Some women have no trouble conceiving, but then can't hold on to the pregnancy. Don't despair. Miscarriages are often followed by a normal pregnancy. However, if you've had two consecutive losses, *insist on seeing a fertility specialist before you try again.* The workup and the treatment for repeated miscarriages are essentially the same as for infertility.

Whose Fault Is It?

In most of the world literature, the blame for infertility is invariably placed on the woman. If a king needed an heir, it was up to his queen to provide one. If she couldn't, His Majesty found another queen or upgraded his harem. Although many people in every culture still believe that infertility is a female problem, the truth is that *both* genders contribute equally to the success (or failure) of the reproductive process. Thirty-five percent of cases of infertility are due to female hormonal or gynecological problems; another 35 percent are attributable to the male; both partners are responsible in 20 percent of cases; and the cause cannot be determined 10 percent of the time.

There is no single treatment for infertility that works for everyone, because the problem has so many different causes. It's not like pneumonia for which you take an antibiotic, or angina pectoris relieved by a nitroglycerin tablet. In order to understand the diagnostic workup and therapy, as well as the chance of success, let's briefly review the reproductive process and the contribution made by each of the partners.

The Making of a Baby: The Female Reproductive System

There are several steps that must be successfully completed before a pregnancy can occur. Let's start with the egg. The ovaries, one on each side of the pelvis, contain a reservoir of eggs from which they normally release one or more mature egg every month. The lucky winner is then gathered into the fallopian tube, down which it wends its way to the uterus. There it meets the sperm that's destined to fertilize it, and the result of their union settles down in the wall of the uterus. Nine months later a healthy infant is born.

It sounds simple, but there are several pitfalls along the way:

- The ovary must be healthy, free of infection, malformation, and other disorders, and contain an ample store of eggs.
- The ovary is under the control of various hormones produced by the brain, the most important of which is

follicle-stimulating hormone (FSH). Without enough FSH, there are no mature eggs. The fallopian tubes in which the egg travels to the uterus must be open, and not scarred or infected.

- The lining of the uterus must be prepared to receive and nourish the fertilized egg. This requires adequate preparation by another hormone, luteinizing hormone (LH), secreted by the brain.
- The mucus in and around the cervix (gateway to the uterus) must be hospitable to the sperm and allow it to pass through and reach the uterus for its rendezvous with the egg.

The number and complexity of the potential roadblocks make you wonder how anyone ever gets pregnant! And we haven't yet even discussed potential problems inherent in the male reproductive system.

The Male Reproductive System

In men, the name of this game is the ability to make healthy sperm, get them out of the testes where they're produced and through the network of ducts that leads to the urethra in the penis. The sperm, bathed in testicular fluid, exits the testicles into a series of tiny ducts that empty into a tightly coiled tube fifteen feet long called the epididymis. This in turn leads into a fifteen-inch long cord called the vas deferens. Two seminal vesicles situated nearby make most of the semen in which the sperm will complete its journey, and they open through a duct into the vas deferens near its final portion. Together they form the ejaculatory duct that empties into the urethra. Rhythmic contraction of the muscles surrounding the urethra results in ejaculation. Once liberated, sperm has about two days to do its job. (The window of opportunity for the egg by, con-

trast, is only twenty-four hours. So for everyone and everything concerned—you, your partner, the sperm, and the
egg—it's a race against time!)

In order to make sperm, the testicles need an ample supply of testosterone, the male hormone that also creates the
desire to have sex and an erection. So both hormonal and
psychological factors enter into play. Once the sperm is produced, every single duct through which it travels before being
ejaculated must be open so that it can flow through them. The
sperm itself must be active, able to swim vigorously "up-
stream" toward the uterus, and there must be enough of them,
even though it only takes one to do the job.

The specialist must evaluate each step in this saga of fertilization, determine what has gone awry, and decide how to fix
it. Let's start with the evaluation of the woman.

The Female Fertility Evaluation

You'll first undergo a thorough history and physical, with specific emphasis on your menstrual history:

- Are your periods painful? (This is often associated with
  ovulation but may suggest endometriosis, an important
  cause of infertility. See Chapter 11.)
- Have you had any pelvic infections or sexually transmitted diseases that may have scarred the uterus or the
  fallopian tubes?
- What medications are you taking?
- Is your thyroid function normal?
- Are you diabetic or anorexic, or do you have tuberculosis or some other infection?
- How much do you smoke and drink? (Cigarettes and alcohol can impair fertility.)

- Did you ever use contraceptives, and, if so, what were they, and when did you stop them? (Hormonal imbalance may last for several months after stopping the Pill.)
- The gynecologic exam will focus on a search for infection of the vagina, cervix, or fallopian tubes. You'll also have a cervical smear.
- You will undergo a hormonal profile: FSH and estradiol level on day 3 of your menstrual cycle are critically important. If your ovaries are not maturing their eggs, the brain makes more FSH in an attempt to stimulate them to do so. So the less active the ovary, the higher the FSH level, an important diagnostic indicator of infertility.
- Other hormonal analyses include the progesterone level measured at the end of your cycle, and thyroid and prolactin concentrations.
- Be prepared to have a "postcoital test." This is similar to a Pap smear and is done about two to three hours after intercourse at midcycle. Its purpose is to assess the interaction between the sperm and the mucus in the vagina. The mucus is sometimes toxic to the sperm. This cervical smear is usually also analyzed for the presence of *Chlamydia* and *Ureaplasma,* two common infectious microorganisms that may be hard to diagnose but that can contribute to infertility.

If all the above are normal, you might require a biopsy of the lining of the uterus to see whether it can nourish a fertilized egg. You also might have a hysterosalpingogram (HSG), the tubal X ray taken after the injection of radiopaque dye. It highlights the uterus and reveals the presence of fibroids and polyps and any deformity of the uterus, and indicates as well whether or not the fallopian tubes are open. If the doctor suspects endometriosis, he or she may also do a laparoscopy or hysteroscopy.

It sounds like a lot, and it is. But there's a 95 percent chance that this workup will reveal the cause of your problem.

Assessing a Male's Fertility

Testing for male fertility is easier. It starts with an analysis of your semen. The doctor collects the specimen and examines it within two hours. He or she counts the sperm and looks at them under the microscope to see how active they are (motility) and whether or not their shape is normal. This is usually done two or three times to ensure accuracy. If you live far from the clinic, you will have to provide your specimen on site.

If your sperm is normal, you can go home. If the postcoital test reveals the presence of *Chlamydia* or *Ureaplasma* organisms, you will be given an antibiotic. If any abnormality of the sperm are detected, you will be asked whether you've ever had any radiation to or near the testicles, or been treated for venereal disease, especially gonorrhea or chlamydia, or have some other generalized illness such as diabetes, alcoholism, liver or kidney trouble, or a history of mumps that was complicated by inflammation of the testicle (where sperm is made). Your testicles will be examined carefully, and the presence noted of varicose veins involving the ducts that carry the sperm (spermatic cord), your prostate will be assessed, and a search will be made for any other genitourinary disorder. Finally, your testosterone hormone level will be measured. Any of the above can impair the ability of sperm to fertilize an egg.

There's one fact every man should know about sperm. It doesn't do well in high temperatures. That's why men whose testicles have not descended from the abdomen (where they develop) into the cooler environs of the scrotal sac outside the body don't make viable sperm. So if you want to make a baby, don't take a hot bath before intercourse, and don't wear tight shorts that keep the testicles too close to the body, where they are warmed by its higher temperature.

So What Do We Do About It?

After the fertility workup, husband and wife will be offered the appropriate therapy. Before going into specifics, let me give you some commonsense tips about intercourse. Everyone relishes the pleasures of making love, but did you know there are optimal positions to increase the chances of a "hit"? If you've had trouble conceiving, beg, borrow, or steal a manual that describes the different coital positions and those that favor fertilization. Women should make sure that their vaginal cream or lubricant doesn't contain a spermicide. You'd be surprised how many women are unaware that the nonoxynol-9 they're using for protection against herpes and other infections also kills sperm! And men, even if your wife isn't using nonoxynol-9, make sure that your condom isn't impregnated with it, as some are! Remember, too, that douching after intercourse may be hygienic, but it is deadly for sperm.

Now let's go through the treatments available for the most common potential infertility problems in both partners.

If your own gynecologist hasn't already done so, the infertility specialist will put you through the ritual of temperature testing in order to determine if and when you're ovulating. That's very important because you have only twenty-four hours in which to act after the egg is released! Here's how it's done: You take your temperature first thing in the morning, before you get out of bed and before eating or drinking anything, or even brushing your teeth. Ovulation, the critical release of the egg, occurs in midcycle. When you have been taking your temperature in this way for a few months, you'll note that about fourteen days before each period, your temperature rises by 1 degree Fahrenheit (0.5 degree centigrade). Now here's the important thing to remember: That rise in temperature occurs twenty-four hours *after* ovulation, so have sex every thirty-six to forty-eight hours starting *the day before*. (Sex every day might well deplete the sperm count.)

You can buy a kit at a drugstore to help you determine somewhat more accurately exactly when you're ovulating. There are several brands and they vary in price; some contain more tests than others do.

If you have an *ovulation problem,* you may need medications to stimulate the ovary to mature and release the egg. These *"fertility pills"* are usually prescribed to be taken by mouth first and then by injection, if necessary. They are powerful hormones that require careful monitoring. Start with clomiphene (Clomid), which has a structure similar to estrogen. It works in a very ingenious way. When it reaches the brain from the bloodstream, it attaches itself to the estrogen receptor sites there and fills them up. When these sites are taken, the brain concludes that there is now too little estrogen left in the blood and initiates a series of hormonal changes that result in the increased production of FSH. This causes the ovarian follicle to mature its eggs. Clomiphene is not expensive and is taken orally for five days each month. It may cause hot flashes, breast discomfort, and migraine-like headaches. The dose is based on your response. You can be examined by ultrasound to see how the eggs are maturing. When one of them is ready, it can be sucked out of the ovary (under local anesthesia in an operating room) to be used in in vitro fertilization (see below).

Researchers report that taking oral contraceptives for one month, then stopping them, increases the subsequent chances of fertilization! Presumably, the birth control pills temporarily suppress ovulation, allowing the ovaries to rest. This increases the prospects of making mature eggs the next time round.

In another recent study, Viagra, of all things, when taken as a vaginal suppository, helped infertile women too. The presumed mechanism of action is increased blood flow to the lining of the uterus, thus enhancing its hospitality to the fertilized egg.

If you have any *physical problems in the uterus,* such as fibroids, polyps, adhesions from previous infection or surgery, or some congenital abnormality, they may have to be surgically corrected. Blocked fallopian tubes can often be opened by the surgeon, but when that's not possible, and there is no way the egg can get into the uterus, your best bet may be in vitro fertilization (IVF). The egg is removed from the ovary and mixed with the sperm in a laboratory dish where fertilization can occur under "ideal" conditions. A few days later the embryo is transferred to the woman's uterus, where it continues to grow.

Endometriosis (see Chapter 11), affects at least 10 percent of all American women and about 40 percent of those who are infertile. Endometriosis may predispose to infertility by causing pelvic adhesions and abnormal ovulation and by blocking the fallopian tubes. It can be treated by laser surgery or hormones that suppress menstruation.

If your vaginal mucus blocks the entry of the sperm into the uterus, your only option may be *artificial insemination by your husband (AIH),* in which the sperm bypasses the vagina and is injected directly into the uterus.

Why sperm is abnormal is not always clear. If the problem is *Chlamydia* or *Ureaplasma* infection, an antibiotic will solve the problem. Sometimes there is a deficiency of testosterone that can be replaced; repairing a varicocele (dilated veins around the ducts that carry the sperm) can help occasionally. When autoimmune factors are thought to play a role, the sperm can be purified by a technique called sperm washing. Some men with a low sperm count are also treated with clomiphene, but I have never seen it work.

If the cause of infertility is some trouble with the sperm, chances are the couple will require IVF. Sperm is injected into the egg, sparing it the arduous journey to the uterus. There are two new breakthroughs in IVF technology that have been successful when other methods have failed. The first is a technique called ICSI (pronounced *icksy*). It stands for "intracytoplasmic sperm injection." It is revolutionary because *only one sperm is needed.* Using microscopic techniques, a single sperm is drawn up into a very thin glass tube whose tip is inserted into the egg. And imagine! For men who are unable to ejaculate, there is now the testicular sperm aspiration (TSA) in which a needle is introduced directly into the testis, from which the sperm is removed and then injected into the egg by the ICSI method.

When more than one cause of infertility is found, the treatment is more complex. When all else fails, or in the 5 to 10 percent of cases in which no cause is discovered, most couples turn to IVF, which often works. If your husband's sperm can't be used, you may want to consider artificial insemination by a donor (using frozen sperm from a sperm bank) who has been carefully screened and found to be free of disease.

Some couple fear that IVF increases the risk of fetal abnormalities. That is possible because conventional IVF techniques are associated with an increase in the number of multiple pregnancies. However, in the ICSI procedure, where there is only one sperm and one egg, no such increase can occur. And there's even more good news about IVF. It can help you have a baby the natural way too. In a recent study, 21 percent of women who gave birth with an IVF procedure became pregnant on their own later. Doctors are not sure why, but presumably the reduced emotional stress after one delivery made it easier for them to conceive on their own.

WHAT AN INFERTILE COUPLE SHOULD INSIST ON

If you've had problems conceiving, insist on a referral to a fertility specialist.

Millions of apparently healthy couples in the United States are infertile. Careful evaluation reveals that the problem lies equally with the man and woman, and sometimes both contribute to it. In some 10 percent of cases, the cause of the infertility remains an enigma.

Infertility is not a single disease; it may be due to one or more anatomic, infectious, or hormonal problems that must first be identified in both genders, and then treated.

The most common causes of infertility in women are failure of the ovary to release a mature egg, hormonal deficiencies, endometriosis, previous pelvic infection, vaginal mucus that is hostile to sperm, and structural abnormalities of the genital tract. In men a decrease in the sperm count, a lack of its motility, and other abnormalities contribute to the couple's infertility.

Insist on the necessary tests to discover and correct the underlying disorder. If these methods do not help, there are new, powerful tools that involve mating selected sperm and egg in a laboratory dish and implanting the fertilized egg into the uterus. These techniques have met with a high rate of success. *Insist on having all the methods explained to you.*

21

IRRITABLE BOWEL SYNDROME

You Are Not Alone (Although Those Around You May Wish You Were!)

Some 10 to 20 million adult Americans have a "nervous stomach," with such symptoms as chronic "indigestion" or "heartburn," nausea and vomiting, bloating, stomach distension with frequent belching, flatulence, constipation and/or diarrhea (the latter rarely at night and most often associated with meals), and the feeling that there's something left after they've finished a bowel movement. There is often mucus in the stool that appears as long, ropy strands. Nature calls them to "go" or "fart" so frequently and unpredictably that their lives are focused on their gut—and the location of the nearest toilet, just in case. These symptoms are mild in some, and debilitating in others.

Doctors give this condition a variety of names such as "irritable bowel syndrome" (IBS), "functional GI [short for gastrointestinal] disorder," "spastic colon," or "mucus colitis." Whatever you call it (I prefer IBS), this disorder is responsible for almost half of all the visits we make to our doctors' offices with digestive complaints. It is said to be the second most frequent cause of absenteeism from work in this country (after the common cold).

No one knows what causes IBS, and there is no cure for it. The term "nervous stomach" is a misnomer because being nervous has nothing to do with it. The condition is so poorly understood that those who have it go from doctor to doctor looking for an answer and a cure. They get neither. They are subjected to repeated colonoscopies, stool analyses, barium X rays, CT scans and MRIs of the abdomen—all of which are invariably "normal." Most of them end up being told by their doctors, "I have great news for you. Your bowel is completely normal. You have nothing to worry about. You don't have lactose intolerance, Crohn's disease, or ulcerative colitis, diverticulitis, and you're not going to get cancer." But despite this clean bill of health, you continue to ache, cramp, fart, and run to the john all day. Doctors expect you to feel secure in the knowledge that your misery is "nothing serious" and won't shorten your life.

Misery loves sympathy as well as company. It's ironic that once your family and friends hear the doctor's "good news," they stop giving you the sympathy you need. After a while, they often conclude that you are probably a hypochondriac.

The frustration of patients with IBS used to be true, too, for those with mitral valve prolapse, fibromyalgia, and chronic fatigue syndrome. For years, anyone (mostly women) who complained of heart palpitations, chest pain, and panic attacks and checked out normal was reassured. Those who didn't accept the "good news" and continued to be distressed by the way they felt were referred to psychiatrists. When the invention of the echocardiogram made it possible to view the interior of the heart, these individuals were found to have a deformity of the mitral valve in the heart. The condition was given a name (mitral valve prolapse), the symptoms were explained, and presto, countless "neurotic" patients became respectable. We're still waiting for a diagnostic breakthrough in fibromyalgia and chronic fatigue syndrome, but these disorders have for the most part also become "legitimate." And so will IBS.

Although the cause of IBS is still a mystery, most doctors agree that its symptoms are the result of a breakdown in the normal communication between the brain and the bowel. Someone with IBS has chronic belly pain, spasm, constipation, and diarrhea because the nerves supplying the gut are either hypersensitive or sluggish. When they send fewer signals to the bowel, the stool passes more slowly down the intestinal tract and the result is constipation; when the nervous activity is excessive, the stools are frequent and liquid.

Although a disorder of nerve function accounts for many of the symptoms of IBS, no one knows why it happens to some people and not to others or why it fluctuates. Like so many other mysterious maladies, the onset of IBS sometimes follows some stressful event such as divorce, bereavement, or a poor report card. However, the symptoms continue long after the event itself is gone and forgotten. Chronic stress does not cause IBS, but it can worsen symptoms. Although there is no cure for IBS, the quality of life of those who suffer from it can be improved.

Diagnosing IBS

If you have the constellation of symptoms characteristic of IBS, you must be sure that they are not due to something else. *Insist* on every test necessary to do so. This is a diagnosis of exclusion that should be made only after everything else has been ruled out. The necessary tests are a complete blood count to include a sedimentation rate, liver profile, stool analyses, and colonoscopy or flexible sigmoidoscopy.

The following conditions mimic irritable syndrome:

Lactose intolerance. Most of us have some deficiency of the enzyme lactase, which digests lactose, the sugar present in milk and milk products. Undigested lactose in the gut can cause some of the symptoms of IBS.

Medication. We are a nation of pill poppers. You name it, we take it—vitamins, food supplements, and scores of different herbs, sedatives, painkillers, tranquilizers, hormones. Every medication is suspect in someone with any chronic bowel complaint. The first things to do is to discontinue every medication that is not absolutely necessary. You'd be amazed how often I've cured diarrhea simply by reducing excessive doses of vitamin C.

Infection. People with the symptoms of IBS often turn out to have unrecognized bacterial, fungal, or parasitic infection. (Viruses usually cause acute and only temporary symptoms.) When the infection, be it an amoeba, *Giardia,* or *C. difficile,* is eradicated, the "nervous stomach" disappears.

Malabsorption. When the pancreas doesn't make enough of its enzymes, undigested food in the intestinal tract can occasionally cause symptoms indentical to those of IBS. The presence of these enzymes is simple to test for, and they are easy to replace, but you first must think of this possibility.

Food allergies or sensitivities account for a surprising number of chronic bowel symptoms. I'm ashamed to admit that a member of my own family was for years diagnosed with IBS until he was found to be sensitive to potatoes. When he eliminated them from his diet, his symptoms cleared up. Any food, no matter how bland or "good" it is for you, can make you sick. Skin testing, as well as trial and error, will usually identify the culprit.

Sprue or celiac disease is a common disorder that mimics IBS. Patients are allergic to wheat, barley, and rye. This condition is especially frequent in those of Irish, English, or Italian ancestry and affects 1 in 200 Americans. It causes bloating, gas, diarrhea, and constipation.

Inflammatory bowel disease (IBD) such as Crohn's or ulcerative colitis can mimic irritable bowel syndrome, but their treatment and outlook are vastly different from IBS.

Other disease of the intestinal tract such as a malfunctioning gallbladder can also cause bowel symptoms. The bottom line is that if you have any chronic bowel problem, you need a comprehensive workup to exclude a host of curable conditions with similar symptoms. *Insist on it* before accepting the diagnosis of "nervous stomach."

Treatment of IBS

After all the other possibilities have been ruled out, and you are left with the diagnosis of IBS, I recommend the following measures:

- Avoid any food that causes or worsens your symptoms, even if you love it.
- Limit your intake of milk and milk products. Eat plenty of foods high in fiber and low in fat. (Fiber makes the stool bulkier, wetter, and easier to pass, thus avoiding constipation.) Wheat bran, oat bran, barley, peas, and a variety of vegetables are all fiber-rich. You can also add fiber supplements to your diet. My favorite ones are FiberCon, Prodiem, and Fibermed. (Although Metamucil is widely recommended, I prefer the others because they contain less sugar.)
- Avoid all stimulant laxatives if you're chronically constipated. Use the osmotic laxatives such as sorbitol or lactulose that draw water into the bowel and make it easier for you to eliminate the stool.
- If you have diarrhea, Imodium, Lomotil, and Pepto-Bismol are useful. Avoid tomatoes and strawberries.
- Develop a bowel routine. Go to the bathroom at the same time every day, preferably after a meal, and give yourself enough time.

- A heating pad or a hot bath may provide relief for abdominal cramps or pain. Antispasmodic drugs such as Levsin, Librax, or Bentyl also help.
- Even though stress and emotional distress are not the prime causes of IBS, they can worsen its symptoms. Seeking professional help does not mean that you're a hypochondriac or neurotic. Ask your doctor about biofeedback, hypnosis, and relaxation therapy, all of which are useful.
- Exercise for at least twenty minutes every day.
- If you smoke, Stop!

WHAT TO INSIST ON IF YOU HAVE IBS

Irritable bowel syndrome (IBS) is a chronic disorder that begins in young adult life and usually becomes less severe with age. It is characterized by irritability of the colon, which fluctuates between overactivity with spasm and diarrhea on the one hand to constipation on the other. There's no known cause, and a complete gastrointestinal workup fails to reveal any structural, physical, or chemical abnormalities. Despite the troublesome and often embarrassing symptoms, IBS does not lead to cancer and does not shorten life. There is no cure or specific treatment, but reassurance, keeping bowels regular, a high-fiber diet, and antispasmodic drugs when needed are helpful.

Do not accept the diagnosis of IBS before you have been thoroughly examined. *Insist on whatever tests or procedures are necessary to exclude a host of other curable conditions that mimic this disorder.*

22

KIDNEY STONES

A Rocky Road

Kidney stones (urolithiasis) have afflicted mankind since time immemorial and have been found in mummies dating back seven thousand years. At least 1 million Americans, most of them between the ages of twenty and forty, suffer a kidney stone attack every year, more whites than blacks and more men than women. When you do, you may experience a level of pain you've never known before. Overall, there is a one in ten chance that you will develop a "rolling stone" sometime during your life, and an even greater chance if a close family member has already done so. Once you've had an attack you can expect to have more in the future. The mechanisms, causes, and treatments of stone formation in various parts of the body such as the gallbladder or salivary ducts are unique. One kind does not predispose you to the others.

Although doctors often refer to it as "*the* kidney," we actually have two of these bean-shaped organs, one on each side of the body below the ribs, toward the middle of the back, just above the waist. A duct or tube called a ureter carrying urine leaves each kidney to connect with and empty into the bladder, which stores the urine. The bladder is a triangular-shaped balloonlike sac with elastic walls. When it contains enough urine to distend it, nerve endings in its wall are stimulated, giving you the all-too-familiar signal that it's time to pee. Muscles in the bladder contract, allowing the urine to flow out of it, into the urethra, and to exit the body.

The kidney is constantly monitoring the water content of the body. If you're in the desert, thirsty and dry as a bone, you won't urinate (or sweat excessively) in order to retain as much water as possible. The kidney also removes certain substances and waste products from the blood circulating through it and excretes them in the urine. (Our other major "exhaust" and detoxification systems are the lung, eliminating carbon dioxide, the bowel, liver, and skin.) The kidney has several other important roles: Its hormones help control blood pressure, prevent anemia, and keep the bones strong.

How Kidney Stones Are Formed

Normally, the various substances in urine are in balance with each other and dissolved in it. Certain chemical "inhibitors" in the urine that prevent its constituents from forming stones are lacking in some people who make such stones.

Medical textbooks list a number of conditions that "predispose" to kidney stones, but take it from me: No matter what else is going on, the most important factor is dehydration, usually the result of not drinking enough water. This is most likely to happen when you're perspiring excessively in hot weather and exercising vigorously.

When you're dehydrated, it's easier for the constituents of urine, especially mineral salts such as calcium, to come out of solution and form tiny crystals. These can combine to end up as stones. Although such stones almost always originate in the kidney, they often leave it and move down one of the ureters and into the urinary bladder. Stones can be classified by their location: When they remain in the kidney, it's called *nephrolithiasis;* in a ureter, it's *ureterolithiasis.* However, most physicians simply refer to them as "kidney stones" regardless of where they are.

The majority of kidney stones are so small that they pass without your even being aware of them. But when they are large enough, they can become stuck in one of the ureters. When that happens, and the stone completely blocks the ureter, urine can't get out. It backs up into the kidney, distending and sometimes damaging it. Furthermore, urine that's prevented from flowing freely stagnates and provides a good breeding ground for bacteria. That's why kidney stones can be associated with infection of the urinary tract.

Many of us, especially women, do not drink enough water. That aversion appears to be lessening. I see people everywhere swigging from disposable plastic water bottles—on the streets, in subways and on buses, in classrooms, arenas, football games, baseball games, board meetings, and doctors' waiting rooms. These bottles have replaced the smoke break! Even though the incidence of kidney stones has been increasing in the past two decades, the next count may well show a reversal of that trend because of this fad.

When Do Kidney Stones Form?

There are other causes of kidney stones in addition to lack of water. The most important are:

- Chronic infection anywhere in the urinary tract alters the environment so that the dissolved minerals crystallize.
- You are more vulnerable if others in your family (in-laws don't count) have kidney stones.
- Chronic obstruction of the urinary tract due to scarring or growths results in stagnation of urine, infection, crystallization, and formation of struvite stones.

- Too much calcium in the urine for any reason leads to the formation of calcium stones. For example, prolonged bed rest causes calcium to leak out of the bones into the bloodstream and eventually the urine, facilitating stone formation. Hyperparathyroidism is another cause of calcium stones. The parathyroid glands produce an excess of their hormone, which sucks large amounts of calcium out of the bones, into the bloodstream, through the kidneys, and into the urine, where it causes stones to form. Some people absorb too much calcium in their diet and it ends up in the urine as stones (this is an uncommon disorder, for which you can be tested). If you take too much vitamin D—say, more than 1,000 mg per day—you can absorb too much calcium and end up with kidney stones. Excessive vitamin C results in increased producion of oxalate and the formation of calcium oxalate stones. Patients with chronic inflammatory bowel disease (Crohn's, ulcerative colitis), or who have undergone bowel bypass surgery for the treatment of severe overweight, are candidates for calcium oxalate kidney stones.
- Certain genetic diseases (such as renal tubular acidosis) alter the chemical environment of the urine, enhancing the crystallization of its constituents. This is most frequently observed in children. Two other rare inherited diseases are cystinuria and hyperoxaluria. In the former, the kidneys excrete too much of the amino acid cystine, which then forms stones. In hyperoxaluria, the body manufactures more oxalate than it can dissolve in the urine.
- Gout leads to an excess of uric acid in the urine and the formation of uric acid stones.

Since almost 95 percent of kidney stones contain some calcium, doctors used to advise patients with these stones to reduce the calcium in their diets. Women who needed calcium to prevent their bones from thinning were in a quandary. Should they take it and run the risk of kidney stones, or avoid

it and suffer fractures from osteoporosis? Happily, newer research has shown that as far as food is concerned, *oxalate* is
the real villain (see below). Its combination with calcium is
what makes the stones; calcium alone doesn't do it.

Kidney stones are painless—until you pass one. In other
words, if they stay in the kidney where they form, you may
never know you have them until they show up in an X ray.
If they are small enough, they can even pass through the urinary system without causing any symptoms. But when a full-
fledged stone starts moving and gets stuck, watch out! It's said
to be the most painful experience you'll ever have. (Recently
one of my male patients in the throes of a kidney stone attack
cried out, "This is worse than childbirth!" His female nurses
and I wondered how he knew!)

Symptoms and Diagnosis of Kidney Stones

Here are characteristic symptoms caused by kidney stones:

- Pain, often described as sharp and colicky, begins suddenly in the back and side where the kidneys are located. As the stone moves down into the urinary ducts,
  the pain radiates toward the groin. It may ease up temporarily when the stone stops moving, but recurs with a
  vengeance once it starts again. The pain is worst when
  the stone is too big to pass easily down the duct, and
  the muscles of the ureter are in continual spasm as they
  attempt to milk it along.
- The urine almost always contains blood, visible under
  the microscope if not to the naked eye. The urine is also
  apt to be cloudy or foul-smelling when there is infection
  in the urinary tract.
- Nausea and vomiting.

- Fever, chills, and weakness, especially when there is accompanying infection.
- Urinary frequency and urgency when the stone reaches the very end of the ureter.

A full-blown kidney stone attack is easy to diagnose. The excruciating pain and blood in the urine are the giveaways. However, to confirm the diagnosis your doctor will usually order an X ray, ultrasound, or CT scan of the abdomen. (The latter will detect virtually every kind of stone. Those that do not contain calcium don't show up on a plain X ray.) Doctors used to suggest an intravenous pyelogram (IVP) in which dye injected into a vein traveled to the kidneys and into the ureters, "lighting them up." If there is a stone, it shows up as a gap in the dye. *Insist on the CT scan if you're offered an IVP.* Stones in the ureter can also be seen by injecting dye directly through the urethra. Be sure to tell the radiologist if you are allergic or sensitive to iodine, a major component of the dye. If you are, you will be pretreated to make sure you tolerate the injection without any ill effect.

How to Prevent Kidney Stones

Read this section very carefully if any of your blood relatives have kidney stones or if you have ever experienced one or more attacks yourself.

Drink at least two quarts of water a day (assuming, of course, that there is no reason such as heart failure for you not to do so). The best way to make sure you're getting enough water is to measure your urine volume. And I mean *measure;* it's too important to guesstimate. Unless you're passing at least two quarts of urine a day, you're drinking too little water!

Try to eliminate any of the risk factors that predispose you to kidney stones. For example, if you're prone to urinary tract infections, nip them in the bud with antibiotics as soon as they start. Don't suffer for days and weeks from frequency, urgency, and burning before you do something about it. Remember that chronic infection makes struvite stones. (And a stone is a stone is a stone. They all hurt.) If you have gout, take allopurinol to keep your uric acid level low so that uric acid stones don't form in the urine (see Chapter 14).

Most stones by far consist of calcium oxalate. We used to assume that the obvious way to prevent them from forming was to cut down on calcium in the diet. Doing so can actually result in *more* stone formation! (Calcium tablets and calcium-rich antacids are another matter. Avoid them if you have these stones.) Reduce the intake of oxalate and maintain or *increase* your consumption of dietary calcium. You won't be able to eliminate all the oxalate from your diet, but you can cut down on your intake by avoiding these foods:

Apples	Grapes
Asparagus	Ice Cream
Beer	Milk
Beets	Oranges
Berries	Nuts
Broccoli	Pineapples
Cheese	Rhubarb
Chocolate	Spinach
Cocoa	Tea
Coffee	Turnips
Cola	Vitamin C
Figs	Yogurt

Here are some other measures that will reduce your risk for kidney stones:

- If you are vulnerable to calcium oxalate or struvite stones, drink lemonade, which is high in citrate—a potent stone inhibitor.
- Certain diuretics (water pills) such as hydrochlorthiazide reduce the amount of calcium released by the kidney into the urine.
- If you're absorbing too much calcium from your gut, you may benefit from sodium cellulose phosphate, which binds with the calcium in your diet and prevents it from being absorbed. The calcium ends up in your stool, not your urine.
- Drinking lots of water and making the urine alkaline can control cystine stones. If that doesn't work, you will need Thiola and d-penicillamine, which reduce the amount of cystine in the urine.
- If prophylactic antibiotics do not prevent recurrent urinary tract infections, you may need acetohydroxamic acid (AHA), a chemical that helps retard the stone formation in chronically infected urine.

If you have an overactive parathyroid gland whose hormone is sucking calcium out of your bones and into your kidney and urine, you may need to have that gland surgically removed.

Treating a Kidney Stone Attack

A silent stone usually needs no treatment, but again, be sure to drink at least two quarts of water a day.

The first priority in a painful attack is pain medication. This is no time to be brave or stoic. There's nothing noble about enduring the agony of passing a kidney stone. *Insist* on whatever painkillers are necessary to provide relief. Drink plenty of water. Up to 90 percent of kidney stones pass on their own, often within seventy-two hours. Strain all your urine because it's important to analyze the stone after it has left your body.

If the stone has slipped out undetected, you should be asked to collect all your urine in a twenty-four-hour period and have it analyzed for potential stone-forming constituents—oxalate, uric acid, calcium, citrate, and others.

If your stone doesn't pass on its own (usually because it's too big and is stuck in a ureter), it will have to be dealt with. You have several effective options by which that can be done:

Extracorporeal Shock Wave Lithotripsy (ESWL). This is probably the least invasive and most frequently used way to deal with a stone that won't pass. Do not take aspirin, NSAIDs (ibuprofen), or other medications that affect blood clotting for about a week before this treatment is scheduled (acetaminophen is okay). Eat a light meal the night before, but nothing after midnight and no breakfast; not even tea, coffee, or water. You lie in a water bath or on a soft cushion; X ray or ultrasound pinpoints the exact location of the stone. Shock waves are then directed toward the stone, shattering it into fragments small enough to pass down and out of the urinary tract. The doctor may insert a stent (a small plastic sleeve) through the bladder into the ureter to keep it open so that pieces of the stone can pass more easily. The procedure doesn't work the first time in 20 percent of cases and requires another session. Don't be a hero. If it's not offered to you, *insist on enough anesthesia to control the pain.*

Lithotripsy can be done on an outpatient basis so that you can go home when it's over and back to work in a day or two. Don't panic if you see blood in your urine during the next few days. It's due to the treatment and to tiny stone fragments that irritate the ducts as they pass through. If you're planning to take part in a beauty contest or show off your body at the beach, be warned that there could be bruise marks where the shock waves were applied.

Ureteroscopy. Don't let these big words frighten you. You now know what the ureters are, and "scopy" is the act of inserting a tube with a light at the end of it. (So gastroscopy means looking into the stomach, colonoscopy into the gut, bronchoscopy into the lungs.) When a stone is lodged somewhere in the middle or lower part of the ureter and isn't moving, your doctor has the option of removing it directly from below. A ureteroscope is inserted into the urinary bladder and up into the involved ureter. No incision is necessary, but you will need some anesthesia. Once the stone comes into view, it's either snared with a small cagelike device or shattered with a laser. You can usually go home later in the day but the doctor will probably leave a small stent behind for a few days to allow the irritated area to drain.

Percutaneous nephrolithotomy (another mouthful) means removing a stone (lithotomy) from the kidney (nephron) via the skin (percutaneous). This technique is not done as often as the other two, but may be needed to remove a stone sitting in the kidney that's too large for the shock treatment. You are hospitalized for one or two days. The surgeon makes a small incision in the back and inserts a "sheath" directly into the kidney. A nephroscope (you can probably figure out what that does) is inserted into the kidney through this little hole. The stone can be removed intact or shattered and its pieces taken out through this instrument. The difference between this procedure and shock waves is that the stone is not allowed to make its way out after being fragmented; its pieces are removed. A small drainage tube is left in the kidney for a few days after the procedure.

WHAT TO INSIST ON IF YOU HAVE KIDNEY STONES

At least 10 percent of us will develop a kidney stone during our lifetime, and 1 million Americans suffer an attack every year. Be prepared for a very painful experience. You're especially vulnerable if you're a woman or if other family members have them. Most stones pass on their own. If they don't, there are several ways to remove them by minimally invasive treatments.

Prevention and treatment depend on the composition of the stone. So if you have one, it's important to "catch" it in order to have it analyzed. The most common kidney stone is calcium oxalate. Patients used to be advised to reduce their calcium intake. This is unnecessary, and in fact may lead to more stones. The major offender is the oxalate found in such foods as beets, chocolate, coffee, cola drinks, nuts, rhubarb, spinach, and tea.

Other types of stones are composed of uric acid (in persons with gout who have high uric acid levels), struvite (found in those with chronic infection of the kidneys) and those caused by a few rare metabolic and genetic disorders.

The key to the prevention and treatment of all kidney stones is drinking enough water to produce at least two quarts of urine a day.

If you are diagnosed with a kidney stone, *insist on a CT scan of the abdomen for confirmation as well as to determine its size and location. Most important, insist on adequate painkillers to control the severe pain that is usually associated with passing a kidney stone.*

23

LYME DISEASE

It Can Really Tick You Off

If you're tired, achy, have frequent headaches, and generally feel out of sorts—all for no apparent reason—chances are your doctor will first tell you that you have a "virus that's going around" or you're "under stress." If your symptoms don't clear up, and you keep complaining, the testing will begin, looking for evidence of low thyroid function, a hidden infection, liver or kidney problems, or cancer. If the search fails to provide an answer, the diagnostic possibilities to be considered will include more exotic or controversial disorders such as fibromyalgia and chronic fatigue syndrome. At this point, and preferably sooner, *you and your doctor should also consider Lyme disease,* especially if you live in high-risk areas in the Northeast and mid-Atlantic states (Massachusetts to Maryland), the upper Midwest (Minnesota and Wisconsin), or the Far West (California and Oregon). *You* may have to initiate this thinking; I'm told that *the average patient with Lyme disease sees five doctors before being correctly diagnosed!*

Lyme disease is so named because it was first described as such in Lyme, Connecticut. This infection strikes about ten thousand people every year and has been doing so since the

1800s, even though what makes it "tick" was only discovered in 1975 by doctors at Yale Medical School.

Lyme disease is caused by a bacterium called *Borrelia burgdoferi* (no relation to the wonderful store in New York where my wife and I buy our clothes). This nasty little bug is harbored by several animals, notably the white-footed mouse and the white-tailed deer, as well as by birds. For some reason, it doesn't make them sick. If the story ended there, everyone would be happy. Alas, it doesn't. Enter the tick. When it feeds on these animals looking for their blood, it picks up the *B. burgdorferi*. When it bites *you* looking for *your* blood, it introduces the bacterium into your body and gives you Lyme disease. (This same tick also picks up other organisms responsible for such other diseases as babesiosis, which resembles malaria, and ehrlichiosis, whose symptoms closely mimic those of Lyme disease.)

Lyme disease can be transmitted either by the adult tick (usually in the fall), but more often it's transmitted in the spring when the tick is in the nymph stage. Because the adult tick is much easier to see, you're more apt to remove it before it can infect you. The nymph, on the other hand, is no larger than a pinhead and very often escapes detection, giving it enough time to do its dirty work. That's why more cases of Lyme disease occur in the spring than in the fall.

Don't panic if you find a tick on your body. Most of them are not infected and so can't give you Lyme disease. Also, it takes twenty-four to forty-eight hours for an infected tick to get the bacterium into your body. In other words, it's got to sit on your skin for a while before it can successfully infect you.

So the requisites for your getting Lyme disease are ticks, a plentiful supply of animals that host *B. burgdorferi*, and leaving yourself vulnerable to being bitten. You'll never get Lyme from infected blood, urine, air, water, sex, or from contact with infected animals (unless you bite them like a tick does!).

Do You Know That You Have Lyme Disease?

The diagnosis of Lyme disease is easier to make if you become sick several days after a tick bite. The problem is that more than half the people with Lyme *do not recall being bitten*. That's because the nymph ticks are so tiny, the size of a poppy seed and not easily seen unless you're looking hard and carefully for them. After it bites you, the infected tick usually leaves its signature, a bull's-eye rash that appears three to thirty days later, usually between five and seven days. The rash varies in size and can last for several weeks. It's a great diagnostic help when present, but it may not be, or may not have the classic bulls-eye appearance. So if you develop fatigue, low-grade fever, headache, sore throat, joint pains, chills, muscle aches and pains several days after being bitten by a tick, suspect Lyme regardless of whether or not there was the typical rash.

If the diagnosis is missed in the first early stage of the disease, the fatigue and the aches and pains continue. You then enter the second stage. In some cases, palpitations and heart pain develop if the bacteria have inflamed the heart muscle. When they've attacked the nervous system, you may develop facial paralysis, drooping eyelids, or meningitis (severe headache, stiff neck, and fever).

Hopefully by this time someone will have thought of Lyme. Unless you're treated, you enter the late stage of the disease when you develop swelling of your joints and arthritis (that's why Lyme disease used to be called Lyme arthritis); a leathery red rash may appear on your skin; you may have chronic pain in various parts of your body; and when *B. burgdorferi* has affected the brain, the result is confusion. Older persons may then be misdiagnosed as having Alzheimer's.

How to Confirm the Diagnosis

Let's suppose that you saw the tick, weren't sure about the rash, but developed some of the symptoms of the early stage of Lyme disease. Although the diagnosis is very suggestive, most doctors will want some objective evidence. Removing a tick is not proof positive because it may not have been infected; or it may not have been on your skin long enough to deliver the Lyme bacterium. Finally, symptoms similar to those of early Lyme disease can be caused by several others conditions. The strongest clinical finding is the rash, and even that may vary in appearance. So for all these reasons, your doctor will probably run some blood tests to confirm his or her clinical impression. *Insist on these tests if they're not offered to you.*

Blood Tests for Lyme Disease

When the body is attacked by any organism, it responds by producing antibodies. The three most commonly used laboratory tests for the diagnosis of Lyme disease are ELISA, IFA, and the Western blot. They identify in different ways the antibodies to the specific bacterium that causes the disease. A Lyme antibody test may come back positive, negative, or, frustratingly, equivocal.

A *positive* antibody test indicates that you've had Lyme disease sometime previously, but it doesn't tell you whether your infection is current. That's because once you've had Lyme, the antibodies remain with you and you will always test positive. A positive test is only meaningful if you also have typical or suspicious symptoms. Also, you can get Lyme disease more than once. Unlike many diseases, this bacterial infection does not confer immunity.

Just as a positive test doesn't necessarily prove that your symptoms are due to *acute* Lyme disease, a *negative* test doesn't mean that you don't have it. It may simply be that the laboratory did not detect the antibodies. That can happen when the infectious agent hides within the cells or so alters its makeup as to interfere with antibody production; or the blood was taken during the first two weeks after infection and there hasn't been enough time for the antibodies to be produced. So if you suspect that you have Lyme and the test comes back negative, have it repeated in two to four weeks. *If everything else points to the diagnosis of Lyme disease and your doctor thinks you should be treated despite the negative blood test, your insurance company may not reimburse you. They are wrong! Insist on it.*

An *equivocal* test means either that the level of antibodies was not high enough to clinch the diagnosis or that whatever antibodies were detected reflect some infectious agent other than that which causes Lyme. Such antibody crossovers sometimes occur.

Remember that blood tests for Lyme should not be done for routine screening in healthy persons, but only when the infection is strongly suspected.

Most doctors start with the ELISA Lyme test. If it's positive or equivocal, you should then have the Western blot, a more specific assay. There are other more sophisticated tests such as the recombinant Lyme test and the polymerase chain reaction (PCR), but these are not widely used. Others are still in research. At the present time, the best way to make the diagnosis of Lyme disease is with a careful history, physical exam, and an ELISA test which if positive is followed by a Western blot.

How to Prevent Lyme Disease

All you have to do to prevent Lyme disease is to avoid being bitten by a tick. That's easier said than done. Ticks are seemingly everywhere—in lawns, gardens, old stone walls, wood-lands and wherever deer and white-footed mice live or visit. These ticks don't fly, jump, or fall off a tree. You have to make direct contact with them in order to become infected. They bite not only humans, but also your dogs and cats, birds, and any other animals that happen to be available.

Once the tick attaches itself to your skin, it moves to a creased or protected area such as the groin, the back of the knee, the navel, armpit, ear, or the scalp, where it starts drilling for your blood and in the process leaves you with *B. burgdorferi*.

For Protection Against Ticks

- Have your grounds sprayed with an insecticide in late May (to get rid of the nymph forms) and in September (against adult ticks).
- If your dogs are vulnerable to tick bites, discuss with your veterinarian having *them* vaccinated against Lyme disease. My vet tells me that a canine vaccine made by Merck using recombinant gene technology has fewer side effects than the older products and will protect your pet (and therefore you) for about a year. However, Fido may still carry ticks in his hair.
- Cover all exposed surfaces of your skin when you're in any area where ticks are present.
- Wear enclosed boots.
- Clothing should be light-colored so that you can spot ticks on it. Look for them on your clothes and skin as soon as you come indoors, then wash your clothes and spin them in the dryer for at least twenty minutes.
- If you sit on the ground or a stone wall, use a blanket. If your hair is long, tie it back when you're gardening.

- Use DEET or other insect repellents on your skin and clothes if you will be working or picnicking in overgrown areas.

If You Find a Tick

Remove it at once but don't panic. Not all ticks are infected, and even if they are, it takes hours for them to transfer *B. burgdorferi* to you. Don't grab the tick with your fingers. Use tweezers whose points come together gently. Grasp the tick by its head, not its body in order not to leave its "fangs" (the head and mouth parts) to do the dirty work in you. Pull the tick steadily outward and away from your skin. You don't need to apply alcohol, jelly, a hot match, a lighted cigarette, or anything else. After you've removed it, drop it in a container of alcohol (which kills it) for identification later. Finally, apply alcohol (from another container) or some other disinfectant to your liberated skin.

Check the site where you removed the tick every day for the next month for the appearance of a rash.

How to Treat Lyme Disease

Treatment, in a word, consists of antibiotics. There are four categories available: tetracycline, penicillin, cephalosporins, and macrolides. All of them either kill the bugs if the dose is high enough or interfere with their ability to reproduce. The three most widely used drugs are doxycycline (a tetracycline that should not be taken by pregnant women or by children because it stains the teeth), amoxicillin (a member of the penicillin family and best for pregnant women) and ceftin (a cephalosporin). All three are given orally for three weeks. In the late stages of the disease, especially when there are cardiac or neurological complications, you may require intra-venous therapy with ceftriaxone (also a cephalosporin) for four weeks or longer. The most popular macrolides are clarithromycin (Biaxin) and azithromycin (Zithromax).

The drug that's best for you depends on how well you've tolerated it in the past. Obviously, you can't use any to which you're allergic or that upset your stomach. But regardless of the antibiotic, the success of the therapy depends on how soon you start it. Do so as soon as the diagnosis is confirmed and within three weeks after the infection.

Since any antibiotic kills the friendly bacteria in your body that keep fungus infections at bay, you should have some yogurt or acidophilus tablets every day.

Patients often call me terrified because they've just removed a tick and demand an antibiotic right away. That's neither necessary nor recommended. Treatment should begin only after the onset of the rash or other symptoms of Lyme disease—and not any sooner. I want to emphasize again that most tick bites turn out to be false alarms either because the ticks were not infected or because they weren't feeding on you long enough to transmit the disease before you removed them.

What About the Lyme Vaccine?

The FDA approved a vaccine against Lyme disease at the end of 1999. Although it's given to humans, it works on the tick, not on them. Antibodies to the vaccine get into your bloodstream, and when the tick feeds on you, it gets more than it bargained for—not only your blood, but the antibodies too, and it's the antibodies that kill it.

You need three shots. The first two are given a month apart, the third eleven months later. All three vaccinations are almost 80 percent protective, but two of them are only 50 percent effective. The cost is under $100 per shot.

Lyme vaccine has been tested and shown to be safe in *healthy* persons between the ages of fifteen and seventy. Don't take it if you're older or younger than that or are pregnant. It's also not advised for anyone with arthritis or certain forms of heart disease.

Weigh the pros and cons very carefully before you decide to get the shots. No one knows how long they will protect you. You'll need frequent boosters, but no schedule has yet been determined. And the safety of repeated shots has not yet been established either.

Despite the fact that there is no conclusive evidence as yet that the vaccine can be harmful, there have been reports of "complications" after its administration. The FDA believes that most of them are minor and probably not due to the vaccine. Nevertheless, before you take the vaccine, check with your doctor as to the status of the studies looking into its safety.

Protection by the vaccine is neither long-lasting nor complete; taking it may give you a false sense of security. What's more, the ticks that transmit Lyme can give you other infections too, so you still have to continue to exercise the same precautions you'd take against Lyme disease. Another downside to the vaccine is that it results in the same antibody formation as that induced by the bacteria. The ELISA test cannot distinguish between them, but the Western blot can. So if you've been vaccinated against Lyme disease, let your doctor know. You can then go directly to the Western blot if necessary.

Given all these caveats, who should consider vaccination?

- Healthy persons between the ages of fifteen and seventy
- Those living in areas where ticks and the animals that harbor them are abundant
- Individuals whose work or other activities call for them to spend much time outdoors

- Anyone who's had previous uncomplicated Lyme disease and continues to be vulnerable to exposure

---

WHAT TO INSIST ON IF YOU HAVE LYME DISEASE

Lyme disease is a common infection in various parts of the United States. The great majority of those infected never have any problem if treated early. However, the diagnosis is often missed because, aside from the telltale rash, its symptoms resemble those of many other disorders. In some cases, the disease can become chronic and its symptoms difficult to eradicate. If you have been bitten by a tick or live in a tick-infested area, keep looking carefully for the appearance of the telltale bull's-eye rash. Consult your doctor as soon as possible if you see it. If you're not sure of the rash and develop achy muscles and joints, sore throat, enlarged glands, and other flulike symptoms, *insist on a blood test for Lyme disease. If the first one is positive, insist on the Western blot to confirm it*. If you're at high risk for developing the disease, ask your doctor about the vaccine.

24

MENOPAUSE

His and Hers

The term "menopause" is derived from *mens*, the Greek word for "monthly," and *pausis,* meaning "cessation." Hence, menopause refers to the termination of a woman's monthly periods. Strictly speaking, since men do not have menses, there is really no such thing as male menopause despite all the hoopla about it. However, if you take the broader view that menopause is the effect of aging on one's hormones, you can make a case for male as well as female menopause. Let's deal with the women first.

Female Menopause

Given the ever-longer life span in this country, an American woman can expect to be menopausal for about a third of her life. So it behooves you to understand the impact of menopause, and what you should do about it.

When they reach their forties, women begin to make less estrogen, the main female hormone. Its production continues to decrease gradually for several years, during which time periods become irregular and insomnia, fatigue, mood swings, and hot flashes develop. The interval during which the periods begin to taper and estrogen production wanes is called the perimenopause. Then, sometime between the ages of forty-eight and fifty-five, and in one percent of those under 40, the periods stop. One year after your last one, you are officially menopausal.

How you feel while all this is happening, and indeed during the rest of your life, is unpredictable. Some women are troubled by the signature symptoms of menopause—the hot flashes and flushes, night sweats, depression, irritability, dry vagina, and loss of libido. Others barely notice them. However, regardless of the severity of the symptoms, bad things are taking place in the body that you won't feel until later. Thus, you may be developing osteoporosis with brittle bones that break easily, as well as hardening of the arteries (arteriosclerosis), which can result in heart attacks or strokes. The lack of estrogen affects organs everywhere in the body.

There is an ongoing major debate among health professionals and between women and their doctors concerning the need for and safety of hormone replacement therapy (HRT). Despite all the rhetoric and passion, there is no consensus. Here are the major positions on the question:

Pro:

The advocates of HRT (of which I am one) make a very simple case. They believe that since, aside from the whale and the elephant we are the only mammals with a menopause, nature's decision to cut off a woman's estrogen supply in her middle years is clearly an aberration. A woman so deprived doesn't feel nearly as well and is more vulnerable to all manner of problems to which she was resistant when her hormones were flowing. That being the case, they argue, let's simply replace what's missing. They point out that the results of doing so are more than subjective well-being, although feeling good is important. HRT does reduce by 30 to 40 percent the risk of bone fractures from osteoporosis; it may decrease the number of heart attacks (although this observation has recently been questioned); it may lower the incidence of stroke, blindness, tooth loss, and diabetes; it definitely keeps the skin looking younger and healthier and the vagina moist; and some believe it may even modify the course of Alzheimer's disease. So as far as the proponents of HRT are concerned, it's an open-and-shut case: every woman should have it except for those who for some reason, such as a history of an estrogen-dependent cancer or a predilection for clot formation, cannot safely take estrogen.

Con:

The opponents of HRT are equally passionate and persuasive. They have an innate respect for nature and choose not to tamper with its decision to confer the menopause on middle-aged women. In their opinion, prescribing medications from a drugstore converts a natural phenomenon into a disease. Just as the proponents of HRT tout its virtues, so do the naysayers emphasize its downside: The increased risk of breast, ovarian, and uterine cancer, bloating, nausea, headaches, blood clotting, gallstones, migraine headaches, breast tenderness, and when progesterone is added to the estrogen, the return of the periods. They point to the large number of women who stop taking these replacements because of the many unpleasant side effects. The naturalist camp feels strongly that a healthy lifestyle that includes diet, exercise, and weight-loss can minimize the impact of osteoporosis and reduce the risk of the other consequences of menopause.

If You Opt for HRT

There are many different forms of estrogen among the available preparations. You can get them as pills, cream, patches, injections, and vaginal inserts. Tablets are the most popular, and Premarin, a conjugated estrogen made from pregnant mares' urine is probably the most widely used. Start with the lowest effective strength and work your way up as necessary. The usual maintenance dose is 0.625 mg a day but no two women are alike. You usually need more if your ovaries were surgically removed. That's because even after menopause, the ovaries continue to make a small amount of estrogen, which is not available after the glands are excised.

If you still have your uterus, do not take "unopposed" estrogen—that is, without adding progesterone. Estrogen alone increases the risk of cancer of the uterus. Progesterone drastically reduces that danger.

Topical HRT is becoming increasingly popular because it eliminates some of the side effects of oral estrogen. Also, when absorbed from the skin, estrogen enters the circulation without first going to the liver. This is an important advantage for anyone with liver problems. These patches are changed either once or twice a week, depending on the brand.

If your main problem is vaginal dryness, and you are not keen on taking estrogen supplements, you can use a vaginal cream that works more quickly locally than do either the Pill or the patch.

The complementary school of medicine takes a position somewhere between the "estrogen yes" and "estrogen no" camps. Holistic physicians agree that HRT does have beneficial effects, but they do not believe that most females need the high doses prescribed by conventional doctors. They point out that Asian women have a much lower incidence of menopausal symptoms such as hot flashes, as well as fewer estrogen-dependent tumors such as breast cancer. They believe that's because instead of taking estrogen supplements, these women consume a diet rich in phytoestrogens, natural estrogen-like hormones. When the body stops making estrogen and the estrogen receptors to which this hormone is bound are empty (resulting in all the symptoms from which menopausal women suffer), these phytoestrogens take over. They become bound to the estrogen receptors, where they act as weaker versions of the hormone. However, they are potent enough to do the job.

The phytoestrogens with the greatest estrogen effects are genistein and daidzein, both present in soya and its compounds. Women who take soy supplements have far fewer hot flashes and are less likely to develop osteoporosis than those who are not on any hormonal supplements. Soybeans contain all eight essential fatty acids and so are a better source of protein than is milk, yet do not have the latter's fat or cholesterol. There are several other plant phytoestrogens sold in health food stores. Among them are dong quai (Chinese angelica), wild yams, black cohosh, and milk thistle. Discuss them with your doctor especially if for any reason you cannot safely take HRT.

One aspect of HRT that's not sufficiently addressed by its proponents is the duration of treatment. Based on the current available information, I am recommending to my patients that they start HRT within five years of the onset of menopause, and unless there is some compelling reason not to do so, to terminate it after 10 to 20 years. Do so gradually, and don't be surprised if you develop hot flashes, even if you never had them before!

Male Menopause

Pro:

No one denies the existence of female menopause; the only argument is what to do about it. The controversy surrounding male menopause is more seminal because there are many who do not believe that there's any such thing. Those who think there is point to the fact that as men age, their blood level of male hormone, testosterone, decreases. This may not be apparent from the total testosterone reading. However, free testosterone, the portion of the hormone not bound to protein, decreases markedly. According to them, these low levels account for the diminished potency, decreased libido, depression, weight gain, fatigue, and loss of muscle and bone mass that are characteristic of "change of life." Replacing the waning testosterone supply can, they say, reverse most of these symptoms.

Con:

Nonsense, say the doubters. There's no such thing as male menopause. The arguments listed above are purely speculative. They attribute most of the symptoms associated with male menopause to "midlife crisis," the consequences of all the physical and psychological factors that come together at that time in a man's life. These include the fear of aging, marital problems, the empty-nest syndrome when their children leave home, awareness of their own mortality as their parents and many friends die, the failure to achieve lifelong goals and the realization that they may never attain them, the onset of other medical problems such as heart disease, high blood pressure, diabetes, tumors, hearing and vision loss (and the side effects of the drugs to treat them). These all contribute to the depression and impaired self-image that some men experience. What they need in order to restore their well-being is not a testosterone supplement, but a program of regular exercise, counseling, abstinence from smoking, reduction of alcohol intake, and when necessary, Viagra! Furthermore, those who do not believe in the existence of male menopause warn that testosterone supplements may increase the risk of prostate cancer.

Your Options

If you feel like hell and think it's because you're "getting older," see your doctor and have your free and total testosterone levels measured. If both values are too low, you may benefit from supplementation.

There are several ways to obtain whatever testosterone you need—orally, by injection, patch, or pellet. Most of my patients use the patch. Avoid pills because they can hurt the liver.

WHAT TO INSIST ON IF YOU'RE MENOPAUSAL (MALE OR FEMALE)

Female menopause usually begins in the late forties, and is due to the great drop in estrogen production by the ovaries. The resulting side effects range from night sweats to osteoporosis and easily broken bones. No two women handle estrogen deprivation the same way. Some feel miserable; others are just fine.

There is no agreement among doctors (or women) about the need for hormone replacement therapy (HRT). Some are staunch advocates; others deplore its use. *Insist that your gynecologist discuss all the pros and cons of HRT with you.*

Phytoestrogens, present in plants and certain foods such as soybeans, have estrogen-like effects that are weaker than the hormone itself. Some doctors believe they should be used instead of estrogen, and are safer too. The jury is still out on this question. *Insist on all the facts about HRT and phytoestrogens before deciding.* If you do take estrogen, make sure you also use progesterone, since unopposed estrogen predisposes to uterine cancer. This warning does not apply to phytoestrogens, which can safely be taken alone. *Insist on having hormone levels checked to determine proper doses.*

The existence of male menopause is controversial. Some doctors believe that the behavioral changes observed in some middle-aged men are due to a reduction in their testosterone level. They recommend testosterone supplements. However, you should *insist on having a free-testosterone level drawn before you accept hormonal replacement.* Other doctors deny the existence of a male menopause and attribute the behavioral changes in middle-aged men to personal and career problems.

25

MIGRAINE

The Mother of All Headaches

We all get headaches now and then, mostly when we're over-tired, tense or anxious, after a hangover, from lack of sleep, are offered sex ("not tonight, dear, I have a headache"), have an upset stomach, sinus trouble, a sprained neck, arthritis of the cervical spine, experience the side effect of some medication, or after grinding our teeth or clenching our jaws during the night. That's the short list. For such "benign" headaches, most people take a couple of aspirin or Tylenol, go about their business, and usually feel better in an hour or two. But headaches can also be due to serious health problem such as glaucoma (increased pressure in the eyes), high blood pressure, and even a brain tumor. So if they're frequent or persistent, see your doctor.

Migraine is not just an ordinary headache. It's all consum-ing. It doesn't kill you, but when you're in its throes, you may wish it did.

The incidence of migraine has increased 60 percent in the past ten years. One American in ten now suffers from it. It can occur at any age and in both men and women, but affects three times as many women (most of them premenopausal) as men. (Migraine in children produces recurrent cyclical vomiting but no headache.)

Here's what a typical migraine attack is like: There is sometimes a warning. Minutes, hours, or even a day or two before
the full-blown headache, you develop a "prodrome." You feel
very tired, lose your appetite, are moody for no apparent reason, and are sensitive to bright light or loud sounds. In 20
percent of "migraineurs," there is another type of prodrome:
an "aura" of flashing lights, zigzag lines, stars or shimmery
sheets, blurring of vision, blind spots, or tunnel vision (you
can only see straight ahead and not from the sides). You may
be unable to speak clearly; you feel confused; there may be
weakness of an arm or leg, or numbness or tingling in your
face.

These symptoms would ordinarily raise fears of a stroke,
but they are old hat to a migraineur, who knows from experience that they are the forerunners of migraine misery. As
soon as the aura starts, the experienced migraine sufferer usually makes a beeline for a dark room, shuts the door, lies
down and waits for the inevitable headache. Then, anywhere
from ten to forty-five minutes later, the migraine strikes with
a vengeance. You are enveloped by a severe throbbing,
pounding, blinding pain on one side of your head—around
the eye, the forehead, ear, jaw, and temple.

Although the term "migraine" is derived from the Greek
word *hemikrania,* meaning "half a head," the symptoms
spread to engulf both sides in one-third of cases. Most migraineurs also have nausea, occasional vomiting, diarrhea,
and increased urination. They can't bear light or noise; they
feel cold and look pale.

Unlike the run-of-the-mill tension headache that clears up
within a couple of hours, this one lasts anywhere from several hours to as long as two or three days. Forget about work,
school, or even talking on the telephone. When you're in the
throes of a migraine, all you want to do is lie still with your
eyes shut, waiting for the attack to pass. And after it's over,
you're wiped out.

The onset, symptoms, duration, and frequency of migraine

vary. In some people they occur several times a week; in others they only strike every few weeks, months, or even years.

The Migraine Mechanism

Migraine was first described in about 3000 B.C., and it has since affected such people as Julius Caesar, Sigmund Freud, Vincent van Gogh, Lewis Carroll—and my beautiful daughter. This disorder has been the subject of intense research for many years, yet its cause remains a mystery. For hundreds of years, and until quite recently, migraine was believed to be a purely vascular phenomenon—narrowing followed by widening of the arteries in the head. However, newer imaging techniques and a better understanding of the chemical changes within the brain suggest that migraine is a brain disorder. The changes in blood flow, though important, play only a secondary role. It's believed that some process inside the brain triggers the migraine attack by altering the concentration of various chemicals (neurotransmitters)—serotonin, norepinephrine, and dopamine—that leads to the release of pain-causing substances.

Some researchers believe that a migraine "generator" in the brain stimulates the nerves supplying blood vessels in the face, scalp, spinal cord, and the membranes covering the brain. These nerves first constrict the arteries, resulting in a decreased amount of oxygen to the brain (this would account for the symptoms that resemble a stroke—difficulty with speech, confusion, and visual changes). Then, in order to restore the blood supply, other arteries in the brain dilate, leading to the release of pain producing substances called prostaglandin from the blood cells and tissues in the area. The combination of dilated arteries and circulating pain-inducing chemicals is thought to account for the blinding migraine headache. But since the brain does not sense pain, the ache in the head originates in the tissues covering it, as well as in the muscles and blood vessels around the scalp, face, and neck.

Migraine Triggers

Most migraineurs know what brings on their headache: Straining at stool, fasting, low blood sugar, high altitudes, a falling barometer, a sudden change in temperature, fatigue, glaring or flickering lights, or motion sickness. Chemicals in more than one hundred foods have also been implicated: Tyramine and phenylethylamine in various alcoholic beverages, cheese, meat, seafood, peas, pickles, olives, sauerkraut (always look for them on every food label); tannin in apple juice, coffee, red wine, and tea; sulfites in wine; monosodium glutamate in your Chinese food; various other chemicals in chocolate, yogurt, and nuts.

Hormones are also important. Half of all female migraineurs will tell you that their headache is related to their menses, usually during the first three days. Such headaches rarely have an aura. Menstrual migraine commonly disappears during pregnancy, when the periods stop temporarily. However, in some women they may first appear during pregnancy or even after menopause.

A similarly confusing picture exists with regard to oral contraceptives. Some women develop migraine when they start the Pill; in others, that's when the headaches clear up.

Preventing Migraine

If you know what brings on your migraine, try to avoid it. You'll have more success doing so if you keep a diary. Of course, not every trigger is preventable. You can't stop a barometer from falling, but you can use some other form of birth control if the Pill provokes an attack. You can also avoid chocolate, red wine, or any other food or beverage that you know is the culprit. Here are some additional steps you can take:

- Exercise regularly (but warm up gradually because sudden aerobic exercise can precipitate a migraine).
- Mind-body techniques, biofeedback, yoga, transcutaneous electrical nerve stimulation (TENS), and tai chi help.
- Follow a diet low in fat and rich in complex carbohydrates (even if you don't have migraine).
- Avoid oral contraceptives, especially if you smoke or have a family history of stroke.
- Estrogen replacement is a crapshoot—it helps some women, and makes matters worse in others.
- Over-the-counter nonsteroidal anti-inflammatory drugs (NSAIDs) such as ibuprofen prevent attacks in 20 percent of migraineurs. Stronger doses that require a prescription are even more effective.
- Beta-blockers, used for treating high blood pressure, angina, and heart rhythm irregularities, reduce the frequency of migraine. I prescribe them for virtually all migraineurs. But these drugs slow the heart rate, lower blood pressure, can cause fatigue, and diminish your sex drive. Avoid them, too, if you have chronic lung disease.
- Calcium channel blockers such as verapamil (the most widely prescribed for this purpose), diltiazem, and nimodipine, which are also used for the treatment of a wide variety of cardiac problems, are as effective as the beta-blockers. But they can lower blood pressure, slow heart rate, and cause constipation.
- Antiseizure drugs used by epileptics (Depakene, Depakote) are also approved by the FDA for the preven-

tion of migraine. Women should not use them in the childbearing years. I prescribe these drugs only if the beta-blockers and calcium channel blockers don't work.

- Another group of cardiac drugs, the angiotensin-converting enzyme (ACE) inhibitors, is under investigation for the possible prevention of migraine. These drugs, of which captopril is the prototype, are generally safe and are used for the treatment of high blood pressure and certain forms of heart disease. At this time, it's too early to recommend them for preventing migraine.
- The older tricyclic antidepressants such as amitriptyline (Elavil) can prevent migraine. I haven't found the newer selective serotonin reuptake inhibitors (SSRIs) such as Prozac, Zoloft, and Paxil very effective and they occasionally cause headaches. However, children in whom cyclical vomiting is a migraine symptom can safely take them in small doses.
- When I was in medical school, ergotamine was virtually the only drug available to abort migraine. It does so by constricting dilated arteries. Some physicians still use it to prevent predictable attacks such as those that occur regularly with menstrual periods. The main problem with ergotamine is that you can become dependent on it. Also, it's dangerous to constrict blood vessels in someone with coronary artery disease, high blood pressure, and narrowed arteries anywhere in the body.
- Vitamin B_2 (riboflavin) in a dosage of 400 mg a day has been reported to reduce the number of migraine attacks. It has no downside and is worth a try.
- Some migraineurs who harbor *H. pylori* in their stomachs (the bacterium associated with ulcers and stomach cancer) report a decreased frequency of attacks after the bug is eradicated with antibiotics. Get rid of *H. pylori* anyway, regardless of what it does for the migraine. You're better off without it in your gut.

- There have been several reports attesting to the effectiveness of feverfew, an herb that has been approved in Canada for the prevention of migraine. There's no harm in trying it, unless you're pregnant. Make sure the preparation you're using has the word "Parthenolide" written on the label.

Treating the Attack

We've come a long way in the treatment of migraine over the millenia, even though we still don't fully understand its basic causes. Archaeologists tell us that people were plagued by migraine as far back as the Stone Age and that therapy then consisted of cutting away a piece of the skull. This approach was later refined to drilling a hole in the skull to liberate the "evil spirits." Records from the ninth century describe a popular British prescription of the time that consisted of "the juice of elderseeds, cow's brain [they were obviously unaware of mad cow disease!], and goat's dung, all dissolved in vinegar." Other inventions have included purges and bloodletting, applying a hot iron to the painful areas, and even inserting a clove of garlic through an incision in the area of the temple. Happily, these have all been abandoned in favor of more effective, modern therapy.

- When treating migraine, try a nonprescription medication first. Use narcotic medications only as a last resort; they can leave you addicted, since migraine is a chronic problem. A good over-the-counter drug with which to start is Excedrin Extra Strength (a combination of acetaminophen, aspirin, and caffeine). Chances are you'll respond within two hours. You may take two Excedrin every six hours.

- A nonsteroidal anti-inflammatory drug (NSAID) is equally good first-line therapy. Remember that high doses of these agents can hurt the stomach lining, so watch for belly pain and black stools (evidence of bleeding). If the migraine is bad, the NSAIDs can be injected. One particular preparation, ketorolac, is very effective, but I avoid prescribing it because of the risk of gastrointestinal bleeding.

- Ergotamine, introduced in the late 1940s, constricts the dilated blood vessels through its action on serotonin. The downside in using this drug is that it can cause nausea and vomiting; it does not relieve any migraine symptoms other than headache, and it can cause dependence. I don't recommend it unless all else fails.

- Dihydroergotamine (DHE) is related to ergotamine but does not cause dependence. It is available as a nasal spray, and I sometimes prescribe it for patients in whom other treatments give only temporary relief.

- The development of a group of drugs called triptans in the early 1990s was a major advance in the treatment of migraine. The first one, sumatriptan (Imitrex), has been followed by a number of me-too preparations: zolmitriptan (Zomig), naratriptan (Amerge), rizatriptan (Maxalt, my current favorite), and several others. The triptans increase serotonin levels in the brain and narrow the dilated, pulsating arteries. These drugs work quickly, especially the newer ones such as Maxalt, and they don't leave you groggy. Take them at the earliest sign of trouble. They are available in several forms: oral preparations, wafers that dissolve under the tongue, by injection, and nasal sprays. Try the various brands and delivery routes to see which one works best for you. Injections act most quickly, but they may hurt; the sprays bypass the stomach and relieve pain faster than tablets, but you can't take them when your nose is stuffy, and they may also leave a bad taste in your mouth. The favorite of many patients is the Maxalt wafer that dissolves in the mouth.

All the triptans can cause a variety of side effects, most of which don't compare in severity to the migraine headache. However, since they constrict the blood vessels, they can cause strokes and heart attacks in someone with arteriosclerosis, vascular disease, high blood pressure, coronary artery disease, or poorly controlled diabetes. Avoid them too if you have severe asthma. Since SSRIs, antidepressants in the Prozac family of drugs, increase serotonin, don't use them along with the triptans, which also raise the concentration of serotonin in the brain. Pregnant women should not take triptans.

- The same botulinum toxin that can kill you if you ingest it in tainted foods is diluted many millions of times and injected directly into the scalp muscles in order to paralyze them so that they can't respond to the nerve signals that throw them into spasm. (The same toxin also eliminates unsightly wrinkles and ends excessive perspiration when injected into the armpits.)

In my opinion, none of the following measures are major players in the treatment of migraine. I am listing them here for the sake of completeness.

- Bromocriptine is an ergot derivative that must be taken cyclically for about ten days each month. Don't use it soon after you've had a baby because it can cause high blood pressure, seizures, and strokes at that particular time.
- If you happen to have a low level of magnesium, its intravenous replenishment may help your migraine. I wouldn't bother with the oral form, which isn't well absorbed, and can give you diarrhea. It's not very effective either.

WHAT TO INSIST ON IF YOU HAVE MIGRAINE

The two major aspects of medical care to insist on if you suffer from migraine are a *confirming diagnosis* to make sure your headaches are not due to some other cause, and then access to the *new therapeutic agents* now available.

The most frequently prescribed migraine medications at this time are the triptans, which can be taken by mouth, injection, or nasal spray. They should not be used by anyone with vascular disease, since the constriction they produce can result in a heart attack or stoke. *If you're suffering from migraines and nothing has helped, insist on a triptan.*

There are several alternative medications—some old, some new—that may be effective in both preventing and treating migraine. Feverfew is the best known in this group.

26

MITRAL VALVE PROLAPSE

Smoke but No Fire

Mitral valve prolapse (MVP) is the most common heart valve "abnormality," affecting between 5 and 20 percent of the population. It occurs more frequently in women and is usually first diagnosed between the ages of twenty and forty.

There are several scenarios in which you may learn that you have MVP. Here's a common one: You're a young woman. During the course of a routine physical, the doctor lays down his stethoscope and solemnly tells you, "I hear a click in your heart. Sounds like you have mitral valve prolapse." You're terrified, because although you don't know what it means, it is, after all, the heart, and that can't be good. Before you can ask him what it's all about, he adds, "We'd better get an echo to confirm it."

"Please," you beg, "let's do it as soon as possible."

If your doctor is a cardiologist, he probably has an echo machine right there in his office. He obliges, and does the test immediately. Some $700 later, your worst fears are confirmed. You do indeed have mitral valve prolapse.

Panicked, you ask, "Doctor, what does it mean? Will it shorten my life? Can I have any children? Do I need to take medication for it?"

The doctor reassures you. "This is a very common finding. Most people with mitral valve prolapse live a normal life without any problems."

You're happy that "most" people do well, but you're worried about what happens to the rest. An hour ago you were a healthy young woman; now, without any new symptoms, you have suddenly become a "cardiac patient," at least in your own mind.

The doctor was right: Your mitral valve will probably never endanger you, but you will always be convinced deep down that you have a "heart condition." You may never be quite the same again.

Here's another clinical situation that, unfortunately, is also very common. A patient, again usually a young woman, complains to her doctor that she has panic attacks. For no reason whatsoever, while watching TV, or at the movies, or shopping at the supermarket, she suddenly feels very anxious. Her heart starts pounding, and she breaks out in a cold sweat. The attack lasts several minutes and ends as abruptly as it began. She tells the doctor that she also has chest pain from time to time. It's not associated with effort; she can just be sitting around when for no reason she feels a pressure in her chest. Like her panic attack, the pain subsides spontaneously. But she's worried because her mother had a heart attack at age sixty and these symptoms sound very much like her mother's.

The doctor does a thorough physical and finds everything, including an electrocardiogram and chest X ray, completely normal, except that when he listens to her heart with his stethoscope, he hears a click. He orders an echo, which reveals mitral valve prolapse. He reassures his patient, but she reacts as you did in the first scenario. She suspects that the doctor may not be telling her "everything" in order to spare her, and she begins her pilgrimage from one cardiologist to another looking for the "truth." They all reassure her, but she's unconvinced.

Both doctors are correct. MVP almost never shortens life,

although it can sometimes cause symptoms that impair its quality. The reaction of both women in the hypothetical cases I've described is understandable. We fear what we don't understand. That's why I sometimes regret that we ever discovered the existence of mitral valve prolapse. In the days before the echocardiogram was available, I probably wouldn't have mentioned the click to you, since I didn't know what it meant. Or I might have said, "You have a click. I often hear it in healthy people. It doesn't mean anything, and the only reason I'm telling you about it is that some other doctor may mention it." I'd have given the second woman, the one with anxiety, palpitations, and chest pain, a thorough cardiac workup—ECG, stress test, risk factor analysis (cholesterol, smoking, blood pressure, family history)—and after finding everything normal, I'd have assured her that her symptoms were not due to her heart. I'd have prescribed an antianxiety medication and also perhaps a beta-blocker such as popranolol to alleviate the heart pounding, and sent her on her way. The medication would help, and she'd learn to live with her symptoms—without fear. That's still all we usually do today anyway after we make the echo diagnosis of MVP. The only difference is that many patients in this generation live in fear with a cardiac diagnosis.

What Is Mitral Valve Prolapse?

The mitral is one of four heart valves. It lies between the left atrium (which receives fresh, oxygenated blood from the lungs) and the left ventricle (which pumps the blood out to the body). The mitral valve, so called because its shape resembles that of a bishop's miter with two peaks, separates these two chambers. When the left ventricle is empty after its last contraction and ready to receive blood from the left atrium, the mitral valve opens, allowing the blood to flow into it. When the left atrium is empty, the mitral valve closes. When the ventricle below it contracts, the blood it contains flows out to the body and not back to the left atrium. So that's the job of this two-"leaflet" valve—to open and let blood flow through it, and then close, sealing itself off.

When the valve is diseased, usually because of rheumatic fever in childhood, the leaflets either fail to open widely enough to allow all its blood to enter the left ventricle (a condition called mitral stenosis) or don't shut tightly, allowing blood to leak back from the left ventricle (mitral regurgitation or insufficiency). Mitral valve prolapse is neither of these two disorders. In MVP one or both of the valve flaps or leaflets are too large, so that the valve doesn't close evenly with each heartbeat. This imperfect closing causes the valve to balloon back slightly into the left atrium when the heart contracts. This creates a click, which the doctor hears with the stethoscope. In some cases of MVP, there may also be a leak of blood back into the left atrium. The magnitude of the leak can be determined with an echocardiogram.

Mitral valve prolapse often runs in families. Its gene, if there is one, hasn't yet been discovered. Before the advent of the echocardiogram, which allows us literally to look inside the heart, we had no idea what caused the click or the murmur that sometimes accompanies it.

The management of MVP depends on its clinical presentation. Patients fall into one of three categories:

- No symptoms. This is true for 60 percent of cases. The diagnosis is suggested by the click with or without a murmur that the doctor hears in the course of a routine exam, and is confirmed by the echocardiogram.
- Minimal symptoms such as slight shortness of breath on exertion and perhaps occasional "palpitations." Again, there is a click and the murmur is apt to be somewhat louder. The echocardiogram indicates MVP with more of a leak across the valve—something that bears watching.

- Many symptoms: patients experience attacks of rapid or irregular heartbeat or palpitations; chest pain that comes and goes for no apparent reason and not usually associated with exertion; panic attacks. unexplained fatigue; and even migraine headaches.

Doctors have wondered for years why there is such a wide spectrum of symptoms in MVP. Why are some patients totally asymptomatic and others plagued by panic attacks, migraine, fatigue, and a host of other symptoms? By what mechanism does this mildly and trivially malformed heart valve leaflet that does not even affect cardiac function cause panic attacks or palpitations?

Here is the answer: The "abnormality" of the mitral valve is only a marker for a condition that affects the entire body. The main problem lies not with this valve or the heart, but with the autonomic nervous system (ANS) of the body. Unlike the voluntary nervous system which we can control (we move an arm or a leg or smile or grimace at will), the autonomic nervous system functions independently. It regulates the heart rate, makes sure you're breathing the right number of times per minute, causes you to sweat when it's hot and shiver when it's cold, determines the level of your blood pressure— these are all things we don't do on a conscious level. Thank goodness for the autonomic nervous system! Imagine what life would be if you had to remind your heart to beat or your lungs to breathe! The ANS also controls the production of chemicals called catecholamines, which you probably recognize by their other names, epinephrine and adrenaline. In some patients with MVP, the ANS suddenly pumps more adrenaline for no apparent reason. That's okay when you need it, such as when you're in a fight, running away, or scared. But patients with MVP may be sitting perfectly still when *wham*, out comes the adrenaline. The result? A rapid heartbeat, panic, stress, headache, all the symptoms that adrenaline can produce. These symptoms stress you and trigger the release of even more stress hormones. None of this is due to the prolapsed mitral valve itself.

Treatment of MVP

Now that you appreciate what MVP is all about, you can better understand that how to deal with it depends on its manifestations in your particular case.

If you have the click (with or without a slight murmur) but no symptoms, and the echocardiogram does not indicate a significant leak across the valve, forget about it. You don't need any treatment. When you see a new doctor, tell him or her that you have uncomplicated MVP. Until quite recently, doctors used to prescribe antibiotics to all patients with MVP to be taken before dental work or any other invasive procedures. This was to prevent infection of the mitral valve in the mistaken belief that this valve was a potential breeding ground for any bacteria that entered the bloodstream when your teeth were cleaned. This is not the case. *You do not need antibiotics in simple MVP.*

If you have a click and *a significant murmur of mitral regurgitation,* documented by an echocardiogram, you may or may not have symptoms. If you do, they are most likely to be shortness of breath on exertion. This happens when the leak across the mitral valve is large enough to strain the left ventricle and cause the heart to weaken. Treatment consists of medications that improve heart function, such as digitalis, ACE inhibitors (captopril), and diuretics. If symptoms become worse and do not respond to therapy, the mitral valve may have to be surgically repaired or replaced. But I want to emphasize that leaks of such magnitude are the exception. The great majority of those cases do not need any treatment. However, *they do require antibiotic prophylaxis* when you go to the dentist, or are having some operative procedure to prevent infection of the leaky valve.

MVP, with or without a leaky valve can be associated with symptoms of autonomic nervous system dysfunction. Although they are not life threatening, they often require treatment.

The Specifics of Treatment

- Exercise. Do not be afraid to participate in a regular fitness program. It will make you feel better. Remember—*you are not a cardiac*.
- Diet. Cut down on sweets, caffeine, and stimulants such as weight-reduction pills and nasal decongestants that can accelerate your heart rate or induce anxiety.
- Anxiety and panic attacks respond to antidepressants, antianxiety drugs, and benzodiazepines. The right therapy can cut the frequency and severity of these attacks by 60 to 80 percent.
- If you have palpitations, irregular heartbeats, and pounding of the heart, *insist* that your doctor establish the exact nature of the rhythm disturbance. But just as the toothache goes away when you get to the dentist, these cardiac symptoms are not always there when you are with your doctor. In that case, ask for a Holter monitor or an event recorder. You wear the former for twenty-four hours, during which time your electrocardiogram is continuously recorded. Any irregular beats will be captured for later analysis. If the attacks occur unpredictably, you're better off with an event recorder. You keep it for a couple of weeks and whenever you "feel something", you push a little button on the machine and it records a run of your heartbeats.
- There are several medications that can control these rhythm disturbances. Remember, however, that the pur-

pose of treating them is to make you comfortable. They are rarely a threat to you, and I have found that reassurance is the best medication of all. However, if you do need something, you can either have a beta-blocker (popranolol, atenolol) or a calcium channel blocker such as dilitiazem or verapamil.

WHAT TO INSIST ON WHEN YOU HAVE MITRAL VALVE PROLAPSE

Mitral valve prolapse (MVP) is a common heart valve abnormality, affecting up to 5 percent of the population. It is more often present in women, but can also occur in men. The disorder is characterized by an enlargement of one or both cusps of a valve that separates the upper and lower chambers in the left side of the heart. The condition runs in families and is usually diagnosed between the ages of twenty and forty.

The diagnosis of mitral valve prolapse is suggested by the presence of a click heard with the stethoscope. The electrocardiogram is usually normal. If you're told you have such a click, *insist on an echocardiogram.* There is sometimes a heart murmur associated with MVP. Unless it is significant, reflecting an important leak across the valve, no treatment is necessary. Antibiotics are no longer prescribed prophylactically unless the murmur and leak are significant. *Insist on a second opinion if you are told to take prophylactic antibiotics because of a click.*

(27)

MULTIPLE SCLEROSIS

When Your Nervous System Short Circuits

Multiple sclerosis (MS) is the most common chronic neurological disorder of younger adults, affecting about 330,000 Americans. It usually strikes between the ages of twenty and forty, it is twice as common in women as in men and on occasion runs in families. Every day, two hundred new cases are diagnosed. Statistically, the disease shortens life by only five years but it can dramatically affect its quality. Within fifteen years of its onset, half of those afflicted are unable to walk without assistance.

Nerve fibers in normal individuals are wrapped in and protected by a sheath of a fatty material called myelin much like electrical wires are insulated. This makes it possible for the nerve to transmit impulses speedily and smoothly. In multiple sclerosis, random segments of nerves in the brain and spinal cord lose this myelin (which is why MS is called a demyelinating disease.) Portions of the nerves that are now "exposed" can no longer transmit messages normally.

The clinical features of multiple sclerosis are unpredictable. Although forgetfulness or confusion sometimes occurs, most mental faculties usually remain intact. Typically, however, bowel and bladder function are impaired, sexual activity is af-

fected, and balance, coordination, and vision often deteriorate. The severity and nature of the symptoms vary from patient to patient because the nerve involvement is sporadic.
They can be so subtle that the diagnosis is often not apparent
for many months.

I remember one couple and their twenty-six-year-old son
who came to see me because the son had had a variety of un-
explainable "mishaps." First he had trouble focusing with his
left eye; a change in glasses helped for a while. When he kept
dropping his knife and fork during meals, everyone thought
he was drinking too much wine. Then one morning, obviously sober, he lost control of his coffee cup and his fingers
began to tingle. The family finally consulted me after he
slipped and fell down the stairs because his right leg had felt
"awkward." He had multiple sclerosis.

The symptoms of MS wax and wane dramatically and unpredictably and the overall course of the disease is unpredictable. They may be debilitating for months and then
suddenly improve—for weeks, months, and even years in
"remission." This is followed for no apparent reason by an
abrupt relapse ("exacerbation"). Some of my patients have
had only a few "crises" years apart and have been able to lead
virtually normal lives, while others became crippled and required wheelchairs relatively early on.

The diagnosis of MS is not difficult when the symptoms are
typical. The most common ones relate to perception of sensation: You don't appreciate temperature change, touch, or
even pain; you're dizzy and unstable because the soles of
your feet don't transmit messages to your brain telling it
where they are; you may see double, or your vision is blurred
or dimmed; you have trouble distinguishing one color from
another; your speech is slurred; your movements are clumsy
and you're poorly coordinated; you may become incontinent
of stool or urine. In addition to all of this, you're extremely
tired.

In order to be secure with their diagnosis of MS, most neu-

rologists look for two attacks or exacerbations to have occurred at least one month apart, each lasting at least twenty-
four hours. There must also be more than one area of the
nervous system involved by the "demyelinating" process, occurring more than once and not due to any other neurological disease.

When you describe these symptoms to your family doctor
or internist, he or she will usually refer you to a neurologist
whose focused evaluation may reveal additional diagnostic
findings. The MRI is the best technique currently available to
detect the evidence of MS. It is more accurate than the CT
scan, and you should *insist on it* if you are suspected of having MS. Remember, however, that the MRI is not foolproof.
Other diseases can result in similar changes, and "abnormal"
areas can be present in healthy older people. By the same
token, the MRI is normal in about 5 percent of patients
proved to have MS by other tests, or whose lesions are in the
spinal cord and not the brain. *Insist* on a careful exam, and
whatever other tests are necessary to confirm the diagnosis of
MS beyond a doubt.

When the clinical picture is in doubt and the MRI is inconclusive, other tests should be done. These include an analysis
of the spinal fluid, procedures called evoked potentials, and
blood analyses.

The spinal fluid of most patients with MS contains increased amounts of IgG antibodies as well as a variety of proteins resulting from the breakdown of myelin, evidence of an
autoimmune response in the nervous system, indicating that
the body is turning against itself for some reason. This type of
response occurs in a variety of other diseases ranging from
thyroid trouble to lupus and rheumatoid arthritis, and is ab-
sent in 10 percent of patients with MS. So such spinal fluid
findings, though suggestive, are not proof positive of the diagnosis. They must be interpreted along with the clinical picture and the MRI findings.

Evoked potentials detects the short-circuiting of the in-twenty to forty times. Some neurologists speculate that the disease may be triggered by viruses (such as the human herpesvirus 6) or bacterial infections. People of Scandinavian heritage are especially vulnerable to MS.

I have long believed that diet plays an important role in the development of MS, probably because I was influenced by one of my teachers in medical school, a researcher named Roy Swank. He noted that during World War II the incidence of MS decreased in occupied countries that were deprived of meat and dairy products—except for the dairy farmers among them who produced and ate their own meat and fat. After the war, when these foods once more became available, the number of cases of MS rose to their previous high levels.

Dr. Swank kept track of 144 patients with MS for thirty-four years. He concluded from analyses made in his laboratory at the Oregon Health Sciences University in Portland that those who, over the long term, followed a low-saturated-fat diet—avoiding meat, whole milk and its derivative products, as well as palm and coconut oils—and who consumed lots of mono- and polyunsaturated fat lived longer and had fewer symptoms of MS than did those who dined with abandon.

Other researchers also believe that there is a link between MS and saturated fat, and have made the additional observations that omega-3 fatty acids found in fatty fish, such as salmon and tuna, are protective. Given the paucity of treatments for MS, I have over the years advised my patients with MS to try to follow such a dietary regimen despite the lack of confirmatory data. A fatty diet may not cause MS but it does appear to influence its course.

Preventing and Treating MS

There is no way to prevent or cure multiple sclerosis, but patients can improve their symptoms by taking certain steps.

volved nerves. The test focuses on vision, hearing,
extremities. It takes about two hours to evaluate all th
a neurologist or neurophysiologist usually interprets
sults. Again, these procedures are not specific for M
must be interpreted in the context of all the other findi

All these steps must sometimes be taken to confirr
without the shadow of a doubt. *Insist on them whenever*
essary. This disease is too serious for you to permit short

What Causes MS

There are many theories about what causes MS. Most MS experts believe that it is an autoimmune disorder, possibly induced by a virus. Whatever the reason, the body's defense
mechanisms go haywire and produce large numbers of antibodies and white blood cells in response to some perceived
but nonexistent threat. These antibodies then attack, inflame,
and destroy the protein in the perfectly healthy myelin
sheaths that envelop nerves in the brain and spinal cord.
Women with MS who smoke are substantially worse, possibly
because of some toxic effect of tobacco on the immune system.

Environmental factors also play a role, as evidenced by the
fact that the disease is more common in cold climates. The
farther away you were born from the equator, north or south,
the more likely you are to develop MS. However, the
causative agent, whatever it is, apparently takes root in the
first fifteen years of life. If you move to a more temperate climate before age fifteen, the danger of developing the disease
is reduced. If you move after fifteen, you're as vulnerable as
if you had stayed in the colder climate all your life.

The disease runs in families. Twenty percent of patients
with MS have some blood relative who has it too. If it's a first-
degree relation (parent, child, or sibling), your risk increases

High temperatures temporarily slow the already impaired conduction of electrical impulses in the diseased nerves. So avoiding exposure to heat, whether it be outdoors, in a tub, or the result of too much exercise, helps. Conversely, since cold increases the velocity of nerve impulses, air-conditioning is a must and exercising in cold water is especially effective. Physical therapy can maintain muscle strength and improve coordination and balance, while occupational therapy helps MS patients cope with such daily chores as dressing, eating, and even getting to work.

If you are diagnosed with MS, *insist* on referrals to the appropriate support specialists—dieticians, physiotherapists, and a good neurologist to monitor the medications described below.

There are two types of medications for MS patients: Those that ease its symptoms and others that slow down the progress of the disease. Here's what you can do to try to improve the quality of your life:

- Amantadine (Symmetrel), pemoline (Cylert), and antidepressants such as Prozac can lessen fatigue.
- Baclofen (Lioresal) and tizanidine (Zanaflex) relieve painful muscle spasm and stiffness.
- Ditropan or Detrol help control your urinary bladder.
- Constipation will respond to a bulk laxative such as Metamucil, and if that doesn't work, move on (no pun intended) to Dulcolax or milk of magnesia.
- Facial pain that affects some MS patients can be treated with carbamazepine (Tegretol), phenytoin (Dilantin), divaloprex (Depakote), or amitriptyline (Elavil). If the pain persists and makes chewing difficult, the nerves in the area can be surgically blocked.
- Exacerbations can be shortened and the severity of the symptoms reduced by oral or injected steroid hormones. However, these should be used in the smallest dose and for the shortest time possible, because over the long

term they can cause many undesirable and dangerous side effects.

- If you do not respond to steroids and your symptoms are very severe, ask your doctor whether you would benefit from plasma exchange. In this procedure your blood is removed and its red cells separated from the fluid (plasma). They are then mixed with a synthetic fluid and returned to your body. This presumably eliminates harmful substances in the plasma that can aggravate the disease. However, plasma exchange is not often done for more than three months after the onset of symptoms and is not a major form of therapy.

Influencing the course of the disease is more difficult than treating its symptoms. However, there are several agents being used for this purpose and research is ongoing to find others:

- Beta interferon-1A (Avonex) or beta interferon-1B (Betaseron) are the first choices for patients with more than one severe attack per year, or who don't recover from flare-ups, or in whom the MRI shows the development of new lesions on the nerves. However, these agents do not reverse the damage. Higher doses of these drugs may prevent permanent disability.
- Another drug, glatiramer acetate (Copaxone) is an alternative to the beta interferons. It works by blocking the immune system's attacks on myelin and has shown promise in decreasing the likelihood of permanent disability and appears to have fewer side effects. Ask your doctor about it.

WHAT TO INSIST ON IF YOU HAVE MULTIPLE SCLEROSIS

If you develop numbness or tingling anywhere in your body, especially if it is accompanied by double vision, *insist on seeing a neurologist as soon as possible.* These symptoms may suggest multiple sclerosis.

If the history and the physical exam point to MS, *insist on an MRI of the brain and possibly a spinal tap for confirmation.* Once the diagnosis is made *insist on referrals to the appropriate support specialists*—dieticians, physiotherapists, and a good neurologist to monitor medicine and keep you abreast of the latest therapies.

The field is rapidly changing, and new treatments are in the works.

28

OSTEOPOROSIS

Bone Up on This

Osteoporosis is a disorder in which the bones become brittle and break easily. (*Osteo* stands for "bone"; "*porosis* means "full of holes.") It affects at least 25 million people in this country, 80 percent of whom are women. After age fifty, females have a one in two chance of some day experiencing an osteoporosis-related fracture. By age seventy-five, 90 percent of them have brittle bones just waiting to break.

Falling and fracturing a bone, especially a hip, is the greatest threat to survival and the commonest cause of disability after age sixty-five. About 1.5 million people have such accidents every year. Among the more than 300,000 who fracture a hip and end up in hospital, as many as 36 percent die within twelve months. Nor will life ever be the same for those who survive; 25 percent end up in a nursing home unable to care for themselves and require permanent "assisted living." A woman's chances of fracturing her hip, with all its dire consequences, are as great as her chances of developing cancer of the breast, uterus, and ovary *combined*.

The good news is that if you act early enough in life, you can greatly reduce your chances of developing osteoporosis.

And should you do so, there are steps you can take to halt or reverse its progress.

Despite the enormity of the problem, the subject of osteoporosis usually generates a yawn in both genders and at all ages. Youngsters and men don't think it will ever threaten them; premenopausal women feel that they're too young to worry about it. The elderly believe that once they have it there's nothing to be done about it. They're all wrong. Here's why:

- Males are *not* immune to osteoporosis. One in every three hip fractures occurs in men, although at a later age than in women, and a third of them do not survive longer than a year. One man in five will fracture his hip by the time he reaches the age of eighty.
- Children receiving long-term steroid therapy for asthma or severe allergies can develop osteoporosis.
- Women can avoid developing significant osteoporosis if they start preventive measures (described below) while they're still in their teens and continue them through middle age and beyond.
- There are several new medications that can arrest and reverse osteoporosis even after the disease has begun.

This chapter spells out the latest and best ways to deal with osteoporosis—no matter who you are and no matter how old or how young.

The Life of a Bone

The beating heart constantly reminds us of its presence; our thoughts, emotions, and dreams make us aware that the brain never sleeps; the immediate response of our muscles to virtually every demand we make on them is evidence of their ongoing biological activity. Every other organ system—the intestines, the bowels, the kidneys, the respiratory tract—is constantly sending signals. By contrast, our bones are usually silent. We rarely think about them until we break one, or we become arthritic, or we see a skeleton. Most people consider bones to be inanimate and lifeless structures akin to an internal Erector set.

This is a very misleading view. Bones are as dynamic as any other organ. They store and then release on demand many of the chemicals and minerals necessary to sustain life. There are thousands of biological reactions constantly in progress in bones as they continuously remodel themselves.

Calcium is what gives bones their strength; it is their major mineral and supports a scaffold of collagen. It is constantly either being deposited in bones or sucked out from them. They need extra calcium when we're young in order for us to grow; we add more than we lose before age forty. The more calcium we eat and the more we exercise over the years, the larger the amount of it enters and remains in our skeleton. However, by age forty, bones lose 0.5 percent more calcium each year than they receive. At 50, that net loss increases to between 1 and 3 percent a year.

Here's what determines whether you will have enough calcium in your bones after age 40:

- How much calcium you eat at any age and whether it's being normally absorbed from the intestinal tract. The more you consume, the more there is available for your bones. It's like money in the bank. If you've been depositing it all along, you can draw upon it when you need it later on.
- If you're active, and especially if you regularly perform weight-bearing exercises, your bones keep calling for calcium to maintain their strength. On the other hand, when you're bedridden, calcium seeps out of your bones and leaves them thin and brittle.

- Before menopause, women make enough estrogen to promote positive calcium balance—that is, to lay down more calcium than they lose. However, as they approach menopause, the ovaries secrete less estrogen and bones begin to give up some of the calcium they had previously stored. That's why females lose so much bone at menopause. Those who've had a shorter exposure to estrogen throughout their lives—because their periods ended early, or they had their ovaries surgically removed for any reason, or their menses were always sparse (all associated with estrogen deficiency)—are especially prone to osteoporosis.

- Too much parathyroid hormone (produced by a hyperactive parathyroid gland or one with a tumor) sucks large amounts of calcium out of the bones, weakening them.

- An excess of steroid hormones due to hyperactive adrenal glands (Cushing's disease) or taken as medication (an oral or injected daily maintenance dose of 10 mg of prednisone is enough to do it) causes calcium loss from bone. Some drugs such as Dilantin (used by epileptics on an ongoing basis to prevent seizures), excessively high doses of thyroid supplement for many years and chronic use of barbiturate sleeping pills can all thin your bones.

- Vitamin D helps your stomach absorb the calcium you eat. When you're deficient in this vitamin, the calcium does not enter your body.

- Osteoporosis runs in families. If your mother had it, chances are you will too unless you work at preventing it.

- Use of tobacco results in calcium loss. So all else being equal, smokers are more prone to brittle bones than are nonsmokers.

- Slim or petite women (under 125 pounds) are especially prone to osteoporosis. (One of the very few advantages of being overweight!)

- More than three glasses of wine a day (or the equivalent) predisposes to thin bones.
- Males are less vulnerable to osteoporosis because they're not estrogen-dependent. They also have greater bone mass than do women because they're generally more physically active and so have usually deposited enough calcium over the years. However, there are circumstances that override these protective features in men. The most frequent ones are alcoholism and decreased testosterone levels (during treatment for prostate cancer, or after surgical removal of the testes, which make testosterone, or if the testes were damaged by mumps). Men with chronic lung disease (asthma or emphysema) are five times more likely to have osteoporosis, and that risk is increased to nine times if they're being treated with oral steroids. Short and thin males with a small body frame are also more vulnerable (as are small, thin women).
- Those of the Caucasian or Asian race are at higher risk than persons of African descent. Although Japanese women have as much osteoporosis as American women, they suffer fewer hip fractures, presumably because they so often sit on the floor with their knees flexed, creating stronger hip muscles, better balance, and fewer falls.
- If your hair turned gray in your twenties, or was half-gray by the time you were forty, your chance of developing thin bones is four times higher. This is true for both men and women. (Don't bother dyeing your hair. Nature is not easily fooled.)

Any given combination of these risk factors makes you a candidate for osteoporosis. Unlike arthritis, which causes your joints to ache and become swollen, osteoporosis does not usually result in any symptoms until fairly late in the game. Your first clue may be a sharp pain in a bone after an unsuspected fracture following a trivial injury or fall, or even only a vigorous cough. Also, as the vertebrae in the spinal column continue to lose calcium, one or more of them can collapse, leaving your back rounded (affectionately described as a "dowager's hump"), and shorter than you used to be.

How to Prevent Osteoporosis

It's never too early to start preventing osteoporosis. Don't wait until your periods come to an end. Ensure an adequate calcium intake (1,000 to 1,500 mg per day combined dietary and supplemental) and continue appropriate physical activity throughout your lifetime. Adolescents need between 1,200 and 1,500 mg of calcium daily; if you're pregnant or breast-feeding, aim for 2,000 mg. Premenopausal women between the ages of twenty-five and forty-nine should have at least 1,000 mg. If you're postmenopausal and taking estrogen sup-plements, you need at least 1,000 mg, and 1,500 mg if you're not on the hormone. Every woman over the age of sixty-five should be taking 1,500 mg daily—regardless. If you're receiv-ing ongoing steroid therapy at any age, be sure to have at least 1,500 mg a day. Is there an upper limit for calcium in-take? I'm not sure, but I'd keep it below 2,500 mg per day.

Fewer than 25 percent of children and adolescents con-sume as much calcium as they need, and its deprivation early in life is an important cause of osteoporosis at menopause. Three eight-ounce glasses of low-fat milk fortified with vita-min D daily provide 900 mg of calcium (some brands of calcium-fortified milk have 500 mg per glass). Other calcium-rich foods are cheese (one ounce of hard cheese has 200 mg of calcium, more than cream cheese or cottage cheese); fish (salmon, sardines); and dark green vegetables. Broccoli is es-pecially good (but not spinach, Popeye notwithstanding), be-cause in addition to calcium, it contains oxalate, which prevents calcium from being absorbed.

If you're avoiding calcium-rich dairy products (because

you're lactose-intolerant, or your cholesterol level is high, or you're cutting calories to lose weight), take calcium supplements. There are many different ones on the shelves of your health food store or pharmacy—powders, pills, and chewable tablets. Choose one that also contains vitamin D, of which you need 600 to 800 units per day. (Vitamin D increases the absorption of calcium from the intestinal tract.) Read the labels carefully because calcium content varies significantly in these products. Be sure calcium content is expressed as "elemental" or "as calcium." I recommend calcium citrate because along with its calcium, it increases iron absorption from food and is less likely to cause constipation.

If you're younger than sixty, take your calcium supplements between meals because you absorb calcium best when your stomach is empty but contains some acid. However, after age sixty, the stomach doesn't produce acid unless there's some food in it. Since you need some acid to absorb calcium, take these supplements with your meals. They're not all equally well absorbed. (To check yours, put the tablet in a glass of white vinegar. It should dissolve within thirty minutes.)

Although calcium is their major mineral, bones need others as well, notably potassium and magnesium. Their best sources are fruits and vegetables, and you can get even more magnesium from fish and whole grains. It's not necessary to take supplements.

Exercise Protects Your Bones

Whichever arm you favor probably has 5 percent more bone than does the other. Postmenopausal women can increase their bone density between 2 and 8 percent per year by doing the right kind of exercise on a regular basis. That means weight-bearing exercises, walking or jogging at least a mile a day, dancing, step aerobics (good for premenopausal females, but they can cause fractures in older women with osteoporosis), and tennis. I don't advise weight lifting for anyone with significant osteoporosis. Young female athletes who exercise very strenuously secrete less estrogen, as a result of which their periods stop, leaving them prone to osteoporosis.

Be sure to have a complete physical exam before embarking on any exercise program. Increase the level of exercise gradually; don't get carried away.

Tai chi classes are springing up all over the country. A recent study revealed that seniors who perform these exercises (or yoga) have better balance and 50 percent fewer falls.

While you're eating all that calcium and exercising, limit your alcohol intake. Too much reduces estrogen levels, as does tobacco in any amount.

Diagnosing Osteoporosis

Look for the earliest signs of osteoporosis if you have any combination of the risk factors listed above. For example, you're obviously a candidate if you're female and had a total hysterectomy in your thirties, so that you haven't been making estrogen for some time, or if you're in your late forties and are no longer menstruating. Remember, too, that osteoporosis is a silent calcium thief. This precious mineral seeps out of your bones without your knowing it until something breaks. Don't wait for that to happen. Unless your back has become rounded and you are shorter than you used to be, there may be no obvious tip-off to the fact that your bones are thin and breakable. A routine X ray won't show it until it's too late. So every menopausal woman, regardless of whether she's taking estrogen, and indeed anyone who's at risk for osteoporosis, needs a bone density test (densitometry). You may have to ask for it because many primary physicians don't tell you about it. The most accurate bone density test is called a DEXA (dual energy X-ray absorptiometry). It measures the calcium content of bone. Double X-ray beams of low intensity are focused on a combination of vulnerable bones, usually the hip and one or two others such as the wrist or the spine. The test takes only five minutes and costs about $250, of which Medicare currently reimburses about half. *Insist on a densitometry every year or two.* It's quick and painless and exposes you to no more radiation than you'd pick up during a six-hour airplane flight.

Treating Osteoporosis

There are several steps you can take to reduce your chances of breaking any of your bones if you have osteoporosis:

Since your spine is vulnerable to collapse (some 500,000 vertebral fractures occur every year), try to maintain good posture. Look at a picture of a grenadier guard standing outside of Buckingham Palace. See how he keeps his head high, chin in, and shoulders back. Avoid leaning over when working at your desk or reading. If you're picking something up, bend from the hips, not the waist. Many cars now have lumbar supports in the front seat. If yours doesn't, put a rolled-up towel in the small of your back.

There are several books available with advice for seniors as to how to reduce their risk of falling. You may have to redesign your home to protect yourself. For example, make sure your staircase is properly lighted and equipped with handrails; your shoes should have low heels and nonslip soles; get rid of anything on which you can trip, such as slippery throw rugs, grandchildren's toys, and electrical cords.

Until quite recently, the only two options for treating osteoporosis were the same as those to prevent it—eating more calcium and/or taking estrogen replacement therapy. Times have changed. You now have several effective, well-tolerated, and affordable choices to deal with osteoporosis after it has set in:

- There is still considerable debate as to whether or not estrogen replacement therapy (ERT) prevents heart attacks, strokes, and Alzheimer's, but there is universal agreement that it does minimize and improve osteoporosis. Every woman should discuss the pros and cons of ERT with her doctor. *Insist on enough time to do so.* Starting estrogen early in menopause, regardless of what the bone densitometry test shows, reduces later bone loss by half.

- Alendronate (Fosamax) is a major breakthrough in the fight against osteoporosis. It's not a hormone, but it acts on bone in very much the same way as does estrogen. There are two main types of bone cells involved in the laying down and seeping out (resorption) of calcium *Osteoclasts* promote calcium loss; *osteoblasts* deposit it. Estrogen and Fosamax both inhibit the action of the osteoclasts. Fosamax halves the risk of fractures, especially of the spine. Its main drawback is that it often causes stomach pain, especially if you have previously had any gastric or food pipe problems. You must be very careful when you take Fosamax. Swallow it with a full eight-ounce glass of water first thing in the morning before eating anything and then do not lie down for at least 30 minutes before breakfast. The usual dose is one 10-mg tablet a day. However, I prefer the 70-mg tablet that you take only once every seven days. This long-acting preparation is just as effective as the daily dose and has fewer side effects. Fosamax continues to work on bone for some time after you stop taking it. Using it with estrogen results in even greater protection. I recommend this combination to women who are not improving with either agent alone. If you're taking both, use only 5 mg of the Fosamax daily and a small dose, such as 0.3 mg, of Premarin. Men with osteoporosis can benefit from Fosamax too, but I haven't found any who have agreed to take female hormone.

- Risedronate (Actonel), chemically similar to Fosamax, is as effective with fewer digestive side effects.
- Calcitonin (Miacalcin), a hormone made by the thyroid gland, is not as effective as either estrogen or Fosamax. Like them, it inhibits the osteoclasts that cause calcium loss from bone. It comes in a nasal spray, and aside from giving some stuffiness and nasal irritation, it is safe and has few side effects. Men with osteoporosis can take it too.
- Raloxifene (Evista), a synthetic estrogen, is the latest advance in the war against osteoporosis. This drug results in a significant increase in bone density and has the additional benefit of protecting against breast cancer. However, it is not quite as effective for osteoporosis as estrogen or Fosamax. It has some of the beneficial actions of natural estrogen (it protects against calcium loss) without the undesirable consequences (possibility of breast cancer). Unfortunately, Evista does not control menopausal symptoms such as hot flashes. You should also be aware of some important precautions if you're taking Evista. It increases the risk of clot formation within the veins, especially in someone confined to bed, as do estrogen replacement and birth control pills. So if you know you're going to be immobilized in this way, perhaps because of impending surgery, *stop the Evista 72 hours before the operation.* Unlike some of the other antiosteoporosis drugs, *Evista should be taken only by postmenopausal women, not men; do not use estrogen with it. Stop the Evista if you become pregnant; it can harm the fetus.*

WHAT TO INSIST ON IF YOU'RE A CANDIDATE FOR OSTEOPOROSIS OR ALREADY HAVE IT

Osteoporosis (brittle bones that break easily) is a major cause of death and disability. Although women lacking in estrogen at and beyond menopause are most vulnerable to osteoporosis, men and even children can also be affected under special circumstances.

Osteoporosis is usually silent for most of its course and first makes itself known after a sudden fracture following a fall, or when bones in the spinal column collapse, causing a rounded back (dowager's hump), loss of height, and bone pain.

If you're vulnerable to osteoporosis, *insist on bone densitometry,* a simple radiological examination that measures the density (and hence the calcium content) of bone. Medicare and most insurance plans reimburse, at least partly, for this procedure.

Prevention is the key to dealing with osteoporosis. Consuming enough calcium and vitamin D is critical during childhood, adolescence, and adult life. In addition, regular weight-bearing exercise over a lifetime can also lead to the deposition of more calcium on the bones, so that when the lack of estrogen causes this mineral to seep out, the bones will have enough left to prevent easy fracture.

Treatment options consist of estrogen replacement for women, a high intake of calcium, regular exercise, and any of the newer drugs (Fosamax, Miacalcin, and Evista). Men are not candidates for estrogen or Evista. *Insist that your doctor take the time to discuss with you all your treatment options.*

29

OVARIAN CANCER

Seek and Ye Shall Find

Some years ago a fifty-five-year-old woman consulted me because for the past weeks she had felt bloated and was having cramps in her belly. These symptoms were unlike anything she'd ever experienced. They occurred frequently, occasionally awakened her at night, and were neither worsened nor improved by any specific food. I thought that she probably had gallbladder disease, given her age and gender. However, a sonogram of the abdomen, the gold standard for detecting disease of that organ, was normal. We then looked with an endoscope directly into her stomach, and it, too, was "clean." I suggested that she might have lactose intolerance and advised her to avoid milk and dairy products for a while and to let me know how she was feeling.

Two weeks later she phoned to say that she was no better and asked whether her symptoms might be due to ovarian cancer. "You'll probably laugh at this, Doctor, but I had an aunt who died with ovarian cancer a few years ago. She also had belly pain and her tests too were normal. She didn't consult a gynecologist because her uterus had been removed several years earlier, she was sixty years old, and she had no 'female' problems. By the time someone thought of ovarian cancer, it was too late. Please humor me and give me the name of a good gynecologist."

From the title of this chapter, you can probably guess what happened next. The gynecologist to whom I referred her, found (and cured) an ovarian cancer.

This was a lesson I never forgot. Since then I have diagnosed this malignancy many times—sometimes early enough to cure—because of my "better safe than sorry" approach to any woman with ill-defined abdominal or pelvic complaints.

Ovarian cancer strikes one of every fifty-five women; more than 25,000 will develop it some time during this next year and almost 15,000 will die—more than from cancer of any other reproductive organ. Even though 95 percent of ovarian cancers are curable if detected before they spread beyond the ovary, the actual survival rate for five years or more is presently less than 50 percent. That's because there is no single reliable screening test for its early detection and most of these tumors present late in the disease. The ovaries are situated deep inside the pelvis and are not easy to feel; the Pap test of the cervix doesn't detect this cancer either. So you've got to look for it—very carefully—in order to find it. Unfortunately, doctors don't recommend the kind of in-depth exam that's necessary to make the diagnosis unless they or their patients strongly suspect it. The red flags that should alert you to ovarian cancer are persistent and unexplained painful intercourse, bloating, extreme fatigue, unusual vaginal bleeding, a feeling of pressure in the pelvis, swelling of the abdomen, and chronic stomach pain, gas, or indigestion. But frankly, when these are present, the tumor has probably already spread.

The following are at special risk for ovarian cancer:

- Postmenopausal women in their late fifties and sixties. If you've been taking estrogen replacement therapy, your chances are more than doubled. Not every doctor is convinced that this is true, but many are.

- Females of North American or North European descent, particularly Ashkenazi Jews (from central and eastern Europe).
- Women who test positive for the BRCA 1 or BRCA 2 genes. The presence of the BRCA 1 mutation means that you have a 20 to 40 percent chance of developing ovarian cancer during your lifetime (and a 50 to 85 percent likelihood of breast cancer); the BRCA 2 mutation confers a 15 to 20 percent chance of cancer of the ovaries (and a 55 to 85 percent likelihood of breast cancer). You should be tested for both these genes if there is a family history (mother, sister, daughter) of either ovarian or breast malignancy. (About 5 percent of Ashkenazi women have mutations of both these genes.)
- If you've already had a malignancy of the uterus, colon, or breast, you should suspect ovarian cancer if you develop otherwise unexplained abdominal symptoms.
- A family history (mother, sister, daughter) of ovarian, breast, uterine, or colon cancer increases your lifetime chance of developing ovarian cancer. If one such relative had ovarian cancer, your risk is one in twenty; with two or more, it's one in fourteen.
- The greater the number of periods you've had during your life, the greater the risk. Women who fall into this category include those who have never had a baby or had their first one after age thirty, whose periods started before age twelve, and/or whose menopause didn't set in until well after age fifty.
- Unsuccessful use of fertility drugs such as clomiphene may be associated with the germ cell of ovarian cancer.

You are at *reduced* risk for ovarian cancer if your tubes were tied, or you used oral contraceptives for at least five years, breast-fed your infants (because periods usually stop during breast-feeding), or were a longtime user of aspirin. Recent research suggests that aspirin may decrease the risk of ovarian cancer by as much as 40 percent.

When and How to Look Especially Carefully for Ovarian Cancer

Be sure to make every one of your doctors—internists *and* gynecologists—aware of a positive family history of ovarian cancer. In every such case, they should do a thorough recto-vaginal pelvic exam every year as part of the routine physical. It should also be done in every woman who has any unexplained chronic abdominal or pelvic symptoms.

If for any reason you and/or your doctor think there's even the *slightest* possibility of ovarian cancer (family history, physical findings, puzzling symptoms—remember, you don't have to be sure) then you should *insist on the following:*

- A bimanual pelvic exam via the vagina *and the rectum* that focuses on the ovaries, together with a complete evaluation of the abdomen. The former may detect cysts or other growths on the ovary; the latter may explain intestinal symptoms.
- A blood test called the CA 125 to measure the level of a protein that is elevated in the presence of ovarian cancer. But be careful about interpreting its results, because it may also be increased by uterine (endometrial) and other cancers, and it may be falsely elevated in healthy women too and lead to unnecessary surgery. A CA 125 reading by itself is not diagnostic, one way or another.
- More and more MRIs and CT scans of the pelvis are being performed for ovarian cancer screening. Unfortunately, they are expensive. You may also have a transvaginal sonogram (the sonic probe is inserted into the vagina) and a color ultrasound Doppler (which looks at the blood vessels in the ovary), both of which can detect ovarian cysts and are especially useful when combined with the CA 125 analysis. However, they can miss early ovarian tumors.

If you have a positive family history, one or more of these tests should be done every six months, starting at age thirty-five. It sounds like overkill, but it's worth it. *Insist on it.*

In the final analysis, when the diagnosis of ovarian cancer seems like a real possibility, laparoscopy and/or surgery may be the only way to make the diagnosis.

The Different Kinds of Ovarian Tumors

Most ovarian tumors are not malignant. If your doctor feels something or there's a suspicious finding on the ultrasound, don't panic; it's probably benign. However, only a biopsy is conclusive. But unlike the simple skin or breast biopsy, biopsy of the ovary requires a laparoscopy or exploratory surgery. And it can be risky. An early stage I tumor can spread, leak fluid, and be converted to a more advanced stage. To avoid this, some doctors simply remove the ovary (or the suspicious cyst) to avoid this complication.

There are three main kinds of ovarian tumors, each of which develops from a different ovarian cell. They are:

- Epithelial tumors, accounting for 85 to 90 percent of all ovarian cancers. There are several subtypes in this category, each of which reflects a different cell on the surface of the ovary. Most of them are benign, but some are cancerous.
- Germ cell tumors, of which there are also several subtypes. They are more likely to occur in girls and younger women. The term "germ" does not refer to a bug of any kind, but to early cells that later form within the ovary. Most of these tumors are benign too, and account for only 5 percent of all ovarian cancers. The surgeon removes the benign tumor, leaving the rest of the ovary intact.

- Stromal tumors originating in the tissue that holds the ovary together and that makes female hormones. Most of these are also benign and constitute only 5 percent of all ovarian cancers.

Ovarian cysts are collections of fluid in the ovary that are usually but not always benign. They come and go and are a normal phenomenon of the ovulation process. Such cysts must be checked from time to time to make sure they haven't enlarged due to a malignancy.

Tumor Staging

If your doctor suspects a tumor (because he or she felt "something" during the pelvic exam, or there is a suspicious finding on one of the imaging tests such as the transvaginal sonogram, MRI, or CT scan), additional procedures must be done as follow-up. *Insist on them.* The safest and most definitive is a biopsy of the tissue in question. If it's benign, you're home free and clear. But don't panic if you're one of the 5 to 10 percent of American women who require a biopsy because of a suspected ovarian tumor. Only 13 to 21 percent of them turn out to be malignant. However, the fact is that most of these biopsies end up requiring laparoscopy or exploratory surgery.

"Staging" a tumor defines how far it has progressed. The stages range from 1 to 4—the lower the number, the earlier it is and the better the outlook.

- A stage 1 tumor is limited to the ovary. Some 25 percent of women diagnosed with ovarian cancer are found to be stage 1.
- A stage 2 tumor involves other organs but is still in the pelvis.

- A stage 3 tumor has spread outside the pelvis and involves the lining of the abdomen and the lymph glands.
- Stage 4 is the worst news. The cancer has metastasized to distant organs such as the liver.

Treatment of Ovarian Cancer

There are several ways to treat ovarian cancer, and ongoing research is finding new ones all the time. *Insist on being told all your options before you commit yourself to any one.* If you have any questions or doubts, *insist on a second opinion.* You may also call the National Cancer Institute at 800-4-CANCER or go to the Internet and ask an expert at a website such as *cancersource.com, cancerfact.com,* or *oncology.com.*

The best treatment depends on your age, your general health, your personal preferences, and most important, the stage of the disease. You have three main options: Surgery, chemotherapy, and radiation.

- Surgery is usually the best option in stage 1. Both ovaries and tubes, the uterus and all visible tumor are removed. If the cancer is epithelial and not especially aggressive ("low malignant potential"), only the malignant ovary and its fallopian tube are removed (especially if you're premenopausal and want to have a family someday). Epithelial tumors may recur after surgery, so it's not uncommon for the surgeon to perform a second operation after a few months to make sure that everything is "clean." If the tumor has recurred, chemotherapy and radiation are usually recommended. Malignant germ cell and stromal tumors are also removed surgically and then treated with chemotherapy.
- You are a good candidate for chemotherapy after surgery if your cancer has progressed beyond stage 1. Such ther-

apy consists of a combination of anticancer drugs given in about six cycles, with rest periods in between. Side effects such as nausea and vomiting, hair loss, sores in the mouth and vagina, loss of appetite, and increased vulnerability to infection (because these drugs weaken your immune system) can make you miserable. Happily, they're only temporary, and there are ways to minimize their severity, so don't reject chemotherapy because of them. It can be life-saving. One of the most widely used chemotherapy agents is Taxol (especially in women whose cancers have recurred); also widely used are combinations of carboplatin or cisplatin and cyclophosphamide.

- Radiation's high-energy X rays kill cancer cells. This is not the main form of treatment for ovarian cancer, but is used in some cases.

The Ultimate Prevention

I'm often asked by women who consider themselves to be at high risk for ovarian cancer whether to have their ovaries removed while they're still healthy. If you have two or more first-degree relatives, or first- and second-degree relatives with ovarian cancer, *you should be examined for the BRCA 1 and 2 genes*. If you test positive, I recommend prophylactic removal of the ovaries by age thirty-five unless you are planning to have more children. This surgery can be done by video laparoscopy (without a major incision), leaving the uterus intact. You should then take hormone replacement therapy. However, be aware that 2 percent of women who've undergone such prophylactic oophrectomy develop a malignancy in the lining of the abdomen (the peritoneum) that looks just like an ovarian cancer. So even after your ovaries have been removed, you should still have a physical exam and CA 125 test once or twice a year.

WHAT TO INSIST ON IF YOU HAVE OVARIAN CANCER

There are 15,000 deaths every year in this country from ovarian cancer. Although early detection can cure 95 percent of cases, most women die from this malignancy because there is no single test to detect it before it's too late. *You must have a high index of suspicion for it and pay special attention to your family history.* For example, if one or more first-degree relatives (mother, daughter, sister) had ovarian cancer, your risk is significantly increased.

Always suspect ovarian cancer if you develop a constellation of unexplained symptoms in the pelvis or abdomen—gas, bloating, fatigue, a change in your menstrual pattern, stomach pain or distension, or pain or pressure in the pelvis. But look for it before these symptoms appear.

The most useful, though by no means foolproof, steps to take are regular, careful *rectovaginal* exams by your gynecologist, a CA 125 blood test, vaginal ultrasound, or pelvic CT or MRI. *Insist on whatever combination of these diagnostic procedures is necessary to clarify any unexplained symptoms, especially if there is a family history of ovarian cancer. Also insist that any suspicious findings be biopsied. Remember, however, that biopsy may involve some form of surgery.*

The treatment of and the outlook for ovarian cancer depend on its stage when discovered. Your best chance for cure is a stage 1. The tumor should always be removed, followed by chemotherapy with or without radiation.

If you're at high risk for ovarian cancer, consider prophylactic removal of both ovaries before age thirty-five.

(30)

PARKINSON'S DISEASE

Shaking Hands

Parkinson's is the fourth most common "neurodegenerative" disease of the elderly. The average age at which it starts is fifty-seven years. Along with Alzheimer's, it's one of the most dreaded afflictions, affecting one in every hundred men and women over sixty-five. (There is a similar neurological disorder of childhood and adolescence called juvenile Parkinson's, as well as *secondary Parkinson's,* which is due to the adverse action of certain drugs—the sedative tranquilizer haloperidol (Haldol), prochlorperazine (Compazine) for the treatment of nausea, metoclopramide (Reglan) for gastric mobility problems, and a variety of "recreational" substances, such as the street drug called N-MPTP.

Parkinson's disease is as old as the hills. James Parkinson, an English physician, first described it as a disease entity in 1817, and referred to it as "shaking palsy." The first breakthrough in treatment did not come until about fifty years ago when scientists examining patients who had died with Parkinson's disease found that their brains were deficient in cells found in an area of the brain called the substantia nigra. These cells produce a chemical called dopamine, a neurotransmitter that helps send messages from one part of the brain to another. The symptoms of Parkinson's disease are due to dopamine deficiency. The man who made this key observation won the Nobel Prize in medicine.

It seemed logical to expect that giving the missing dopamine to patients with Parkinson's would cure the disease. It didn't work out that way because the brain is very selective about what it allows to enter it, thus protecting itself from potentially harmful chemicals circulating in the bloodstream. However, researchers found that a naturally occurring substance called dopa, related to but different from dopamine, could penetrate this "blood-brain" barrier. Unfortunately, the amounts necessary to be of any help were so toxic that dopa was abandoned as a possible therapeutic agent.

Enter Dr. George Cotzias, a neurologist friend of mine working at Cornell Medical School some forty years ago. He found that a specific form of dopa called levodopa did cross the barrier into the brain where it was converted to dopamine. More important it improved the symptoms of the disease. To this day, levodopa (referred to as L-dopa) remains the basic treatment for millions of patients with Parkinson's disease. It does have side effects, but they're tolerable.

Diagnosing Parkinson's

There is no specific test for Parkinson's. However, its symptoms are so classical that the diagnosis is easily made from the history and the physical exam alone. The onset of the disease may be subtle. In about 80 percent of cases the earliest clue is a mild tremor of *one* hand, arm, or leg, in that order of frequency. However, the jaw, tongue, or eyelids (but not the voice) can also "tremble." A key characteristic of this tremor is that it improves when you reach for something and it disappears during sleep. It is also more pronounced when you're tired or upset. (Don't panic if your hands tremble a little. Many older persons develop a little "shake" that doctors call "benign essential tremor." Unlike the tremor of Parkinson's, benign essential tremor is *worsened* by movement, it affects *both* hands, it is not accompanied by any of the other symptoms of Parkinson's described below, and it never progresses to anything more serious.

The earliest symptom of Parkinson's disease may be stiffness, not tremor. These patients move very slowly and with difficulty; their muscles are chronically tense and rigid, leaving them achy and tired; the face is often expressionless, voice low, monotonous, and often stuttering. These individuals have a short attention span, they can't concentrate, and their memory is poor. They tend to shuffle when they walk; their steps are short; they keep their arms flexed at the waist and don't swing them. The phenomenon of "freezing," a sudden inability to continue walking, is a special problem. Balance is often so poor that they may run a little when starting to walk so as not to fall. It's as if they were chasing their center of gravity. Patients with Parkinson's are vulnerable to fractures, especially of the hip because they do fall so easily. The handwriting is small and difficult to make out; there may be trouble swallowing and sleeping. Constipation is common; it may be difficult to empty the bladder; the scalp is apt to be abnormally oily. Many of these patients are depressed, and half of them eventually become demented. In the end, many are totally dependent on a caregiver to feed them, dress them, and, in fact, for total support.

In addition to the obvious symptoms, your doctor may record a sharp drop in blood pressure that leaves you dizzy when you get up from the sitting position (postural hypotension)—all evidence of malfunction of the autonomic nervous system over which we have no control.

It's not a pretty picture, but if you're diagnosed with Parkinson's, don't give up. Parkinson's progresses at an unpredictable pace; some patients continue to function satisfactorily for many years. Keep trying to cope, because not only may your symptoms not worsen seriously or quickly, but equally important, there are some significant treatment breakthroughs in the works.

Always insist on access to a specialist when you need it. Most primary physicians and general internists do not have the necessary expertise to deal with many aspects of Parkinson's and its complications. The more important anti-Parkinson's drugs have potentially serious side effects. Their optimal dose and scheduling vary from patient to patient. Finding the right one for you is extremely important and often requires an expert opinion.

Because of the multitude of symptoms, patients with Parkinson's disease have complex needs. *Insist on seeing whatever specialists are necessary (such as physiotherapists, psychiatrists, speech therapists, and nutritionists), to provide the support that* can improve the quality of your life. Do not allow yourself to be dismissed and left in limbo because you have an "incurable" disease.

Treating Parkinson's

Levodopa is a useful and important medication but improves symptoms only partially. What's more, the longer you take it and the higher the dose, the greater are its debilitating side effects. That's why many doctors delay prescribing it for as long as possible. There are several other less toxic drugs that can be used instead of levodopa in the early stages. Levodopa is added when the disease has progressed. Combination therapy makes it possible to administer levodopa at a lower dose and with fewer side effects.

Other medications that can ease the Parkinson's burden include:

Agonists. The term "agonist" refers to any chemical or drug that enhances the effects of another. *Dopamine agonists* increase the effectiveness of whatever small amounts of dopamine the brain continues to produce. An effective agonist reduces the amount of levodopa required.

The older dopamine agonists, bromocriptine (Parlodel) and pergolide (Permax), are less effective than the more recent preparations, pramipexole and ropinirole. In a recent study of 268 patients with early Parkinson's, ropinirole alone was successful for five years. So if you have recently been diagnosed *insist that your doctor discuss with you the option of delaying treatment with levodopa and first trying one of these dopamine agonists.*

Dopamine agonists can cause such troublesome side effects as a drop in blood pressure when changing position (postural hypotension), and a variety of behavioral complications ranging from confusion to delirium. Still, they're worth trying.

Amantadine (Symmetrel), a medication widely used for the treatment of mild cases of Parkinson's helps the remaining cells in the substantia nigra in the brain release their dopamine. Try amantadine alone, and, when it is no longer effective, combine it with levodopa, whose actions it enhances. The usual dosage of amantadine is 100 to 300 mg a day. Although it's usually well tolerated, this drug can cause confusion, as well as swelling of the legs.

There is an interesting sidelight to the amantadine story. Several years ago doctors in Russia who were evaluating its possible use in Parkinson's observed that patients to whom they gave the drug and who also happened to get the flu recovered more quickly from their viral infection. Further research has confirmed that amantadine is effective against type A influenza. This drug, and others related to it, are now part of the armamentarium against the flu—an example of how the same agent can work in different ways in totally unrelated illnesses.

In addition to dopamine, the brain makes another neurotransmitter called *acetylcholine*. The two balance each other in healthy persons because there are enzymes in the brain that prevent either of them from accumulating. However, someone with Parkinson's needs all the dopamine he or she can produce. So medications that prevent the enzymatic action against dopamine improve Parkinson's disease. These include selegiline (Eldepryl), tolcapone, and entacapone. When given to patients who are still making some of their own dopamine in the early stages of the disease, these drugs may be all that's necessary for a year or two. And continuing them thereafter makes a little levodopa go a longer way. But it's a double-edged sword because the antienzyme medications may aggravate the side effects of levodopa.

In Parkinson's patients whose dopamine supply is reduced but who have normal amounts of acetylcholine, the imbalance between these two neurotransmitters aggravates their symptoms. Drugs that decrease the concentration of acetylcholine can therefore be useful. There are several such *anticholinergic agents*. Those most common prescribed are trihexyphenidyl (Artane) and benztropine (Cogentin). They reduce tremor and muscle stiffness, but can cause dry mouth, blurred vision, constipation, urinary retention, and confusion.

You can maximize the effectiveness and decrease the side effects of levodopa by adding carbidopa, a medication that prevents its breakdown in the liver. The combination of carbidopa and levodopa in a preparation marketed as Sinemet is the most widely used anti-Parkinson's medication. It comes in several fixed dosages and should be taken fifteen to twenty minutes before meals to make sure it is fully absorbed. Start with the lowest strength, containing 25 mg of carbidopa and 100 mg of levodopa, and increase the dose every week or so until you're getting maximum benefit with the fewest side effects. Most patients need to raise their maintenance Sinemet dose from time to time because the brain's limited production of dopamine continues to decline. Most individuals eventually require 100 mg of carbidopa and 1,000 mg of levodopa in divided doses every few hours, and some need as much as 200/2,000 daily.

carry a gene that stimulates the formation of dopamine-producing cells. Three months later these monkeys were making normal amounts of neurotransmitter and had lost their Parkinson's symptoms. The results are encouraging and plans are under way for human trials.

What Else Can You Do?

In addition to what your doctor can do for you, you must manage your lifestyle to help yourself function normally for as long as possible.

Regular exercise keeps your muscles strong, flexible, and moving, and stimulates your circulation. It also helps control weight and ensures a good night's sleep.

The best way to reduce muscle stiffness and tremor and to slow the spontaneous movements that plague you is to walk, jog, stretch, or swim as often as possible. Check with your doctor before starting any such program and always rest when you become tired. Begin and end every workout with stretching, bending, and breathing exercises that a physio-therapist can show you how to perform.

Exercise your face, jaws, and voice. Drinking through a straw is a good way to strengthen the muscles of the lips, mouth, and throat.

The right diet helps prevent both weight gain (due to re-duced physical activity) and weight loss (the result of the con-stant involuntary muscle movements that burn up calories). Here are some important dietary tips:

- Cut your food into smaller portions that are easier to chew.
- To avoid constipation, eat lots of fiber, the best sources of which are whole grains, fruits, and vegetables, and drink at least eight glasses of water a day.

- High-protein foods may interfere with some anti-Parkinson's medications and should not be taken together.
- Sucking on hard candy, lozenges, and sour balls, or chewing gum, reduces excess salivation and drooling.
- Patients with Parkinson's often clamp the jaws shut during sleep and bite their tongue. Ask your dentist to fit you with a mouth protector to prevent this from happening.

Here are some other sensible steps you can take:

- You're better off in a shower than a tub bath. Sit on a stool while showering.
- Buy a raised toilet seat with arm rails to help you get off the john.
- Buy soap on a rope so that you can pick it up more easily if you drop it.
- Modify your home environment to reduce the risk of falling. For example, don't have your floors waxed. Don't put throw rugs on the bathroom floor because you can slip on them. All carpets should either have a skid-proof backing or be tacked to the floor.
- Use a cordless phone that you can carry from room to room so that you don't have to rush to answer a call. Install a speakerphone and use a headset that allows you to talk hands-free, especially if you have a troublesome tremor. Install an intercom system or a portable walkie-talkie to communicate with others in your house.
- Don't walk on bare floors in socks, slippers, and stockings. Wear low-heeled shoes with nonskid soles.
- Picking things up off the floor can throw you off balance. Buy an inexpensive "grabber" with which you can pick them up.
- Don't be shy about using a cane.
- Turning in bed is easier if you wear silk pajamas and have satin sheets.

- High-protein foods may interfere with some anti-Parkinson's medications and should not be taken together.
- Sucking on hard candy, lozenges, and sour balls, or chewing gum, reduces excess salivation and drooling.
- Patients with Parkinson's often clamp the jaws shut during sleep and bite their tongue. Ask your dentist to fit you with a mouth protector to prevent this from happening.

Here are some other sensible steps you can take:

- You're better off in a shower than a tub bath. Sit on a stool while showering.
- Buy a raised toilet seat with arm rails to help you get off the john.
- Buy soap on a rope so that you can pick it up more easily if you drop it.
- Modify your home environment to reduce the risk of falling. For example, don't have your floors waxed. Don't put throw rugs on the bathroom floor because you can slip on them. All carpets should either have a skid-proof backing or be tacked to the floor.
- Use a cordless phone that you can carry from room to room so that you don't have to rush to answer a call. Install a speakerphone and use a headset that allows you to talk hands-free, especially if you have a troublesome tremor. Install an intercom system or a portable walkie-talkie to communicate with others in your house.
- Don't walk on bare floors in socks, slippers, and stockings. Wear low-heeled shoes with nonskid soles.
- Picking things up off the floor can throw you off balance. Buy an inexpensive "grabber" with which you can pick them up.
- Don't be shy about using a cane.
- Turning in bed is easier if you wear silk pajamas and have satin sheets.

- If your handwriting is small and difficult for others to read, write on oversize sheets of paper with a large felt-tip pen.
- Buy clothing with Velcro closures. Buttons are the nemesis of Parkinson's disease.

WHAT TO INSIST ON IF YOU HAVE PARKINSON'S DISEASE

Parkinson's disease is a chronic neurological disorder of unknown cause that affects older persons. It is due to a decrease in the number of brain cells that produce a chemical called dopamine. The disease is characterized by tremor, progressive muscular rigidity, and involuntary jerky movements. Emotional and behavioral problems frequently develop in the later stages. Patients may eventually become totally bedridden and require complete care. However, the rate of this progression varies greatly, and some persons with Parkinson's can go for years with only minimal symptoms.

If you've been told you have Parkinson's, *insist on having the diagnosis confirmed by a specialist.* The proper dosage and combinations of drugs to treat Parkinson's are critical. *Insist on access to a neurologist with special expertise and interest in this disease who's keeping up with the rapid advances in therapy. You may also require physiotherapy, preferably in a setting where specialized equipment is available. Insist on that too. Patients with Parkinson's often have gastrointestinal problems that may require consultation with a specialist. Insist on it.*

Several medications can improve the symptoms of Parkinson's disease. The most important is levodopa, which is converted into the missing dopamine in the brain. Other drugs can be taken along with levodopa to enhance its action and minimize the severity of its side effects.

Insist on being seen and examined by your doctor at regular intervals. That's the only way he or she can tell whether or not your medical regimen needs adjustment.

31

PHLEBITIS

Oy Vein

You wake up one morning with pain in the back of your leg. It's tender to the touch and slightly warm. The painful area is pink and there may be reddish streaks on the skin. You can also feel something hard, like a cord, in your calf. Your leg feels heavy, and you're more comfortable when you try to elevate it. What the devil could this be? You don't remember hurting yourself, and there was no hint of trouble after you arrived home from your overseas flight a couple of days ago.

Theoretically, your symptoms could be due to anything from an insect bite to a blocked artery. The leg is made up of muscles, joints, bones, veins, and arteries (all covered by skin), and any of these could be affected. Well, there's no use pampering yourself, so you get dressed and go to the office, hoping that whatever this is will go away. But it doesn't, so you stop at your doctor's office on your way home from work. She examines you, tells you she thinks you have phlebitis, orders some tests to make sure of the diagnosis, and prescribes some pills. She advises you to stay home for a couple of days.

What's this all about, you ask? If your doctor were to take the time to explain it to you, this is what she would tell you:

There are three main kinds of blood vessels: Arteries carry blood away from the heart and deliver oxygen and other nutrients to every part of the body; veins that transport this "used" blood back to the lungs where its oxygen is replenished; and capillaries, the network of vessels that connect the veins and the arteries. Phlebitis is "inflamation of a vein." It can happen anywhere in the body but occurs most frequently in the legs. Women are much more likely to have phlebitis than are men.

Some veins flow near the surface (they look blue and you can see them best in your legs when they're dilated—varicose veins). Larger veins deep in the body are not visible. Veins anywhere can become inflamed. If they're superficial, you have superficial phlebitis; when the deeper ones are involved, it's (surprise!) deep venous phlebitis.

Clots frequently form in veins that have become inflamed, especially the deep ones. When that happens, you have thrombophlebitis or venous thrombosis.

I will discuss superficial phlebitis and deep phlebitis separately, but that's only for convenience's sake, because although their therapy differs, they are similar processes in different location.

Superficial Phlebitis

The symptoms you experienced—tenderness over the vein, redness of the skin, and maybe a little swelling—are classic for superficial phlebitis. Superficial phlebitis in the legs usually occurs in the following circumstances:

- In the presence of preexisting varicose veins
- In pregnant women because the fetus presses on the abdominal veins, forcing the blood to pool in the legs
- In persons who have been bedridden for any reason

- In smokers
- In overweight individuals
- After a local injury to the leg
- Following a long flight (especially if you have varicose veins)
- In women taking birth control pills, notably those who also smoke. Oral contraceptives with a high estrogen content increase the risk of phlebitis three to twelve times.
- In someone with cancer anywhere in the body, but especially in the lungs or pancreas, because malignancy affects the blood-clotting mechanism
- In association with other disorders that interfere with normal blood clotting such as lupus, heart attacks, and even ulcerative colitis.
- In hospitalized patients suffering from trauma or infection due to an intravenous therapy, or in drug users. (Phlebitis in the arms is otherwise rare.)

Superficial phlebitis is not a cause for major concern. Here's what to do for it:

- Rest until the tenderness and redness clear up. It may take seven to ten days to do so.
- Don't rub the affected area because that may dislodge a clot that happens to be present in a deeper vein.
- Elevate the affected leg whenever possible and apply warm compresses.
- While in bed, move your feet, ankles, and legs frequently to stimulate the circulation.
- Elastic stockings can relieve your discomfort and help the flow of blood up the leg and back to the lungs. Don't wear garters or knee-length stockings.
- Take aspirin or an NSAID for five to seven days to reduce inflamation.
- Drink lots of fluids.

- Once the attack has subsided, remain active. Walk. Avoid prolonged sitting or standing.

That's it. You don't need antibiotics because there is rarely any bacterial infection in superficial phlebitis.

Once the attack is over:

- Resume your normal activities gradually and don't get overtired.
- Get plenty of rest but don't spend too much time in bed.
- Postpone for a few days any travel plans that call for long plane flights or car trips.
- If you're on the Pill, discuss some other form of birth control with your doctor.
- Stop smoking.
- Don't cross your legs when sitting or lying in bed.

Although superficial phlebitis itself is not serious, the catch is that the deep, larger veins are also involved in about 10 percent of cases. When that happens, the situation is more serious, because, in addition to being inflamed, these vessels virtually always contain clots that can break off and travel to the lung, a condition called pulmonary embolism. If you've had deep thrombophlebitis before, always assume that what appears to be only superficial phlebitis has a deep vein component to it—and should be treated as such.

When you have superficial thrombophlebitis, your doctor should perform additional tests to make sure that the deep veins are not involved. *Insist on these tests*—just to be sure.

Testing for Deep Vein Thrombophlebitis

Before the availability of modern, noninvasive imaging procedures, contrast venography was the gold standard for diagnosing deep thrombophlebitis. Dye was injected into the leg veins, and X rays were then taken to indicate the location and size of the blood clot. That's no longer the way to go. *Insist on either a duplex ultrasound or an MRI.* (I prefer the MRI because it's more sensitive, especially for detecting thrombosis in the calf veins.) The problem with the MRI is its cost. Ultrasound, though useful for revealing vein problems in other areas of the leg, is not as accurate for the detection of thrombosis in the calf.

The clot in deep vein thrombophlebitis (DVT) is made up of red blood cells, white blood cells, and platelets. It sticks to the inner lining of the vein and interferes with the flow of blood through it. DVT is potentially serious because if a piece of the clot breaks off, it can travel through the network of veins all the way to the lungs (pulmonary embolism). It can then lodge in one of the pulmonary arteries and cut off the blood supply to an area of the lung. When the blocked vessel is a large one the patient may die. The death rate from pulmonary embolism is about 20 percent. DVT can also result in permanent damage to the vein, so that blood doesn't flow through it properly. It backs up, leaving the legs swollen.

In 50 percent of cases, DVT causes no symptoms. Typical symptoms, when they do occur, are abrupt pain, appearance of swelling in one leg, tenderness, warmth, and redness in the calf. You don't feel the cord as you do in superficial phlebitis because the diseased vein is deep inside the leg. The first signs of serious trouble may be chest pain and cough due to an embolus that has reached the lungs.

DVT has the same causes as superficial phlebitis and can be present without superficial phlebitis.

Treating Deep Thrombophlebitis

The treatment of DVT differs in one major respect from that for superficial phlebitis. You now must have your blood "thinned" in order to prevent the clot from traveling to the lung. Such anticoagulation is the main reason why 300,000 Americans with DVT are hospitalized each year. Since it takes time for the oral blood thinner (warfarin) to reach protective levels in the blood, you will first receive an anticoagulant by injection—intravenous heparin or one of its variations given just under the skin. This begins to protect you quickly. (Sometimes, if a large clot is detected in a major deep vein, you may also be given a clot-dissolver—thrombolytic—such as urokinase or streptokinase.) At the same time as this initial injection therapy is started, you'll be given oral warfarin (Coumadin). A few days later, when the Coumadin level in the blood is high enough, the heparin is discontinued and you can go home on the Coumadin alone.

If you have phlebitis and develop any chest pain or acute shortness of breath insist on a VQ scan, a noninvasive procedure specifically designed to detect blood clots in the lung.

The oral anticoagulant is usually continued for at least six months to protect you against any recurrence of phlebitis. Remember that many drugs and herbs interfere with warfarin. These include aspirin, any of the NSAIDs, ginkgo biloba (widely used for improving memory), garlic, ginger, and a host of others that can leave your blood too "thin" or not thin enough. You need to have a blood test to measure your prothrombin time or INR (measures of anticoagulant effectiveness) checked every few weeks and the dose of your warfarin should be adjusted as necessary. Remember, too, that there's always the danger of internal bleeding when you're taking an anticoagulant. Look for and immediately report the presence of blood in your urine, stool, or sputum, or excessive bleeding of your gums and unexplained nosebleeds.

Sometimes anticoagulants don't seem to work as well as we'd like—usually because the vein clot is very large—and fragments of the clot continue to break off. In such cases, the surgeon may have to insert an umbrella-like filter into the large central vein in the abdomen. This traps any clots on their way from the legs and prevents them from reaching the lungs. Inserting this filter used to require an operation. Today it can be done by threading the device into the vein from a site in the groin. No big deal anymore.

WHAT TO INSIST ON IF YOU HAVE PHLEBITIS

Inflammation of a vein is called phlebitis. It develops most commonly in the legs. It can involve a superficial vein just under the skin that you can see and feel, or a deeper one. Injury to any vein as a result of intravenous drug usage or intravenous therapy in hospital can cause phlebitis. When phlebitis is accompanied by clot formation in the wall of the vein, it's called thrombophlebitis.

Phlebitis of the superficial and deep vein share the same causes. These include injury, prolonged bed rest, surgery, pregnancy, high-estrogen-content contraceptives (especially in women who smoke), malignancy and any disorder that alters the clotting mechanism of the blood.

Superficial phlebitis alone is easily treated with one of the nonsteroidal anti-inflammatory agents and carries little risk. You are advised to rest in bed for a day or two.

Deep vein phlebitis can be life threatening when clots from the affected veins travel to the lungs. This complication, called pulmonary embolism, is associated with a death rate of about 20 percent. *If this diagnosis is suspected, insist on a VQ scan of the lungs.*

Superficial and deep vein phlebitis often occur together. *That's why every case of superficial phlebitis should be checked for the possibility of deep vein involvement. Insist on it.* The best tests are a duplex ultrasound or an MRI.

The hallmark treatment of deep vein phlebitis is thinning of the blood (anticoagulation), which is usually continued for six months or longer after the phlebitis has subsided.

③②

PREMENSTRUAL SYNDROME

Madam President!

The constellation of symptoms that plagues women for about a week before "that time of the month" and eases up shortly after the menstrual flow begins is called premenstrual syndrome (PMS). Every premenopausal woman suffers from it—some more than others—but never when she's pregnant.

PMS has been described from time immemorial in virtually every culture. It has been used to demean and ridicule women and has resulted in a stereotype that has made it more difficult for them to achieve equality in the workplace. The unfortunate decision of the American Psychiatric Association in 1987 designating PMS a psychiatric disorder gave further credibility to the image of the periodically and predictably unstable and hysterical female.

PMS is most troublesome between the ages of thirty and forty-five, and the more children you've had, the more severe it's likely to be. It never occurs before menarche (the onset of menstruation), during pregnancy, or after menopause. PMS is estimated to affect 80 percent of all women, but I can't remember ever seeing a single one who didn't feel a little "different" during those few days before the onset of her period.

At least 150 kinds of symptoms of PMS, most of them behavioral, have been described over the years. Here's a typical scenario. A few days before her period, a woman may become depressed, moody, tense, angry, or just plain ornery. (That's why my male chauvinist friends worry about electing a female the nation's chief executive. "Imagine having her finger on the nuclear button when she's mad at the world!" A simplistic but common attitude.) She may lose interest in activities that she normally enjoys; she may not be able to concentrate, is worn out, and can't sleep. Physically, she may have aches and pains in her muscles and joints; she may feel bloated and gain some weight due to fluid retention; her breasts become swollen and tender, and chances are she'll have headaches too. For some reason, almost every woman I know who has PMS craves sweets during those few days, especially chocolate. In about 5 percent of cases, depression and/or rage is severe enough to interfere with everyday activities. These extreme cases are termed premenstrual dysphoric disorder (PDD).

In recent years the purely psychiatric view of PMS has lost ground among many doctors (including me). Women activists and many physicians have insisted all along that PMS is not a psychiatric disorder, but rather a transitional hormonal phenomenon. For years it was assumed that women with severe PMS secrete different concentrations of estrogen and progesterone than those who breeze through it. As a result, most therapies for PMS have until now focused on trying to modify these hormonal fluctuations by touching them up with a little more progesterone or estrogen. This approach has not really worked; neither have a host of nonhormonal therapies.

Now comes the big news from a recent landmark study of hundreds of women with PMS of varying severity—ranging from those with virtually no symptoms all the way to the most severely debilitating cases. *All were found to have similar estrogen and progesterone levels,* regardless of how bad their symptoms were. So every woman's hormonal profile changes in those few days before the onset of her period, those with bad PMS and those who barely have it. So if it's not the hormones that are the cause, what is? The brain! The hormonal fluctuations that *every* woman has, regardless of the severity of her PMS, triggers the brain to change its chemical profile at that particular time of the month. It's not clear exactly what happens in the brain during that last week of the menstrual cycle, but there is probably a reduction in the level of serotonin—an important mood-altering substance. As a result of this key observation, the emphasis on treating PMS has shifted away from hormonal manipulation to drugs that increase serotonin levels.

Lower serotonin concentrations in the brain may account not only for the behavioral changes of PMS but for the fluid retention, bloating, and weight gain as well. During those few days before the period begins, the adrenal glands that sit atop the kidneys probably make too much aldosterone, a hormone that causes the body to retain salt. Aldosterone production is under the control of the brain, so this is additional evidence of its influence in PMS. The craving for sweets probably reflects fluctuations in insulin production and sugar levels.

There are several other theories to explain why PMS is so debilitating in some women and not in others. These include genetic predisposition (because there is a higher incidence of PMS in identical than non-identical female twins); sexual abuse during childhood (I find it hard to believe that 80 percent of all women have been sexually abused); deficiency of vitamins or minerals (even in so affluent a nation as America?); just plain old-fashioned neurosis (nonsense!) I don't find any of these speculations as convincing as the brain link.

Treating PMS

There are almost as many remedies for PMS as there are symptoms. Some may ease your symptoms; most are placebos. However, there are a few measures that you should take in addition to whatever medications you try. For example:

- Regular aerobic exercise fits in very well with the current theory about the cause of PMS. Walking, jogging, swimming, or biking for twenty minutes to an hour a day five days a week alleviates PMS by stimulating the production of endorphins in the brain. These natural opiates affect behavior, and like serotonin, their production is decreased during the premenstrual phase.

- Cut down your salt intake, since increased amounts of aldosterone are already retaining salt; and salt holds on to water.

- Avoid concentrated sweets because they stimulate the pancreas to make more insulin that in turn causes the blood sugar to fall. A low blood sugar leaves you weak and dizzy. Forget about your usual three regular meals a day with nothing in between. Don't go for more than three hours without eating something. If you do, you will be too hungry to control your craving for sweets, especially chocolate. Have smaller meals and snacks five or six times a day. These should consist of complex carbohydrates such as bread, pasta, cereals, whole grains, fruits, leafy green vegetables, and potatoes. Complex carbohydrates are more slowly absorbed into the bloodstream than is glucose and so don't cause a reactive drop in blood sugar that stimulates insulin production. They may also increase the level of mood-elevating serotonin in the brain.

- Keep away from alcohol, tobacco, and caffeine (coffee, tea, soft drinks) for the duration. Caffeine stimulates the desire for sweets; more than three cups a day can make you nervous and aggravate your emotional symptoms. Alcohol can worsen mood swings, and as for tobacco— well, I don't think I even need to elaborate.

- Learn biofeedback and other stress reduction techniques such as the Relaxation Response (described in Dr. Herbert Benson's book of the same title), yoga, tai chi, and guided imagery. They all reduce stress, probably by increasing the depleted serotonin and endorphin levels.
- Some people with seasonal affective disorder (SAD) become depressed in the fall and winter when the days shorten and there is less exposure to natural light. There is some evidence that increased light also reduces symptoms of depression in PMS. Spend some time outdoors every day to get the needed light. Even if it's cloudy, you'll still be exposed to better light than you will be by staying indoors or shopping in a mall.

Specific Therapy for PMS

- Anything that helps the brain restore the chemicals it lacks improves the symptoms of PMS. That's why antidepressants (selective serotonin reuptake inhibitors, SSRIs) make such a great difference. I recommend Zoloft in a dosage of 50 to 250 mg a day; other doctors prefer 30 mg a day of Paxil or 20 mg of Prozac. However, the problem with the SSRIs, as effective as they are, is that they take time to build up in the bloodstream and so you've got to keep taking them throughout the cycle. Therapy for just a few days doesn't work in time. So they're good for women with severe PMS, especially those with PDD who are sick enough to need these drugs on an ongoing basis. But for those whose symptoms are mild, SSRIs are not a realistic answer.
- Antianxiety drugs such as Xanax (1 to 2 micrograms daily for six to fourteen days before the start of your period) or BuSpar (25 to 60 mg per day for twelve days) will make you feel better too.

- Try 50 to 250 mg a day of vitamin B_6 (pyridoxine) to increase brain serotonin levels. However not everyone benefits from it and higher doses can cause numbness and tingling of the hands and feet.
- Vitamin E supplements (400 to 800 IU per day) may reduce breast tenderness.
- Magnesium, sometimes called the antistress mineral, sometimes helps depression and fatigue. Doses up to 250 mg per day may also control the craving for sugar and ease breast tenderness.
- I recommend 1,500 mg per day of evening primrose oil to relieve mood swings, depression and irritability.
- NSAIDs improve muscle and joint aches and pains. They are available in several doses that you can buy without a doctor's prescription—Advil, Aleve, and Motrin. If you need something stronger, my preference is 500 mg of naproxen twice daily after meals.
- For troublesome bloating and fluid retention, I prescribe a mild diuretic such as 25 mg of hydrochlorothiazide for the few days it's needed.
- Some doctors recommend oral contraceptives, but I've never seen them work.
- Progesterone, estrogen's sister hormone, is popular with women who suffer from PMS. You can take it by mouth or as a vaginal suppository. There is no rationale for its use or any evidence that it has a beneficial effect. Neither do oral contraceptives.
- Danazol (Cyclomen, Danocrine) is sometimes prescribed for PMS, but I do not recommend it. It stops the pituitary gland in the brain from secreting gonadotropin, a hormone that in turn stimulates the ovary to make estrogen. Danazol is effective against endometriosis and reduces the discomfort of fibrocystic breast disease, but it doesn't work in PMS. Avoid it if you're pregnant or on birth control pills. Danazol also interacts with alcohol

and caffeine (which you should not be taking anyway when you're in the throes of PMS).

- An herbal remedy has received a favorable review in a recent report in the *British Medical Journal.* Extracts from the fruit of the "chaste tree" (*Vitex agnus-castus*), which grows in warm areas of Asia, Africa, and America, were found to improve symptoms of PMS in approximately half the women so treated. They were less irritable, had fewer headaches, were not as moody, and their breasts were not nearly as engorged. The active ingredients of the fruit include a mixture of iridoids and flavonoids that appear to have hormonal and neuroactive effects. Natives in the areas where the chaste tree grows have traditionally used these extracts for alleviating symptoms of PMS, but this is the first time that they have been scientifically evaluated. The authors of the study conclude that women suffering from PMS may safely try this preparation. It is available in health food stores.

WHAT TO INSIST ON IF YOU HAVE PMS

PMS affects virtually all women during their childbearing years, but it's most troublesome between the ages of thirty and forty-five. Long considered to be purely an emotional disorder, PMS now has been shown to result from an abnormal response of the brain to the normal hormonal fluctuations in the menstrual cycle. Exercise and the avoidance of salt, alcohol, tobacco, caffeine, and concentrated sweets may ease the symptoms.

The mainstays of therapy for severe PMS are antidepressants that restore levels of serotonin in the brain.

However, they must be taken all month, since a therapeutic level in the bloodstream is necessary for them to work. Antianxiety medications such as BuSpar and Xanax, on the other hand, can be taken while the symptoms are most troublesome and then stopped for the rest of the cycle. Vitamin and mineral supplements, notably B$_6$, E, and magnesium, are useful too. Hormones don't help. PMS disappears during pregnancy and after menopause.

Reject the stereotype of emotional instability because of the symptoms you develop those few days every month. *Insist on the prescriptions that help restore the brain serotonin levels that drop cyclically each month. Insist on your right to run for the White House.*

33

PSORIASIS

Itching to Be Cured

Psoriasis is a chronic skin condition that affects more than 2 percent of Americans. That adds up to millions of people with patches of skin that itch, burn, crack, sometimes bleed, and become discolored and infected. It's only a minor inconvenience for many; but is devastating for some. After all, who wants to dance cheek-to-cheek with a cheek that's sporting pimples, a rash, or a scaly eruption?

What Psoriasis Looks Like

The hallmark lesion of psoriasis is an easily recognizable plaque—a thick red patch of skin covered by large white or silvery scales. The scales flake off easily and when you remove them, the exposed skin bleeds. These plaques vary in size from very small to quite extensive, and can appear anywhere on the body. Although they are most common on the scalp, elbows, knees, and lower back, don't be surprised to find them on the face, palms, soles, chest, arms, legs, toenails, fingernails, between the buttocks, around the groin and genitals, and under the breasts. Psoriatic plaques often develop in the same place on both sides of the body. They usually itch (the word "psoriasis" comes from the Greek word for "itch") and rarely also burn. When they're located near a joint, they may crack and become painful. In approximately 5 percent of patients the joints themselves are inflamed and arthritic (psoriatic arthritis). The nails may develop tiny pits in them, and if more severely affected become loose and thicken or crumble. This manifestation is especially hard to treat. Psoriasis is an equal-opportunity disorder, striking men and women with the same frequency.

There are several different forms of psoriasis and they vary in location, size, and appearance. *Plaque psoriasis* is the most common type. It begins as little red bumps that grow bigger and then form scales. Although psoriasis usually spares kids, a special kind, *guttate psoriasis,* develops in children and young adults, usually after a streptococcal throat infection. Unlike the adult form, which usually begins in the teens and persists for life, guttate psoriasis clears up after a few months.

Psoriasis can be aggravated by stress (is there any disease that stress, tension, and anxiety do not worsen?); medication (beta-blockers, angiotensin-converting enzyme [ACE] inhibitors prescribed for heart problems, lithium and other antidepressant drugs, some nonsteroidal anti-inflammatory drugs); a local injury (new spots may appear within two weeks after the skin is cut, scratched, or sunburned); and in the wintertime, when the air is dry and there is less sunlight. Psoriasis can also improve dramatically and spontaneously, the most common example being during pregnancy—but it always recurs.

Psoriasis is not contagious; there's no way you can pass it on to anyone. Nor is there anything you can do to prevent it; you're either destined to get it or you're not. About one-third of cases are familial.

What Causes Psoriasis?

Scientists have found that inappropriate activity of a particular white blood cell, the T cell, triggers excessive skin cell reproduction. The rapidly growing cells pile up to form the psoriatic plaque.

Since a third of the cases appear to be inherited, researchers have been looking for a psoriasis gene. Although they haven't found it yet, now that the human genome has been mapped, its discovery is a real and foreseeable possibility.

Treatment of Psoriasis

There are many treatments for psoriasis. Some are time-consuming and inconvenient. The fact that there is no cure has led to a laissez-faire attitude among both patients and doctors, who take the position that you simply have to learn to live with psoriasis. Don't accept that advice. There are many different measures to control it, ranging from topical ointments to bathing in the waters of the Dead Sea.

There's no special diet for psoriasis, although most dermatologists will caution you about drinking too much. Eliminating gluten (present in wheat, oats, rye, and barley) improved some patients in one study. Don't wait for long-term studies to prove or refute this observation. Avoid gluten for a couple of weeks and see what happens.

I advise my patients (with and without psoriasis) to eat lots of fish. If you don't like fish or can't afford it, take between three and four grams of an omega-3 fatty acid supplement. Its anti-inflammatory effect may help the skin lesions.

Insist that your health plan grants you access to and continuing care by a skin specialist with expertise in psoriasis, preferably one who keeps up with the latest developments in this area, who is interested in the problem and views it as a challenge. Such a doctor is most likely to be aware of the clinical trials of new and promising treatments that are available. Psoriasis cannot be cured, but an informed doctor can help control it.

Currently, the goal of therapy is to reduce inflammation of the plaques and to stop their cells from dividing rapidly. The response to each of the following measures varies from patient to patient. Your doctor will prescribe what he or she thinks you're most likely to respond to, depending on your overall health status, age, and the severity of the condition.

If one approach doesn't help, go on to another—until you find the right one. Keep at it, because there *is* an optimal treatment or combination of therapies for *you*. The following list is long and varied, but one of these treatments will surely help you. I have divided them into three categories in the order in which you should try them, although they are often combined.

- Topical therapy (medications applied to the skin)
- Treatment with light (phototherapy)
- Oral medication (systemic therapy)

Topical Therapy

There are scores of ointments and creams from which you can choose. Some have been proved effective; others have only testimonial endorsements such as "Hey, remember George, the guy with the terrible psoriasis? Well, he took this secret formula, this Chinese herb, and he's cured!"

The problem with such anecdotes is that we don't know what George's diagnosis really was, what else he was doing that might have had an effect, and what the enthusiastic proponents mean by "cured." We also have no idea how many other Georges there are who didn't respond or were hurt by the "miracle drug." So don't put just anything on your skin because of sensational advertising. Let your doctor do the prescribing.

Here are some of the more widely used products applied to psoriatic skin:

- Moisturizers to loosen scales and control the itch. Try them before you resort to more potent topical agents. A warm bath to which you've added some oils, followed by a pleasant moisturizer can be very soothing. To help remove scales, soak for about fifteen minutes in water containing Epsom salts or Dead Sea salts.

- Topical corticosteroids usually improve psoriasis temporarily and sometimes are quite effective. The preparations vary in potency from high to medium to low. Use the weakest ones on the face, genitals, and groin; save the stronger ones for tougher skin on the palms, soles, knees, elbows and scalp. Betamethasone is especially effective on the scalp. (A mousse is preferable to lotion because it's evenly distributed throughout the scalp.) High-potency corticosteroids such as Temovate and Diprolene are often prescribed first for localized plaques, but they're also useful to treat an acute flare-up. However, these steroids should only be used intermittently because (a) they thin the skin (so don't apply them frequently to areas such as the face or your genitalia where the skin is delicate), and (b) they are absorbed by the body and can raise blood pressure, dilate the blood vessels, and lead to easy bruising. Most important, if you continue to use topical steroids, the psoriasis becomes resistant to them after a few months.

- Calcipotriene ointment (Dovonex), available only by prescription, is a synthetic form of vitamin D_3. (It also comes as a cream, which, though cosmetically more acceptable, doesn't work nearly as well as the ointment.) Try Dovonex if your psoriasis does not involve more than 20 percent of your body surface. Too much can raise the level of calcium in the blood with serious consequences. Also, some patients find it quite irritating; it can cause a rash of its own. (That's all you need with your psoriasis—another rash!) Don't apply it to your face or your genitals. Except for these limitations, Dovonex has a good track record. About 60 percent of patients respond well to it after four months, especially if they've been taking salicylic acid or a corticosteroid along with it. Don't confuse Dovonex with other vitamin D ointments that you can buy over-the-counter. The latter have absolutely no effect on psoriasis.

- Occasionally injecting steroids into a particularly nasty plaque that's not responding to other therapy is effective. But don't do this to multiple lesions and do not use oral steroids.

- Anthralin has been a mainstay in the treatment of psoriasis for more than a century. It works best for thick patches that are otherwise hard to treat. It can irritate normal skin near the plaques and it leaves a purple stain on anything with which it comes in contact—skin, towels, clothes, and bed sheets. (These stains wash off easily with cold water.) Anthralin is applied for ten to thirty minutes a day. Don't use it on inflamed areas.

- Coal tar has also been around for a least a hundred years. This old-timer comes in different strengths; the weaker ones are available over-the-counter, the others only by a prescription. You can use it on the skin, in the bath, or as a shampoo. Unfortunately, coal tar is messy, it smells, it stains, and strengths that are effective can also be irritating. To top it all off, its benefits are short-lived. It can be combined with topical steroids as well as with other forms of therapy such as ultraviolet B (UVB), described below.

- Tazarotene (Tazorac) is a retinoid (a vitamin A–related drug) that's fairly widely used for severe cases, alone or in combination with ultraviolet rays. It requires a prescription. Tazorac is a fast-drying clear gel that's somewhat less effective than the steroids. It's also irritating, dries the skin, lips, and eyes, and raises cholesterol levels (avoid it if you have heart disease or any vascular problems). It's better tolerated when taken together with a midpotency steroid cream. However, if you're of childbearing age, avoid it or take birth control pills, because it can harm the fetus.

- Salicylic acid is not usually used alone. When you have scales that need to be removed, salicylic acid can be combined with a topical steroid, coal tar, or anthralin.

Phototherapy

There are many ways to benefit from solar rays, both natural and artificial. Exposure to the sun for just a few minutes every day does wonders for psoriasis. A little goes a long way, so don't overdo it and get sunburned, because that damages the skin. If you live in a warm climate where there's lots of sun, your dermatologist can tailor a daily sunbathing regimen for you.

If short periods of solar exposure don't help, there are equally good artificial alternatives. Be very careful with them. You can't lie down under artificial sunlight for as long as you like!

The most beneficial rays of the sun are ultraviolet B (UVB). They are effective for moderate to severe psoriasis and used alone are safer than sunlight. They can be generated by artificial light boxes that selectively emit only this wave band. You can receive this treatment either in your doctor's office or, more usually, in a specialized center. However, if you live in a remote area and it's difficult for you to get to a clinic, buy one of these units, learn how to use it, and treat yourself at home under your doctor's supervision. Improperly used, these rays can damage the skin. A newer form of UVB treatment known as narrow band is now available. It contains the most effective wavelengths, and may be more effective than other forms of UVB therapy.

Although some specialists prescribe UVB as first-line therapy for psoriasis, most usually reserve it for tough-to-treat cases or for patients in whom the disease is extensive. You will usually need three treatments a week for two to three months. If the therapy is going well, the doctor may combine UVB wih calcipotriene. This combination yields better results than when the UVB is given alone or combined with coal tar baths and/or anthralin. Once your skin has cleared, you usually need to be "touched up" at intervals to maintain the remission. There are several such UVB treatments, each named after the doctor who pioneered it. The best known are the Ingram and Goeckerman techniques. The latter was developed in 1925 at the Mayo Clinic, where it is still being used, usually in combination with coal tar.

Ultraviolet A, another constituent of sunlight, is usually combined with an oral or topical antipsoriasis medication called psoralen, which leaves the skin more sensitive to the UVA. The combination of psoralen and UVA (called PUVA) is a good short-term therapy with quick results for moderate or severe psoriasis that has been resistant to other measures. It works in almost 90 percent of cases that have failed other treatment and is especially effective when topical calcipotriene is applied *after* each PUVA session. (Calcipotriene is inactivated by the UVA rays, so never apply it beforehand.) You'll need about twenty-five treatments over three months, followed by a maintenance program of about forty treatments a year. PUVA is not without side effects, and if you decide to undergo it, expect some nausea, headache, and fatigue. I don't recommend it for any length of time because it can age the skin, leave it freckled, and, most important, it can cause various cancers of the skin, including the lethal malignant melanoma.

Internal Medications

The worse your psoriasis, the more likely you are to need some form of medicine by mouth or by injection. The following drugs are part of your doctor's armamentarium:

- *Methotrexate,* used for years to treat various forms of cancer, is also helpful in rheumatoid arthritis and psoriasis in much lower doses than those required for malignancies— and with fewer side effects. In patients with psoriasis, it causes the immune system to slow the overproduction of T cells. However, even in these lower doses, methotrexate can damage the liver, affect the blood, and cause nausea, fatigue, loss of appetite, and occasionally mouth sores. Always take folic acid supplements with it, and never use it if you have underlying liver disease or are anemic. Also, women of childbearing age should not be on this drug, and neither should their partners.
- *Cyclosporine* is a well-known antirejection drug that has been used over the years for patients receiving organ transplants. In patients with psoriasis, cyclosporine acts like methotrexate, causing the immune system to slow the rapid turnover of skin cells. It is taken by mouth and is effective only as long as you continue treatment. It's really only used after other methods have failed. It can hurt the kidneys and raise blood pressure. Don't take it if you have a weak immune system that may not be able to bounce back after the cyclosporine is discontinued. Also, don't use cyclosporine if you're pregnant or breast-feeding, or if you have previously been treated with phototherapy.
- *Hydroxyurea* is an oral medication that is sometimes administered along with PUVA or UVB to potentiate their action. It's less toxic than methotrexate and cyclosporine, but it's also less powerful. It can affect the

blood and cause anemia. Don't take it if you're pregnant.

- *Retinoids* are vitamin A derivatives that, like cyclosporine, are last-resort drugs used only in cases resistant to other therapy. They can cause serious birth defects, so don't use them if you're pregnant now or can be in the future, and don't become pregnant for three years after you stop taking these drugs.
- Antibiotics are only used if the psoriasis plaques are infected.

Alternative Medicines

When confronted with diseases that modern, scientific methods can't cure, patients may turn to alternative therapy. So intense and widespread is the interest in these nonconventional approaches that a majority of American medical schools have incorporated integrative medicine into their curricula. That is not because they necessarily endorse it, but they are evaluating them, and preparing tomorrow's doctors to view them with an open mind.

Here are some of these preparations which even some conventional dermatologists have found helpful in treating psoriasis:

- Capsaicin (Zostrix), derived from hot peppers, has been so widely accepted that it no longer belongs in the alternative medicine category. When applied to the skin, it reduces superficial discomfort by acting on the nerves that transmit pain. It also eases itching and scaling. I routinely prescribe it to patients with shingles, painful arthritic joints, and diabetic neuropathy as well as psoriasis. Be sure not to apply it to broken skin, and wash your hands well after using it because it can be very irritating to the eyes, nose and mouth.

- A recent report from Pakistan claims that topical aloe can improve psoriasis. This herb has been around for thousands of years, but I'm not aware of any scientific confirmation of its efficacy in the treatment of burns and minor wounds, as is claimed by so many. However, as my mother would have said, "Harm it can't do you."

- Alternative practitioners swear by milk thistle's ability to improve liver function. Just ask Dr. Andrew Weill. Since there is a theory (never substantiated) that people with psoriasis have trouble clearing "toxins" from the body (toxins, by the way, that have never been identified), there are those who recommend milk thistle for psoriasis. I have not seen any convincing reports of its effectiveness for this purpose.

- Traditional Chinese medicine has a pharmacopoeia all its own with which I have little experience. Many of these preparations consist of mixture of herbs put together by Chinese practitioners. Let me warn you that you can't be sure how or when these herbs were grown, whether there were any pesticides used, or if they're contaminated. There have been reports of toxicity, notably kidney and liver failure, following their use.

- There are areas of the world where you can soak up the sun, bathe in mineral baths, and wallow in mud. The best place to do so, as far as psoriasis is concerned, is the Dead Sea. Some of my patients and many, many Israeli and Jordanian tourist agencies are convinced that a visit to the Dead Sea (on which both countries just happen to border) has salutary effects on psoriasis. As many as 88 percent of cases have been reported to show marked improvement and even complete clearing after such an interlude.

    There's no question in my mind after examining several of my own patients returning from spas located by the Dead Sea that for whatever reason, they often do improve dramatically. Unfortunately, the benefits are not

long-lived. If you can't go there (I am not aware of any third-party payer who will finance a trip to the Middle East for that purpose), the next best thing is to buy a variety of the salts, creams, ointments, and other therapeutic substances shipped by vendors in that area.

The Dead Sea regimen usually consists of gradually increasing exposure to the sun, up to a maximum of three hours a day, and bathing in its waters for an hour a day—all packaged in a nice stress-free vacation far away from home where you're waited on hand and foot.

Aside from the ambience, why does a visit to the Dead Sea work, even if only temporarily? First, there are the sun's rays. Since the area is twelve hundred feet below sea level, where the ozone layer is almost intact, solar rays are high in therapeutic UVA and low in the more powerful UVB. That's what makes it possible to sunbathe safely for many more hours. The water in the sea itself is rich in natural tars and minerals; the baths of dark mud help absorb UV light, and the mud packs themselves stimulate the circulation to arthritic joints.

WHAT TO INSIST ON IF YOU HAVE PSORIASIS

Psoriasis is a chronic skin condition that's probably due to malfunction of the immune system. Red patches with silvery white scales appear virtually anywhere on the body surface. They itch, burn, and hurt, and in a significant number of patients are associated with a form of arthritis (psoriatic arthritis). Most cases of psoriasis are mild and respond to a variety of topical preparations, some of which can be obtained over-the-counter. Such mild forms can be managed by well-trained family practitioners or internists. However, when the psori-

asis is severe and resistant to therapy, sophisticated treatment beyond the expertise of most general practitoners is required.

Combinations of topical medications, including steroids along with various forms of light therapy, as well as the drugs taken internally, require the expertise of a specialist. They are all potentially toxic. Since there is no cure for psoriasis, treatment must be ongoing and modified at frequent intervals. If you fall into that category, *insist on a specialist, in this case a dermatologist, to take charge of your case.*

There may be times when psoriasis becomes resistant to the less expensive therapies and a costly ultraviolet light regimen is required. *If that's what's needed, insist on it too.*

34

ROSACEA

Rembrandt Was Not a Drunkard

The next time you're in Washington, D.C., visit the National Gallery of Art and look for Rembrandt's self-portrait. He painted it in 1659 when he was fifty-three years old. You'll note that his face has a ruddy complexion, as if he'd been out in the sun for too long; there are several reddish blotches on his cheeks, chin, and forehead, and his nose is a red lump. He was clearly an alcoholic. Right? Wrong! Rembrandt was not a drinker. His appearance was due to rosacea, a skin disorder that's sometimes called adult acne. The credit for this observation and diagnosis on this famous artist belongs to Dr. Carlos Espinel, surprisingly not a dermatologist, but a cardiologist, at Georgetown University School of Medicine in Washington.

Even though it affects 5 percent of Americans, not many people are familiar with rosacea. For example, my wife and I attended a reception at Cornell University the other day in honor of a man who had given the school a large amount of money. He was unpretentious, self-made, and of Irish ancestry. As we toasted our benefactor, someone whispered in my ear, "Isn't it amazing that such a boozer has made so much money?"

"I didn't know he's a boozer," I replied. "He certainly isn't drinking tonight."

"You're obviously not wearing your doctor's hat," he retorted. "Look at the guy's nose! You can practically see the alcohol oozing out of it." With a laugh he downed the rest of his Scotch in one gulp and added, "It takes one to know one. He and I are both Irish."

My friend was right about our patron's Irish heritage, but he was wrong about the drinking. The guest of honor was, in fact, a teetotaler. I knew that because he was my patient. The amateur diagnostician by my side had made a very common error of mistaking rosacea for alcoholism. That is not to say that they can't coexist. Thirteen million people have rosacea and some of them probably do have a drinking problem, but the relationship is purely coincidental. The Irish connection, however, is real. A preponderance of rosacea patients in this country (39 percent in one survey) are of Celtic origin (Irish, Welsh, Highland Scottish), which is why this condition is sometimes referred to as "the Curse of the Celts"! However, English, eastern Europeans, and Scandinavians are also prone to it.

Although acne vulgaris, described in Chapter 1, and acne rosacea have very little in common, the distinction between them was not made until 1891. You may go through adolescence without even a blemish and then develop rosacea in your thirties, forties, or even fifties. Here's what it usually looks like: Early on, when you blush, there is a telltale redness on your cheeks, nose, forehead, neck, or chin, singly or in combination. Your eyes may also be bloodshot and feel irritated. At first this discoloration, which looks like you've been out in the sun too long (even if you haven't), comes and goes. However, in time it may become permanent. Later you might develop a network of tiny blood vessels in areas where you have the reddish hue. Unlike the acne of adolescence, there are usually no pimples, but when they do sometimes occur, they are almost always red; whiteheads and blackheads are rare. About 10 percent of patients whose rosacea is not treated develop the characteristic reddish nose that doctors call rhinophyma.

Although rosacea is most apparent on the face, it can also appear on the neck, shoulders, chest, and back. Ocular rosacea, which develops in about half of all rosacea patients, is characterized by inflammation of all parts of the eye—the iris, conjunctiva, and even the cornea. Indeed, corneal ulceration due to rosacea is a common cause of blindness.

With their red faces and bumpy noses, these individuals go through adult life wrongly tagged as alcoholics, a misperception that can hurt them socially and in the workplace. And it's understandable. Supposing you're an employer interviewing a job applicant. You know nothing about him, but he has red cheeks and a bulbous nose. The position is a sensitive, high level one. Unless you happen to be informed about rosacea, who could blame you for thinking twice about hiring him. You're not permitted to discriminate on the basis of age, gender, sexual orientation, race, or religion, but there's no law against not hiring alcoholics. In one survey of four hundred persons with rosacea, 35 percent stated that their skin condition was responsible for their not being hired in a new job or promoted in an old one; 70 percent said that they were embarrassed by their rosacea; 69 percent were frustrated by it; and 56 percent said rosacea had "robbed them of pleasure." To appreciate what living with rosacea can be like, read the biography of J. P. Morgan. He was one of the richest and most powerful men in the world, yet he felt that his rosacea appearance robbed him of much of the satisfaction and pleasure he might otherwise have enjoyed. Princess Diana also manifested rosacea, as does former president Clinton. When you look at Clinton's color photos, or when he appears on TV without makeup, his red nose is diagnostic.

Unlike acne vulgaris, in which an excess of androgens leads to an overproduction of oil and blockage of the sebaceous glands, the cause of rosacea remains a mystery. Al-

though it is more prevalent in women, it is usually more severe in men. That may be because women pay more attention to their appearance than do men, they see the doctor
sooner, and are apt to be treated early enough to slow the
progression of their rosacea. Genetic factors might play a role
since rosacea tends to occur more often among the fair-
skinned, and appears to run in families. But all rosacea suf-
ferers share one attribute—they blush very easily. This may
eventually dilate the blood vessels, causing permanent facial
discoloration.

If you have rosacea, anything that reddens your face will
intensify the symptoms. The most common triggers, all of
which you should avoid when possible, are:

- Hot liquids
- Caffeine
- Sunlight. (Always use sunscreen with an SPF of at least
  15 and preferably higher.)
- Wind
- Hot and cold temperatures, including hot baths
- Spicy foods, especially white and black pepper, hot red
  peppers, paprika, cayenne, oriental mustard sauce, spicy
  nachos, or salsa
- Alcohol
- Stress and embarrassment (easier said than done)
- Overheating—after a strenuous workout or in a steam
  room (worsened by high humidity)
- The hot flashes of menopause (which can be minimized
  by hormone replacement)

Treating Rosacea

Although you'll never grow out of your rosacea, and there's
no cure for it, your symptoms can be improved. Conversely,

they will usually worsen unless you're treated. In addition to avoiding the triggers listed above, and any others you may have identified in your particular case, the following therapy will help:

- Oral tetracycline, 250 milligrams every six hours for three to four weeks and then tapered, is the mainstay of treatment. (Your doctor may prefer a different dosage schedule). I prefer two related antibiotics, doxycycline or minocycline, 50 to 100 milligrams every twelve hours. They're easier on the gut than is tetracycline, and you don't have to take them on an empty stomach. If you can't tolerate any of these, erythromycin is also effective.
- Topical metronidazole (Flagyl) (also sometimes given by mouth), is effective.
- In 1998 the FDA approved Noritrate cream, the first prescription topical therapy for rosacea, applied once a day.
- If and when the dilated blood vessels become prominent and cosmetically embarrassing, they can be obliterated either by fine electric needles or by lasers.
- Avoid any topical preparations that contain alcohol, acetone, witch hazel, menthol, peppermint, eucalyptus oil, or clove oil
- Make sure that whatever you put on your face has "non-comedogenic" written on the label. That means it does not clog pores.
- Use a skin moisturizer every day during cold weather to protect against the drying effects of cold and wind.
- Cover your cheeks and nose with a scarf when you go outdoors in winter. Some of my patients even wear a ski mask. (One of them was viewed with some suspicion as he walked into a bank!)
- I advise my male patients to use an electric razor rather than a blade, and warn against applying any after-shave lotion that stings or burns.

- If you have heart disease, take the lowest possible dose of vasodilator drugs (Isordil, Imdur). They widen blood vessels on your face as well as those in your heart.
- Topical steroids aggravate rosacea over the long term but may be used to reduce redness and irritation twice a day for a week or so.
- Niacin, which effectively lowers cholesterol, usually causes a flush and aggravates rosacea. Use a statin drug instead.
- If you blush easily, clonidine can be useful. But this is a potent blood-pressure-lowering drug, so check it out with your doctor.

HERE'S WHAT TO INSIST ON IF YOU HAVE ROSACEA

Acne rosacea is a chronic skin disorder whose cause is not known. It results in a reddish discoloration of the face and upper body. It's appearance, especially when it involves the nose, falsely suggests alcoholism.

If you have symptoms associated with rosacea, *insist on an early consultation with a dermatologist*, who can prescribe the necessary oral antibiotics (tetracycline and erythromycin) and topical metronidazole (Flagyl) and other creams (Noritrate) to minimize the facial symptoms of this skin condition.

35

SEXUALLY TRANSMITTED DISEASES

How Do I Love Thee?
Let Me Count the Ways

When I was a teenager, the only venereal diseases we knew or cared about were gonorrhea ("a dose" or "the clap") and syphilis ("syph"). Even if we'd heard about the others, we would have assumed that Chlamydia is a girl's name, Herpes a Greek god, and Papilloma a popular Italian song. Even after I became a medical student some fifty years ago doctors were still focusing their attention on syphilis and gonorrhea, the big killers and cripplers at the time. There were as yet no antibiotics to cure them. The fear of syphilis was so great that to this day, even though it is no longer as major a health threat as some of the other infections, most states still require a test for syphilis before they will issue a marriage license. The other STDs were rare, considered to be esoteric, and were referred for treatment to specialists.

Venereal disease (VD), now termed "sexually transmitted disease" (STD), refers to any infection—bacterial, viral, or parasitic—that is transmitted primarily by sexual contact. Although the entry sites are most commonly oral, vaginal, penile, or anal, organisms can penetrate the body through a nonsexual route such as a cut or sore in the skin, and babies can be infected during the birth process.

One of every four people worldwide will one day contract an STD. Aside from AIDS, an estimated 56 million Americans already harbor at least one such infection, and millions more are newly infected every year.

There are some twenty-five different STDs, only a few of which you are ever likely to encounter or even hear about. Many are easily treated and cured; others can stay with you forever. Some cause only minor symptoms, but a few can result in severe illness, serious reproductive consequences, and death.

Here's an overview of the current STD picture in this country:

- Although the infection rates of syphilis and gonorrhea have been declining over the years, there are still over 1 million new cases of gonorrhea and 120,000 of syphilis reported annually (I can't even guess how many are not).
- Forty million people have chronic genital herpes, and there are 500,000 new cases each year.
- Four million men and women contract chlamydia annually in addition to the many millions who already have it, making it the number one STD in the United States.
- The human papilloma virus (HPV) that causes genital warts infects some 40 million American men and women, whose ranks are joined by 1 million new cases every year. Thirteen of the more than seventy types of HPV are present in virtually every cervical cancer and are presumed to cause it.
- There are between 100,000 and 200,000 new cases of hepatitis B every year, some of which end in cirrhosis and cancer of the liver.

- One million Americans are infected by the killer HIV/AIDS virus that strikes an additional 45,000 people in the United States every year.

The Keys to Controlling STDs

Prevention boils down to *everyone* practicing safe sex—heterosexuals, homosexuals, men and women of all ages, of every background, and all income groups. Because of their anatomy, women are more likely to become infected during unprotected sex than are men, but no one is immune. The only prevention that's 100 percent sure is total abstinence; your next best bet is *always* to use a condom—not just once in a while or when you think there is some risk, but every time you indulge—unless you and your partner are monogamous and not infected.

STDs can be transmitted in ways other than vaginal and anal sex, notably kissing, touching, and sharing needles. Condoms won't protect you in those situations.

All pregnant women should be tested for syphilis and hepatitis. (Many countries now vaccinate all women of childbearing age against hepatitis B. I believe the practice should be universal.) Those who test positive should enter a program to protect their infant. If there's any question of possible exposure, pregnant women should also be tested for gonorrhea, have a Pap test, and be offered an HIV exam. Some doctors recommend that women with recurrent genital herpes with sores have a cesarean section in order to protect their unborn child.

If you're hooked on drugs, remember how dangerous it is to share needles. Ask about rehabilitation programs in your area or those that provide clean needles.

A high index of suspicion. STD doesn't only happen to the other guy. If there is *any* possibility that you were infected in a relationship or encounter, inform your doctor and tell *all* your sex partners too. The sooner an STD is diagnosed, the greater the chances of curing it. Don't wait for symptoms; they may take a long time to show up. Even the tests for STD may not become positive for weeks after exposure. Delay means not only less of a chance of a cure for you but the possibility that you will go on infecting others.

The STDs You're Most Likely to Encounter

Chlamydia

Chlamydia is the most common STD in this country, and its numbers are continuing to rise. It's caused by a bacterium called *Chlamydia trachomatis* that infects both males and females during unprotected vaginal or anal sex. Any one of a number of antibiotics can cure chlamydia easily. The problem is that 70 percent of women and 30 percent of men infected with it have no symptoms and are unaware they have it, and continue to infect their sex partners. It's often only after they develop the complications of the disease that they learn they have it. By that time, females may have developed pelvic inflammatory disease with chronic, severe pelvic pain and a 20 percent chance of infertility and a 10 percent likelihood of having an ectopic pregnancy because the *Chlamydia* bug scars the fallopian tubes (an important cause of maternal mortality in this country). If a woman with untreated chlamydia does retain her pregnancy, her baby may be born prematurely, have a low birth weight, and develop pneumonia or conjunctivitis (a threat to vision later in life). Men with chronic chlamydia may develop ongoing infection of the urethra and swollen, tender testicles. Untreated, this can result in infertility.

Symptoms of chlamydia infection, when present, appear anywhere from one to three weeks after exposure. Women usually experience a yellowish-green vaginal discharge or bleeding, painful urination, pain and bleeding during inter-course, and chronic lower abdominal pain; men may develop a burning sensation when they urinate and a whitish mucoid discharge from the penis. The *Chlamydia* bacterium can cause an inflamed rectum and a sore throat from anal and oral sex.

It used to be more difficult to diagnose chlamydia. The older methods were expensive and complicated. Newer tech-niques, now available, are easier, faster, and cheaper, and your doctor can do them in the office as part of a routine checkup.

A single dose of azithromycin will cure chlamydia; so will a seven-day course of tetracycline, 500 milligrams four times a day, or 200 milligrams of doxycycline a day. (If you're preg-nant, avoid these latter two antibiotics because they can dis-color infants' teeth and cause growth problems later in life. Take azithromycin instead.) Continue the antibiotic for the prescribed length of time, even after your symptoms have ap-parently cleared, and be sure to see your doctor two weeks later to make sure you're no longer infected. Penicillin doesn't work.

Remember that gonorrhea, AIDS, herpes, and virtually every other STD can occur at the same time as chlamydia, so if you have it, you should be tested for the others.

Gonorrhea

The gonorrhea (Gc) is caused by a bacterium called *Neisseria gonorrhoeae* that's spread by unprotected oral, vaginal, or anal sex. Despite what some patients have insisted to me, you don't get gonorrhea from a wind that blew on your genitalia, or from lifting a piano, or even from the universally maligned toi-let seat. This little bug loves moisture and thrives in the vagina, penis, throat, rectum, and the eye. Gonorrhea is the only venereal disease that can be transmitted by eye contact. If you scratch your infected genital area and then rub your eye, you may develop ocular gonorrhea, which untreated can lead to blindness. Most cases, however, are spread between penis and vagina, mouth, and rectum as well as mouth to vagina and, rarely, mouth-to-mouth. Pregnant women can transmit it to their babies.

As is the case with chlamydia, Gc is not apparent in most infected women and 20 percent of men. So a woman who has had unprotected sex with an infected man should assume that she has contracted the disease. When symptoms do appear, anywhere from one day to two weeks after exposure, they consist in men of a yellowish pus-like discharge from the tip of the penis accompanied by burning and stinging during urination. Blood may be visible in the urine, the head of the penis may be inflamed and red, and the glands in the groin may swell. Women develop a cloudy vaginal discharge, irritation of the external genitalia, burning on urination, and irregular menstrual bleeding.

Gonorrhea never goes away until you're treated. Women eventually end up with pelvic inflammatory disease involving the fallopian tubes, uterus, and ovaries. Men can develop infection of the prostate gland and testicles. In men it can also result in a septic form of arthritis that affects only one joint, either the knee or the elbow.

Gonorrhea is easy to treat. Penicillin used to be the antibiotic of choice. I know men who would go to the nearest emergency room after a fling for a shot of penicillin just in case. That doesn't always work anymore because many strains of Gc have become resistant to penicillin. However, a wide range of antibiotics will still eradicate it. The most widely used currently, is a single injection of 250 mg of ceftriaxone or 500 mg of ciproafloxacin orally (but not in pregnant women or children). When Gc has spread, more vigorous prolonged treatment is required. Since chlamydia and Gc often coexist, the former should be treated at the same time (see above).

Syphilis

Although syphilis is now much less common than it used to be, there are still 120,000 new cases reported every year. It remains a treacherous infection because you may not know you have it and so can pass it along to others.

Primary syphilis begins as a painless sore at the site of infection (the sex organs or the mouth), and it's easily mistaken for a harmless cold sore. A high index of suspicion at this point can save your life, because after this initial warning, the *Treponema pallidum* that causes syphilis goes into hiding and may not make itself known for weeks or months. At that time it causes a rash anywhere in the body (secondary syphilis). If you don't think of syphilis now, and miss the diagnosis again, the third stage may not appear for years. In the tertiary stage the disease can kill or cripple you, striking anywhere—the heart, the brain, or any other vital organ. Syphilis can be diagnosed with a simple blood test and all three stages are treated with penicillin, the earlier the better.

Genital Herpes

Genital herpes was the big STD villain until AIDS came along. The infection is caused by one of two viruses, HSV-1 and HSV-2, but mostly the latter. Like so many others you may be infected and never know it, or you may develop painful bumps and sores at the site of infection days or weeks after exposure. You get herpes not only from oral, anal, or genital sex but also by touching a sore when there is a break in your skin, or by kissing. It's so benign an infection compared to some STDs that most people don't take it seriously anymore.

That's a mistake because herpes sores are not only painful, and annoying, but present serious problems to the newborn. The infection can flare up or recur at any time and there is no cure for it. The main fact to remember about herpes is that you can catch it or transmit it even when there are no visible lesions. Acyclovir and several other newer antiviral agents have made a big difference in the lives of those infected with herpes. They shorten the duration of the outbreak and reduce its severity when taken early enough, and also delay or prevent recurrences.

HPV

The human papilloma virus (HPV) causes a variety of warts in the genital and anal areas that may appear as soft, pink cauliflower-shaped lesions or hard smooth, yellow-gray ones. This virus attacks both men and women. The wart may be hard to find if it is hidden inside the folds of the vagina. Should HPV affect the cervix, it may lead to cervical cancer. Although there are several treatments for the warts themselves (lasers, freezing, burning), the infection itself cannot be cured and the warts may reappear at any time. Every woman should have an annual Pap test for the detection of early cervical cancer, especially if she has genital warts.

Hepatitis B

Hepatitis B is a viral infection of the liver that strikes at least 300,000 Americans every year. The B virus is one hundred times more infectious than the HIV that causes AIDS; both are spread primarily via infected blood. But there is one big difference: hepatitis B can be prevented by a vaccine, and AIDS cannot. It is the only STD for which there is a vaccine. I recommend it to most of my patients, especially those who are health-care workers or who are vulnerable because of their sexual lifestyle. There is no treatment for acute hepatitis B other than rest. However, the chronic form that causes liver disease, cirrhosis, and cancer in some patients may respond to interferon. (See Chapter 18.)

Trichomoniasis

Trichomoniasis ("trich") is a common, nonlife threatening STD caused by a protozoan organism called *Trichmonas vaginalis*. It affects 2 to 3 million people every year. Many of them have no symptoms; others experience burning on urination, vaginal discharge, abdominal pain, or painful intercourse. Both sex partners should be treated, even if only one is known to be infected. A single dose of Flagyl will often do the trick on the trich.

HIV/AIDS

HIV/AIDS is the deadliest of all the STDs and there is currently no cure for it. Most of those infected will eventually die as a result of the failure of their immune system, which is attacked and compromised by the HIV virus. The result is a loss of resistance and infections such as pneumonia, fungal diseases, and malignancies. Symptoms of AIDS may not appear for months or years after infection, during which time the disease is progressing. There are many new treatments that can delay death and improve the quality of life. If you test positive for HIV, *insist on a consultation with a specialist* to decide when the drugs, notably the protease inhibitors, should be started. (You will find a more detailed description of AIDS in Chapter 2.)

HERE'S WHAT TO INSIST ON IF YOU HAVE A SEXUALLY TRANSMITTED DISEASE

Remember that many sexually transmitted diseases exist together; infection with one means that you might have others. The diagnosis of any STD makes it imperative to search for the others, especially HIV. *Insist on having all the necessary tests.*

36

SHINGLES

Not the Kind You Hang Out

Most bacteria, viruses, and other infectious nemeses of mankind play by the rules. After your immune system finally defeats them, with or without the help of an antibiotic or two, they pack up and leave. Not so the varicella-zoster virus (VZV) that causes chickenpox. This virus usually attacks little children. And as if that weren't shameful enough, after it's had its fun with them, making them miserable for days, covering them with ugly little sores and blisters, VZV doesn't just go away. Secure in the knowledge that for the moment it is invulnerable, that no antibiotic can destroy it, it takes up permanent residence in that same poor kid's body. It migrates from the sores on the skin along nerve pathways to ganglia (nerve centers) alongside the spinal cord. In most cases, the virus spends the rest of its life asleep, in retirement, in its new home and does not cause any further trouble. However, in about 20 percent of its hosts (usually those who have an impaired immune system or are elderly), it "wakes up." Ungrateful for the hospitality that its victim has provided over the years, it retraces its steps down the nerve pathways it ascended years ago. Once again, it causes pain and blisters on the skin, but this time with an even greater vengeance. We don't call this new illness chicken pox. Its new name is *shingles.*

The Shingles Attack

Here's a typical shingles scenario: You wake up one morning with a burning or shooting pain, or numbness, tingling, or itching, in some part of your body—the trunk, back, chest, face, spine, neck, near an eye or an ear—but *only on one side.* You may also feel like you have the flu, with headache, a little fever, even chills and nausea. But the characteristic feature is the localized "sensation" some place where you have not hurt yourself, been scratched, or been burned. Strangely enough, there's nothing to see on the skin. *Serious pain or other unpleasant sensations on your skin without a visible rash and in the absence of a prior injury are the tip-off to shingles.*

Once you suspect shingles, keep a close eye on the affected area. A red telltale, painful rash will appear within a few days, sometimes later. A band or cluster of these "pimples" emerges on the side of the body where you felt the original symptoms. *It virtually never crosses midline.* Within a couple of days, the rash evolves into fluid-filled blisters that dry up and fall off during the next two to four weeks. (If you start treatment with an antiviral medication in time, they will clear up in a week or so.)

Keep the blisters clean. Unless you do, they can become infected. As soon as the rash appears, and preferably before it does, *call your doctor* if you suspect shingles. The sooner treatment is started, certainly within seventy-two hours of the appearance of the rash, the better the results. There are occasional cases of shingles in which the rash never develops and in persons with a severely compromised immune system, the rash may occasionally appear on both sides. However, from a practical point of view, stick with the "one-sided rash" characteristic.

I can't imagine anyone missing the diagnosis of shingles if they're aware of its typical symptoms. Sometimes, however, patients insist that their rash couldn't be shingles because they never had chicken pox. Of course, they have; they just don't remember. It may have been a very mild case, or the disease was not diagnosed. *There's no way to get shingles without having been previously infected* with varicella virus.

If you don't think of "shingles," you may blame the pain and rash on an insect bite, a drug reaction, a fungus of some kind, or some injury of which you were not aware. I have seen cases in which the pain preceding the rash was in the chest, and so severe that the patients thought it was due to a heart attack or pleurisy. In the legs they suspected phlebitis; in the belly they worried about appendicitis or an ulcer.

There is a test your doctor can do in the unlikely event that there is any doubt about the diagnosis. It's call the Tzanck test, and involves scraping one of the blisters, staining it with a special dye, and looking at it under the microscope for the presence of typical cells of a herpes virus infection. It's rarely done.

Can you "catch" shingles? No. Even if you touch one of the weeping blisters? Still no. Can you get shingles from someone with chicken pox? No. There is no direct route from someone else's chicken pox to your shingles. You must have had chicken pox first. If you've never had chicken pox and come in contact with the shingles rash, you can still get chicken pox—but never shingles.

How to Treat Your Shingles—the Seventy-Two Hour Window

The moment you know (or have good reason to suspect) that you have shingles, start therapy. Better safe than sorry. Unless you do, you may be in for a long haul of pain and suffering. If you start taking the right medication and you turn out not to have shingles, you've lost nothing. The therapy is neither difficult nor toxic. *If shingles affects your forehead or your eye, insist on seeing an ophthalmologist.* Shingles in this location can leave you blind.

Until just a few years ago, all your doctor could do for shingles was to prescribe some ointments and painkillers. If things got really bad, you'd then be given steroids. Although steroids are sometimes still used in patients who are not responding well to the newer agents, there is no evidence that they are of any real benefit.

The introduction of specific antiviral drugs has changed the course of shingles and the long-term outlook. These agents don't kill the virus, but they prevent it from reproducing by inhibiting one of its DNA enzymes. Stunting viral replication in this way reduces pain, shortens the duration of symptoms, and improves the long-term outlook.

The fact that the new shingles treatment works is common knowledge among doctors. Nevertheless, the shocking fact is that fewer than 50 percent of patients with shingles see a doctor within the optimal seventy-two hour window of opportunity.

The most widely used drugs to treat shingles are acyclovir (Zovirax), the first one on the market, valacyclovir (Valtrex), and famcyclovir (Famvir). They all shorten the course of the disease and reduce the occurence of its most common complication, postherpetic neuralgia (PHN) described below. Acyclovir is taken orally in a dose of 800 mg five times a day for seven to ten days; famcyclovir, 500 mg three times a day for seven days; and valacyclovir, one gram (1,000 mg) three times a day for seven days. In severe cases these drugs are administered intravenously. They're all effective when started no later than seventy-two hours after the first blisters appear (but the earlier the better). I prefer famcyclovir and valacyclovir because they seem more effectively to reduce the duration and severity of PHN.

Whatever drug you use should be continued until all the blisters have completely healed. That's rarely longer than seven to ten days. These medications are safe, but you should take them in lower doses if you have any kidney problems. Keep the blisters covered and don't expose them to direct sun. Avoid hot showers. Wash only with mild soaps or soap-free cleansers such as Cetaphil and Aveeno. If the blisters become infected, apply a topical antibiotic ointment or cream. Cool, wet compresses of tap water, baking soda, or Burow's solution will relieve the symptoms, as will calamine lotion. If the blisters itch when drying up, try a mild over-the-counter oral antihistamine.

There is no reason not to use a topical preparation along with the oral drugs. Your pharmacist can make one up for you that contains camphor and menthol.

Postherpetic neuralgia (PHN)

Postherpetic neuralgia (PHN)—persistence of severe pain for months and occasionally years after the rash and other symptoms have disappeared—is the most dreaded complication of shingles. It is the result of injury to the nerves by the zoster virus, and develops in about 15 percent of cases overall. However, the incidence reaches 50 percent after age sixty. And the older you are, the longer it lasts. At age seventy-five half the patients with PHN still have pain a year after their shingles started. Such patients are often depressed (and for good reason); they find it hard to maintain social contacts because of their suffering, and some have taken their lives. Although the shingles rash clears up completely even if you do nothing, you run a higher risk not only of PHN but also of neurological complications if the virus attacks an eye or an ear.

The pain itself can be burning, aching, stabbing, or come in bursts. No matter how you describe it, it hurts—bad. The involved area is so sensitive that even a mild breeze or the pressure of a bed sheet can be uncomfortable. You're especially prone to PHN if your shingles affects your forehead or eyes (ophthalmic shingles).

Once you have PHN, it's too late for the antivirals; you need painkillers. First try one of the nonsteroidal anti-inflammatory drugs that are available without a prescription. You can move on to stronger ones if necessary. The next level of pain control is a tricyclic antidepressant such as amitripty-line. Start with a low dose such as 25 mg three times a day and increase it over time to a total dose of 75 mg four times a day. These drugs work by blocking serotonin and adrena-line uptake in the brain and they are usually well-tolerated. However, they can cause cardiac arrhythmias, low blood pres-sure, glaucoma, constipation, and urinary retention in older men. I do not prescribe them to anyone with heart trouble. You can also apply a patch impregnated with the local anes-thetic lidocaine to the affected area of the skin. It's marketed as Lidoderm. I have had success with topical capsaicin cream (Zostrix), although it can cause allergic contact dermatitis, but don't use it while the blisters are still present. You might also try transcutaneous electrical nerve stimulation (TENS), acupuncture, behavioral modification such as biofeedback, and, if necessary, nerve blocks of the affected area. The "lat-est" treatment of which I am aware is something that's been around for thousands of years—honeybee venom! When in-jected directly into the pain sites, it has been shown to afford significant relief throughout a two-year follow-up. It's worth asking about. Most patients require some narcotic analgesia to control their pain.

Unlike other viral illnesses such as the various types of hep-atitis, you *can* get shingles more than once. Up to 5 percent of cases recur. Interestingly, the next time around, the rash does not necessarily appear in the same location as the first one. If you're getting one attack after another, some other her-pes virus may be the culprit, and not the VZV of shingles.

The Chicken Pox Vaccine

A varicella (chicken pox) virus vaccine has been approved for use in healthy children between the ages of twelve months and twelve years. I recommend that kids receive it between ages twelve and eighteen months at the same time as they are given their MMR shot (mumps, measles, Rubella) but in a different syringe and not in the same area. Also, since at least 95 percent of Americans have had chicken pox, I suggest that if you're among the few who haven't, you, too, should be vaccinated, especially if your immune system isn't up to handling this infection. In any event, it will allow you to play with your children and grandchildren who have chicken pox without catching it yourself. This infection is not a great threat to children, but it can be serious in adults.

There are some very vocal opponents to all vaccines, including that against chicken pox. Although most of the medical profession, including myself, does not agree with their objections, I respect their sincerity. In every medication, and indeed in every vaccine, there is a little poison. We must continue to search for safer vaccines. However, the final decision as to whether or not to use a particular vaccine depends on the risk-benefit ratio. For all the reasons that I have mentioned, I believe that on balance, the varicella vaccine is worth having. Although the shot can cause temporary pain and redness, the number of serious side effects has been minimal. During the first twelve months after the vaccine became available, there were 2.3 million shots administered and only a handful of serious medical events were reported, including four cases of encephalitis. However, a causal relationship between the vaccine and these adverse effects was never proved.

WHAT TO INSIST ON IF YOU HAVE SHINGLES

If you've ever had chicken pox, you're a candidate for shingles. Ten to 20 percent of the population will develop it some time in their lives; there are an estimated 600,000 to one million new cases every year. Although you can get shingles at any age, it's most common after fifty, especially if your immune system is impaired by chronic disease such as AIDS or TB, or you're receiving chemotherapy, radiation, or cortisone-type drugs, or are under great physical or emotional stress. The older you are, the more severe the symptoms and the longer they'll last.

VZV has been plaguing mankind since time immemorial, but its heady, carefree days may be numbered. The new safe and effective vaccine against chicken pox means that more kids may become immune to and never get this infection. The VZV will have nowhere to go; no chicken pox means no shingles. There's even hope for the millions of adults who are already harboring this virus. Studies are under way to see whether giving them vaccine will boost their immunity to VZV and prevent shingles.

If you're given the choice as to whether or not to vaccinate your infant, *insist on having it done.*

If you're at high risk because your immune system has been compromised by a serious chronic illness, *and you did not have chicken pox as a child*, ask for the vaccine. Do not be dissuaded because you are an adult. *Insist.*

Even if you only *think* you're developing shingles, based on the symptoms I have described, *call your doctor immediately.* The newer antiviral drugs prevent lots of suffering, and can even save your life. But there is a seventy-two hour window during which you must act. Do not accept an appointment several days later because "It's only a rash and the doctor is tied up with critical cases." You must be seen right away. *Insist.*

There are at least three effective antivirals available. The oldest one, acyclovir (Zovirax), still works. However, famciclovir (Famvir) and valacyclovir (Valtrex) have a better track record in lessening the chances of your developing postherpetic neuralgia, the dreaded complication of shingles. They are expensive but don't settle for anything but the best. *Insist on it.*

If the shingles virus affects an eye or your forehead, ask for a consultation with an eye specialist. Don't be deterred by "We can handle this ourselves." Ocular shingles can lead to blindness. *Insist on seeing a specialist.*

③⑦

STROKE

A Brain Attack by Any Other Name

Stroke is the third leading cause of death in this country. (Heart disease is first, and all cancers combined are second.) Some 600,000 Americans are stricken each year, and 160,000 die. (The death rate is significantly higher in African Americans than it is in whites.) Among stroke victims who survive, 70 percent have some residual disability—physical and/or mental. Although the risk of stroke does increase with age, don't get the idea that it occurs only in the elderly. Almost 30 percent of these patients are under the age of sixty-five.

To "stroke" is "to touch lightly and with affection"— certainly a misnomer for the subject of this chapter. Most every one knows that a heart attack occurs when a coronary artery in the heart suddenly closes, depriving a portion of the heart muscle of its life-sustaining oxygen. That's also what happens in a stroke, except that the diseased artery is in the brain, not the heart. I read the other day that in one survey of patients hospitalized because of a stroke, nearly 50 percent were unaware of the diagnosis; 10 percent thought they'd had a heart attack; the other 40 percent had no clue whatsoever why they were there!

When cardiac muscle is destroyed, the heart doesn't pump

blood efficiently, and its beat may become weak and irregular. By contrast, when brain tissue dies, a wide variety of the bodily functions it controls are affected. There is another major difference between a heart attack and a stroke. In the heart, interruption of the blood supply is almost always due to arterial obstruction. By contrast, a stroke may occur not only when blood vessels in the brain are blocked but also when they rupture and hemorrhage into the cerebral tissue.

The Different Causes of Stroke

Arteriosclerosis (hardening of the arteries) is the chief cause of stroke. Over the years, plaques form within the arteries of the brain just as they do in the heart and elsewhere in the body. When these plaques become big enough, blood flow through the vessel is progressively reduced. The obstruction becomes complete when a thrombus (clot) forms at the site of the plaque. When that happens, the area of the brain nourished by the involved artery is damaged or dies.

A stroke can also occur when the *carotid arteries* in the neck close, shutting off the blood supply to the brain.

A third mechanism can suddenly deprive the brain of blood. A small *clot* originating elsewhere in the body can travel through the body to an artery within the brain, occluding it. The heart is the most common source of these clots (embolic), especially when the cardiac rhythm is very irregular, a condition called *atrial fibrillation* (2 million Americans have this disorder: see Chapter 6). A fibrillating heart does not expel all its blood when it contracts. What's left behind stagnates and forms clots that are squeezed out during a cardiac contraction. Pieces of plaque from the carotid arteries in the neck can also break off, travel "north," and clog a critical vessel in the brain. These various mechanisms by which the blood supply to the brain is blocked (ischemic strokes) account for approximately 80 percent of brain attacks.

The remaining 20 percent of strokes occur when a blood vessel ruptures and bleeds into the brain. This happens after the artery's walls have been weakened by long-standing uncontrolled high blood pressure, or from a head injury, or because of a congenital aneurysm. (An aneurysm is the result of a structural weakness of an artery and can burst at any time. Unfortunately, such aneurysms are not usually detected while they are still intact.) An arterial rupture can occur in the interior of the brain or on its surface. In the latter case, blood collects in the space between the brain and the skull (subarachnoid hemorrhage).

Regardless of how the stroke came about, the brain cells die minutes after being deprived of their oxygen supply. The resulting symptoms depend on the location of the damage within the brain and the bodily function it controls. So a stroke may cause paralysis, visual problems, speech impairment, behavioral changes—indeed anything that depends on a normally functioning brain.

Whether and how well you recover from a stroke depends on the size of the artery involved and its location. A small artery may leave you without any residual symptoms; a large one, critically situated, can cause death or paralysis.

When discussing the subject of stroke, there are four main considerations. How to:

- Prevent it
- Recognize its earliest symptoms
- Treat it
- Deal with its consequences

How to Prevent a Stroke

You can reduce your chances of having a stroke by controlling or eliminating its risk factors. Here are some of the more important ones that you *can* do something about:

- *High blood pressure.* This is the single most common cause of stroke. Untreated hypertension leaves you four to six times more likely to have a stroke by virtue of two mechanisms: It weakens the walls of the arteries in the brain, and it speeds up the formation of arteriosclerotic plaques within them. Hypertension is also very treacherous because it's silent. You can go for years with high blood pressure and not know it until it's too late. (See Chapter 19.)

  The best way to protect yourself against a stroke is to have your pressure checked regularly. If it's high (the diastolic pressure is the lower half of the fraction and should not exceed 85; the top figure—systolic pressure—should be less than 140), do whatever is necessary to lower it. That requires a combination of steps: weight loss (if needed), regular exercise, reducing your salt intake (this applies to some people but not to everyone), and—when the other steps aren't enough—medication. (But even if you end up requiring a blood-pressure-lowering drug, the thinner you are and the more you exercise, the less of it you'll require.) Remember this about blood-pressure-lowering medications: They do not inevitably cause side effects. The early drugs years ago did produce a wide variety of side effects, ranging from weakness to impotence. These days, however, an experienced physician can almost always normalize your pressure without any significant toxicity. So there's no reason for you to be walking around with untreated hypertension.

- *Tobacco*. Stroke is yet another hazard of smoking, presumably because of carbon monoxide and other toxic ingredients. Women who take the Pill and smoke are especially vulnerable to stroke.
- *Transient ischemic attack* (TIA). As you will read below, once you've had such a ministroke, you're in great danger of being felled by a full-blown one. You can greatly reduce this risk by taking one of several blood thinners, ranging from aspirin to warfarin (Coumadin).
- *Too much alcohol*. Booze in moderation protects against heart and brain attacks, but having more than two drinks a day increases the risk of stroke, presumably by raising blood pressure.
- *Drug abuse*. Cocaine has been strongly implicated in both heart and brain attacks.
- *Abnormal blood fats* such as high cholesterol promote hardening of the arteries everywhere in the body. Keeping them as close to normal as possible by means of diet or using one of the statins or some other drug reduces the risk of stroke (as well as heart attack).
- *Overweight*. Obesity predisposes to diabetes, coronary disease, and high blood pressure—all of which are important risk factors for vascular disease and stroke. However, it also leaves you more vulnerable to a brain attack in its own right.
- *Lack of exercise*. Regular physical activity at any age lowers the risk of stroke. We used to think that this required a really exhausting, sweat-producing workout, the kind that leaves you with the agonized expression seen on the faces of people running in the park. All you need to do is walk at a comfortable pace for thirty minutes three or four times a week.
- *Estrogen replacement* in postmenopausal women is believed to reduce the risk of stroke, but this observation has recently been questioned.

- A recent study of 6,000 patients in Europe, Asia, and Australia apparently yielded "phenomenal results" according to the British Stroke Association. Individuals with hypertension who were given a combination of ACE inhibitor and a diuretic benefitted from a 28 percent reduction in all types of stroke. This combination not only reduced the number of strokes, but when they did occur they were less serious, with fewer instances of disability and dementia.

Unfortunately, there are other risk factors that you can't do anything about. But if you have them, you should pay more attention to those that you can modify. Here are the more important ones:

- *Age.* The older you are, the greater your vulnerability. The incidence of stroke doubles every decade after fifty-five.
- *Gender.* Men have an almost 20 percent greater risk of stroke than women (although more women die from it).
- *Race.* African Americans and Hispanics suffer twice as many strokes as do Caucasians, presumably because they are more prone to high blood pressure. What this means is that African Americans and Hispanics need more frequent screening, more careful monitoring, and more effective therapy.
- *Diabetes.* The more poorly controlled the disease, the greater the likelihood of vascular disease and stroke (especially if you also have high blood pressure).
- *Your genes.* If other close family members have had strokes, you're more likely to have one too. But there is more to it than just genes. Family members usually share important modifiable risk factors. So don't let your family history leave you with a nihilistic attitude. Enjoy yourself, by all means, but pay special attention to any correctable risk factors such as smoking, lack of exer-

cise, high blood pressure, and elevated cholesterol level. This will make your genetic "inevitability" a lot less likely.

Risk factors are only a general indicator of vulnerability. However, there is one specific way you can determine whether you are a stroke candidate in the forseeable future even if you haven't had any warning symptoms. A noninvasive sonogram of the carotid arteries in the neck measures their thickness (and therefore the degree of arteriosclerosis). In a recent study of almost 4,500 men and women aged sixty-five and older, those with the thickest arteries had almost five times the incidence of stroke or heart attack than did those with the thinnest walls. When the sonogram detects a partial blockage of the carotids, removing it surgically may sometimes avert a stroke.

Recognizing the Symptoms

It's critical for you to recognize the earliest symptoms of a stroke. Brain damage occurs quickly, and modern treatment, *if started early enough,* can mean the difference between life and death, and whether there is normal function after the stroke or permanent disabilities. Here's what to look for:

- *Sudden* onset of numbness or weakness in your face, arm, or leg, usually on one side of the body
- *Sudden* confusion, and trouble speaking or understanding what's going on around you
- *Sudden* double vision, or trouble seeing out of one or both eyes
- *Sudden* difficulty in walking, trouble with balance or co-ordination, or dizziness
- *Sudden* severe and unexplained headache

Notice that all these symptoms begin suddenly. Unlike a heart attack, which may give warning symptoms such as gradually increasing angina for weeks, a stroke strikes abruptly; you're fine one minute and sick the next. Sometimes symptoms such as double vision or weakness of an arm or leg clear up in a few minutes. If they do, you're still not out of the woods, for then you're probably having a transient ischemic attack (TIA) or what some doctors call a ministroke. This is potentially serious because unless you do something to prevent a recurrence, there's a one in three chance that the next TIA will be followed by a full-blown stroke. If you've had more than one TIA, you're at ten times the risk for stroke anytime in the future.

What to Do If You Suspect a Stroke

It's extremely important to recognize the symptoms *and act immediately. Time is of the essence!* If you suspect that you might be having a stroke (remember, you don't have to be sure; it's better to be safe than sorry) take an aspirin (I advise my adult patients always to carry a couple of 81 mg aspirin in their pockets; it's useful as the initial treatment for both heart attacks and strokes), then call an ambulance or have someone get you to the emergency room of the nearest hospital as quickly as possible. Don't try to drive or get there by yourself, your symptoms can worsen rapidly. When you arrive in the ER, ask someone to notify your own doctor.

In the Emergency Room

You will not (or should not) be kept waiting when you reach the emergency room. Anyone suspected of having a stroke or a heart attack goes to the head of the line. (The bone fractures can wait!) The doctor will perform a focused neurological exam, which, at least initially, consists of looking at you, evaluating how you walk and talk, in order to determine whether you in fact are having a stroke. The next decision is whether it's due to a blockage or a bleed. That's crucial to know because thinning the blood when there's a clot can save your life; it can kill you if you're already bleeding! (Taking aspirin as soon as symptoms appear is safe in the long run because bleeding is much less common than an obstructive stroke.)

The doctor's impression as to whether your stroke is due to clot or hemorrhage must be confirmed before any therapy is started. This is done quickly by means of one of the following:

- CT scan, usually the first test done in the ER to distinguish between a clot and a bleed. The brain is visualized through low-dose X rays.
- Magnetic resonance imaging (MRI) of the brain, a more sophisticated procedure that yields more information about the extent of the damage and its location within the brain.
- Magnetic resonance angiography (MRA), also noninvasive, provides information about the arteries inside the brain.
- Carotid duplex scanning generates sound waves that diagnose blockage in the carotid arteries in the neck.
- PET (positron emission tomography) scanning evaluates brain metabolism and reveals how much of the injured area of the brain is still functioning.

If a clot is diagnosed by whatever test is used, you will be given a clot-dissolving drug such as tPA. It is most effective within three hours after the onset of your symptoms. This breakthrough therapy, the same drug that's used to treat fresh heart attacks, will reduce the amount of damage to your brain. In one study of more than six hundred stroke patients, those who received tPA were 50 percent less likely to end up permanently disabled.

If the cause of the stroke is a clot within a carotid artery, you will be treated with blood thinner or by a "ballooning" of the vessel. A stent (similar to what is done in diseased coronary arteries) may also be inserted, but this is still experimental, or the clot is surgically removed.

If you're found to have atrial fibrillation, the risk of another stroke can be reduced by anticoagulation. You may be given a heparin-type drug injection, which thins the blood quickly, as well as warfarin, a longer-acting oral preparation.

If there has been a bleed in the brain, your doctor may give you medication to reduce the pressure of the blood within it, or even perform a lifesaving operation.

Some centers are conducting clinical trials with hypothermia in stroke patients. The body temperature is reduced for a twenty-four-hour period to between 89 and 91 degrees Fahrenheit. Initial results are encouraging and suggest that such therapy reduces brain damage.

After the Stroke

If your stroke was due to a clot, you should be treated long-term to prevent another one from forming. Your doctor will choose among aspirin or some other drug such as Plavix, Aggrenox (a combination of aspirin and extended-release dipyridamole marketed alone as Persantine), or a full-fledged blood thinner (anticoagulant) such as warfarin (Coumadin). Aspirin and dipyridamole both prevent clot formation by acting on platelets in the blood, but they do so in different ways. Although Plavix can on rare occasions cause serious abnormalities in the blood, it is generally safe and effective. Citicoline is a new drug being used in some centers in the belief (and hope) that it may restore function in some damaged brain cells. It's too early to assess its effect, but if you're offered it as part of a clinical trial, I would be inclined to accept it, although I have no personal experience with it.

When newer techniques in physiotherapy are begun in time, they can reduce the likelihood of long-term complications such as paralysis. If you have weakness of an arm or leg, *insist on being referred to a rehabilitation facility for intensive treatment.*

WHAT TO INSIST ON IF YOU HAVE A STROKE

Stroke leads to brain injury due to interruption of blood flow to the brain. This can result from a clot or hemorrhage. The key to dealing with stroke is to know its risk factors, to control them as soon as you've identified them, to recognize the acute symptoms, and to receive treatment immediately. Unlike yesteryear, a stroke no longer means inevitable and permanent paralysis or death.

If you go to the emergency room with symptoms of a stroke, *insist on an immediate CT scan of the brain.* If the diagnosis is confirmed, and the stroke is found to be due to a clot, *insist on a clot-dissolving drug.*

If you've been left with residual symptoms such as paralysis or weakness of an arm or leg, or speech difficulties, *insist on being referred to a physical therapy facility.* Rehabilitation can make all the difference to the quality of your life.

38

THYROID DISEASE

Gland Central

Who doesn't feel tired now and then, or at some time have trouble losing weight, become constipated, lose too much hair, feel unusually cold, or develop dry skin? Aren't we all occasionally nervous or irritable? Doesn't everyone have trouble sleeping once in a while or experience a racing heartbeat? If you mention these complaints to your friends, even to your doctor, they're likely to reassure you with such remarks as, "It's nothing to worry about. Everyone is constipated [or fat, or tired, or tense] from time to time."

I don't want you to be a hypochondriac. However, you should know that these commonplace, everyday complaints, if they persist, may in fact, reflect a treatable disorder. Over the years I have seen many patients who were either chronically tired and convinced that they were "born that way" or very "high-strung" because "that's my nature." Some of them were right, but most turned out to have either overfunction or underfunction of the thyroid—the gland that sets our "energystat." The appropriate treatment "miraculously" changed their lives. Because thyroid disease is so prevalent and its symptoms often so subtle, especially in the elderly, the American College of Physicians recommends that thyroid evaluation, done by a simple blood test, be part of the routine health examination of all men and women thirty-five years of age and older. I agree. *Insist on it.*

The thyroid gland is shaped like a butterfly and wraps around the front of the windpipe in the lower part of the neck just below the Adam's apple. It's the largest hormone-producing gland in the body and weighs about ten grams. If we provide it with enough iodine in our diet (most Americans do, because many of our foods contain iodine supplements), the thyroid makes two hormones that determine our heart rate, body temperature, the pitch of our voice, muscle strength, blood pressure, bowel function, mood, memory—even our cholesterol level, and how often we menstruate.

Some 13 million Americans, almost eight women for every man, have a thyroid problem and a least half of them are unaware of it. By the time she reaches sixty, one woman in five has an underactive thyroid gland, and so do almost 10 percent of sixty-year-old men. In yet another twist, 8 percent of women develop a thyroid problem after they give birth.

Let's take a closer look at this omnipotent gland, the symptoms caused by its malfunction, how to get to the root of the trouble, and what to do about it.

Despite its importance in determining the quality of our lives, the thyroid gland is not its own master. It secretes its hormones at the pleasure and under the control of your brain. The hypothalamus releases thyrotrophin-releasing hormone (TRH), which in turn signals another part of the brain, the pituitary gland, to discharge its own hormone—thyroid-stimulating hormone (TSH). It is this TSH circulating in the bloodstream that stimulates the thyroid gland in turn to make two of its own hormones—thyroxine (T_4) and triodothyronine (T_3).

The pituitary gland closely monitors the level of these thyroid hormones. When it detects too much in the blood, it makes less TSH. When there's too little, it produces more. The thyroid responds to these TSH signals by appropriately varying its own hormone production.

Several things can go wrong with this elaborate communication system. When it breaks down, you're left with either too much thyroid hormone or too little. In addition to the abnormal levels of thyroid hormone, this gland can also develop tumors, some of which are malignant. Let's now look at each of these three main categories of thyroid malfunction.

Hypothyroidism

Failure of the thyroid gland to make enough of its hormones is the most common form of thyroid disease. That's why more than 11 million Americans have less "oomph" and energy than they should. Most of them are women and the elderly.

Symptoms of Hypothyroidism

The symptoms of hypothyroidism and their severity depend on the amount of its hormones the gland is producing. When the shortfall is minimal, the symptoms are subtle and are apt to be attributed to stress, overwork, fatigue, anemia, or some emotional cause. When the gland is making much less than what the body needs, the full-blown picture of hypothyroidism (myxedema) emerges.

Here are some typical symptoms caused by an underactive gland. Several of them usually occur together. Severe underfunction develops over time, so recognize the telltale symptoms and intervene early.

- You're always tired, even though you get plenty of sleep. You're also a little depressed and don't really know why. Your muscles are weaker, too, despite regular workouts.

- Your bowels used to be regular, but you now tend to be constipated.
- Your skin has become dry and thick, and you sweat less than before; your hands and face are puffy, especially under the eyes; your scalp is dry; your hair is coarse and starting to frizzle, and there's more of it than usual in the basin and bathtub after shampooing.
- Your nails are brittle and they break and split easily.
- You often become moody for no reason. You don't have as much fun with your friends as you used to (or they with you).
- Your voice is of a lower timber. You used to be a tenor; now you're almost a baritone.
- Your memory is not as good as it once was (and you assume that it's because you just turned forty).
- You can't seem to lose weight. Although you've always been on the heavy side, the pounds used to go up and down. Now it's only up—and up. You're really not eating that much either (even though no one believes you).
- You used to love the cold. Now you need an extra sweater even when everyone else in the room is perfectly comfortable.
- The outer third of your eyebrows are becoming sparse.
- Your neck size has gone from 16 to 17, and your son, a first-year medical student, thinks you have an enlarged thyroid gland (goiter). (Hypothyroidism can cause a goiter because as the gland makes less hormone, the pituitary gland produces more TSH to stimulate it. This forces the gland to work harder and enlarge.)
- You'd like to have a baby but can't seem to get pregnant. You did last year and had a miscarriage. Your periods are irregular and the bleeding is heavy. Also you're less interested in sex.

- Your cholesterol has always been normal. Now, although you're just as careful about what you eat, it's been climbing—from 190 to 260 in less than a year. (Low thyroid function is the cause of high cholesterol in 9 million Americans.) That's because when the metabolism slows, the body doesn't burn fat or clear cholesterol as effectively from the bloodstream. The result is weight gain *and* high cholesterol.
- Have you had a baby recently? About 8 percent of women develop an inflammation of the thyroid gland (thyroiditis) soon after they deliver. Then three or four months later they become hypothyroid.
- Your heart rate is slower than usual, and your blood pressure is lower than it's ever been.

Most of these symptoms can be due to low thyroid function. When several of them occur together, you can bet on it.

Causes of Hypothyroidism

- In the United States, the most common cause of hypothyroidism is Hashimoto's disease, an inflammation of the thyroid gland (thyroiditis). The fault lies with the immune system, which for some reason gets its signals crossed, mistakenly identifies the thyroid as a foreign body or "invader," and produces antibodies that destroy it. (Several other important diseases, including diabetes, also result from such immune system malfunction.)
- Treatment of an overactive gland by radiation or surgery. What's left can't produce enough hormones. Or you may have received radiation for cancer of the head and neck. You may also be one of those unfortunate kids who were treated with the now discredited and abandoned practice of radiating enlarged adenoids, or the thymus gland at infancy, or acne, or ringworm of the

scalp. (That radiation left you vulnerable not only to hypothyroidism but to thyroid cancer.)

- Viral or bacterial infection can temporarily damage the thyroid gland and cause temporary hypothyroidism.
- A rare hypothyroid condition in which the gland itself is willing and able to do the job, but the pituitary doesn't make enough TSH to stimulate it to do so, can cause hypothyroidism.
- There is also an unusual rare congenital problem in which there is not enough thyroid tissue at birth or the gland is defective in some way and can't make the necessary hormones.

Diagnosing Hypothyroidism

When the deficiency of thyroid hormone is severe, the skin is pasty and dry; the face and limbs are puffy; the hair is coarse; speech is slow; the heart rate is decreased and blood pressure is low; reflexes are sluggish (when your doctor strikes your knee with the little hammer, your kick is not as brisk).

Any combination of these signs and symptoms suggests hypothyroidism, but the diagnosis must be confirmed by specific blood tests. One in particular, the TSH level, is accurate and relatively inexpensive. When the thyroid gland is making too little hormone, the pituitary gland produces more TSH to spur it on. The normal level of TSH in the blood is between 1 and 4, depending on the lab that's doing the analysis. The more severe the hypothyroidism, the *higher* the TSH level. The other day I found a level of 100 in one of my patients. (Patients have called me and said, "You told me my thyroid is low, but my TSH is high!" So remember, TSH is not the thyroid hormone—it's the whip that's trying to get the horse to run.)

Thyroid function can also be assessed by measuring the level of its hormones, T_3 and T_4, in the blood. But these results can be distorted and rendered falsely high or low by nonthyroid causes such as birth control pills or estrogen supplements. They can also be mistakenly reported as "normal" because the thyroid gland can store a two to three month's supply of hormone and keep sending this reserve out into the bloodstream even when the gland isn't currently making any.

Treatment of Hypothyroidism

The therapy of hypothyroidism boils down to one word—replacement. All it amounts to is taking a little pill every day that in the right dosage causes no side effects. There are several different brands of thyroid hormone available. The key is to stick with the one that works best for you. I happen to prefer levothyroxine, which is the T_4 thyroid. The usual maintenance dose is 100 micrograms a day, but some patients need less and others more. It costs about twenty-five cents a pill. Try to take it at the same time each day. If you miss a dose, don't double up the following day; just resume your schedule.

Levothyroxine takes several weeks to work, so don't expect results right away. It's not like aspirin for headache or insulin for high blood sugar. Also, start at a low dose and work your way up to whatever maintenance level you need. The right dosage is critical—too little won't help all your symptoms and too much can make your heart pound or leave you nervous, irritable, and unable to sleep. Check your thyroid function with a blood test from time to time and adjust the dose up or down as necessary.

Thyroid replacement therapy must almost always be continued for life because hypothyroidism is never cured and never just clears up.

Hyperthyroidism

Hyperthyroidism (an overactive thyroid gland) is less common than an underactive one and affects one in every one hundred Americans, including former president George Bush and Barbara Bush, famous Olympic athlete Gail Devers, and former Senator Bill Bradley. Almost 90 percent of them women. Hyperthyroidism, no matter what causes it, means that there is too much thyroid hormone circulating in the bloodstream. This excess results in a host of symptoms that reflect the acceleration of the body's biological motor.

Symptoms of Hyperthyroidism

Suspect that your thyroid gland is overactive if you experience any combination of the following symptoms for which there is no other explanation:

- You're restless, can't sit still (not because you're taking too much caffeine or other stimulants), and you've become an insomniac.
- You're anxious (and don't know why).
- You have mood swings (again, for no apparent reason).
- You're easily distracted and can't concentrate like you used to.
- You're more tired than usual, and your muscles are weak.
- Your skin feels warm and looks flushed as if you were blushing. It's also smooth and moist. (The body is eliminating increased heat generated by the accelerated metabolism by dilating the blood vessels in the skin.)
- Your hair is fine, silky, and thin.
- You perspire very easily (when no one else is complaining of the heat).

- You have a ravenous appetite, and you're eating more than you ever did, but you're not gaining weight.
- Your neck appears to be fuller below the Adam's apple.
- You have a rapid heartbeat and are experiencing palpitations (without even being excited).You may also have bouts of atrial fibrillation (see Chapter 6), a totally irregular heart rhythm.
- You have skipped beats (you never had any cardiac irregularity before).
- You become short of breath after even slight exertion.
- Your bowel movements are more frequent, usually soft, and you have occasional diarrhea (you normally tend to be constipated).
- Your periods have become irregular or scanty, or have stopped altogether.
- Although you're not as likely to be infertile as a woman who is hypothyroid, you are at risk for having a miscarriage when you do conceive. Should you become pregnant while you're hyperthyroid and do not miscarry, you are very vulnerable to premature labor or having a stillbirth.
- If you're menopausal, chances are you have some degree of osteoporosis.
- People think you're staring at them because your eyes are bulging. You've also noticed blurred and double vision.
- There is a fine tremor in your hands and fingers.
- Your breasts are full and a little tender (all the more surprising if you're a man).

Any combination of these symptoms suggests hyperthyroidism. If your gland is hyperactive, you may develop a *thyroid storm or crisis at any time* during which the pulse becomes very rapid, fever sets in, and you become agitated and possibly even delirious—a prime emergency.

The symptoms of hyperthyroidism are what you'd expect,

because thyroid hormones set the level of activity of every tissue, organ and cell in the body. Too much whips them into a biological frenzy.

Causes of Hyperthroidism

- Grave's disease accounts for 60 to 90 percent of all cases of hyperthyroidism, so for all practical purposes they are synonymous. Typically Grave's disease strikes females between the ages of 20 and 60, although it can affect both genders at any age. The mechanism that causes an overproduction of thyroid hormone is fascinating. For some reason, the immune system produces antibodies that attach themselves to the thyroid cells and stimulate them to make excessive amounts of thyroid hormone. Although we don't understand the cause of this aberrant behavior by the immune system, there does appear to be a genetic predisposition to Grave's disease, since it often runs in families. However, it also occurs without any familial association. People who smoke are at three times the risk of developing this disease, as are patients treated with alpha interferon—for hepatitis and other disorders. It's possible that some infection or other is the cause of Grave's, but the organism that presumably does so has never been identified. Grave's may also develop after a pregnancy, and stress has also been implicated.
- A benign tumor called a toxic adenoma that secretes extra thyroid hormone can cause the classical symptoms of hyperthyroidism. When the tumor is removed surgically, the hyperthyroidism disappears.
- A generalized swelling of the gland called a toxic multinodular goiter can produce excessive amounts of thyroid hormone. This is a more common cause of hyperthyroidism in the elderly than is Grave's disease.

- Taking too much thyroid hormone to treat an underactive gland can leave you *temporarily* hyperthyroid.
- Viruses and other infectious agents can cause inflammation of the thyroid gland and transient hyperthyroidism.
- Amiodarone, a drug that's fairly widely used for the treatment of certain cardiac rhythm disorders, can cause hyperthyroidism (or hypothyroidism) when continued for weeks or months. It clears after the medication is stopped.
- Very rarely, some abnormality of the pituitary gland causes it to make too much TSH, which then stimulates the thyroid gland to produce excessive amounts of its hormones.

Diagnosis of Hyperthyroidism

Your doctor doesn't have to be a specialist, and you don't need to be a doctor, to recognize full-blown hyperthyroidism. The bulging eyes, the tremor, the warm, smooth skin, the rapid pulse, and the irritability are diagnostic. In addition, your thyroid gland may be diffusely enlarged, even as much as five or six times its normal size. When your doctor strikes your knee with the reflex hammer, you really kick!

However, as is the case in hypothyroidism, the diagnosis should be confirmed by blood tests, the most important of which is again the TSH, whose level *falls* dramatically. The reason, of course, is that there is so much thyroid hormone being produced that the gland is sending messages to the pituitary to please "stop stimulating me." The pituitary obeys, and the TSH falls to a diagnostically low level. In fact, it may even be imperceptible.

In addition to the blood tests, your doctor will usually order a radioactive scan of the gland (unless you're pregnant) to be sure that the symptoms aren't due to a hormone-producing tumor in the gland.

Treatment of Hyperthyroidism

There are several ways to treat Grave's disease, depending on your age, gender, general health, personal preferences, and your doctor's preferences.

The most frequently used treatment is radioactive iodine (I-131). You drink it in a glass of water; it's odorless and tasteless, and knocks out thyroid tissue, making it impossible for the gland to produce any of its hormones, regardless of what's stimulating it. It is 90-95 percent successful, but it takes several weeks to work. Until it does, you will be given a beta-blocker such as propranolol (Inderal) to calm you down and, most important, to slow the heart rate. In a few months your enlarged gland shrinks to normal. Unfortunately, I-131 therapy destroys so much thyroid tissue that it eventually leaves you with too little and you become hypothyroid. Such overshoot occurs in almost every patient within ten years after the treatment was given. This complication means you'll need to take a thyroid supplement every day. If that bothers you, make believe it's a vitamin! We used to worry that radioactive treatment, especially in young persons, might lead to cancer of the thyroid later on. Long-term follow-up studies have not substantiated this fear.

If for any reason you prefer not to have the radioactive treatment, there is an acceptable alternative. Two antithyroid drugs, propylthiouracil (PTU), usually taken three times a day, and methimazole (it is long-acting and you take it only once a day), stop production of thyroid hormone. These drugs are used by 30 percent of patients. However, they can occasionally cause a dangerous blood disorder. You must have a blood count every few months just to be sure you're not one of the unlucky 1 percent to whom this happens. Low-dose PTU is the preferred therapy for pregnant women who are hyperthyroid because it doesn't expose them or their baby to radiation. After a year or two, this therapy results in a prolonged remission of the hyperthyroid state in just under half the patients. It can then be stopped. However, symptoms of hyperthyroidism can recur. I like PTU therapy because when it works it's the only one that leaves you with a normal thyroid. By contrast, the I-131 and surgery (see below) both destroy the gland.

Surgical removal of a portion of the overactive thyroid gland is a third option, but is not done nearly as often as it used to be, given the success of the I-131 and PTU therapies. Why risk an operation if you don't need one? But if you're pregnant, and can't take the antithyroid drugs for any reason, then surgery may be a good alternative.

There is great interest in diet and "natural" therapies to treat thyroid disease. A healthful diet is, of course, good for you under any circumstances, but I don't know of any specific one that affects the thyroid gland. It's important for someone with hyperthyroidism to take calcium supplements and vitamin D to rebuild the bone if osteoporosis has occurred (which it often does). Acupuncture, meditation, and other mind-body techniques will make you feel better, but they don't have any effect on the toxic thyroid gland.

Acute Thyroiditis

The thyroid gland can become acutely inflamed as a result of an injury or an infection. These cases are different from Hashimoto's thyroiditis described above in that they almost always clear up on their own without causing either permanent underfunction or overfunction of the thyroid gland. The symptoms of acute thyroiditis usually respond to aspirin and other anti-inflammatory drugs. Sometimes a short course of T_3 hormone or even a steroid hormone such as prednisone is required.

Thyroid Nodules and Tumors

Little nodules in a goiterous thyroid occur in almost 90 percent of women over the age of eighty. They are rarely malignant. However, a *single* such lump may or may not be cancerous—and it's important to determine that as soon as possible. For the record, most of them are benign, but you've got to make sure. Your past history is important. Previous radiation to your head and neck should raise a red flag. However, with or without such a history *if you have any lump in your thyroid gland, insist on an ultrasound test of your thyroid*. This indicates whether the lump is a cyst (and therefore almost certainly benign) or solid. If it's solid and greater than one centimeter, *insist that it be biopsied*. A fine needle is introduced into the lump and thyroid tissue is sucked up, then looked at under the microscope. If it is malignant, the lump should be surgically removed. We used to take out the whole thyroid and all the lymph nodes in the neck in such cases, but that is no longer routinely done. The long-term outlook is usually very favorable.

Have regular follow-up examinations of your thyroid looking for evidence of recurrence and take thyroid hormone to prevent it. Such monitoring should consist of lung X rays and scans for evidence of tumor spread because thyroid cancers, when they do metastasize, go to the lungs.

WHAT TO INSIST ON IF YOU HAVE THYROID DISEASE

The thyroid is the largest hormone-producing gland in the body. It makes two hormones that control the metabolism of every organ, tissue, and cell in the body.

Underproduction of these hormones causes a generalized slowing of bodily functions; excess results in a "hyper" state. Both need treatment. If you're puzzled by your constant fatigue or are "hopping" and irritable for no apparent reason, *insist first on the simple blood test that diagnoses malfunction of the thyroid gland.* It may save you the time and trouble of more extensive investigation.

There is a feedback mechanism between the brain and the thyroid so that when more thyroid hormone is needed, the brain increases production of a hormone (TSH) that stimulates hormone secretion by the thyroid gland. TSH levels can be measured in the blood and are an accurate measure of thyroid function. In the presence of hypothyroidism, the TSH level is high, since the brain is trying to whip the thyroid into making more of the needed hormone. A very low TSH reading indicates that there is too much thyroid hormone—hyperthyroidism. *If only one thyroid blood test is offered or available to you, TSH is the one to insist on.*

Disorders of the thyroid gland occur more often in women than in men, and they increase in frequency with age. The most common cause of hypothyroidism is an autoimmune disorder (Hashimoto's disease) in which the body mistakenly turns on itself and destroys the thyroid. In such cases the TSH level in the blood is high. Treatment consists of thyroid hormone replacement. Although there are several types available, I usually recommend synthetic levothyroxine. This therapy is effective and inexpensive. Whatever type of supplement you're taking, stay with it and *insist that your doctor regularly monitor your response to it.* The dosage may have to be adjusted from time to time. Too much thyroid supplement can result in symptoms of hyperthyroidism.

The most common cause of hyperthyroidism is Grave's disease, also due to malfunction of the immune system. It makes antibodies that mimic the action of TSH and stimulate the thyroid to produce toxic amounts of its hormones. There are three major treatments for hyperthyroidism: radioactive iodine (the most widely used), which eventually destroys the thyroid; antithyroid drugs, taken for a year or two, which cause remission in about half the cases and leave the thyroid gland intact; and surgical removal of the gland. Surgery is a last resort. Along with radioactive iodine therapy, it can cause permanent underfunction of the thyroid gland, so that you need to take supplements.

Nodules of the thyroid can be benign or malignant. Isolated thyroid lumps greater than one centimeter in size should be biopsied. *Insist on it*. Malignant tumors must be surgically removed.

39

URINARY INCONTINENCE

Voiding When Prohibited

Your baby is finally toilet-trained. No more diapers, right? Wrong. Between 11 and 17 million adults, most of whom are female, also need diapers because they cannot control their urine. Doctors call it urinary incontinence. The problem is more common in older people (half of all nursing home residents are incontinent). People who suffer from it spend an average of $4,000 a year treating its complications. That adds up to a total national expenditure of some $30 billion a year, most of which goes for the diapers; the rest is to buy deodorants, disinfectants, products to treat rashes resulting from the chronic contact of urine with skin, antibiotics for treating urinary tract and other infections, and the cost of managing pressure sores that are handmaidens of incontinence. Add to the financial burden the sleep disturbances, impaired sexual activity, depression, and the social impact of incontinence, and you can appreciate why incontinence is a major problem.

Why We Become Incontinent

Here's how one becomes incontinent: The kidneys remove waste from the blood and then excrete it in urine through two tubes (ureters) that empty into the urinary bladder. This bladder is a muscular sac that expands to receive the urine and contracts to eliminate it. Urine flows from the bladder into a single tube, the urethra, through which it is excreted from the body. A muscle (sphincter) wraps around the portion of the urethra that connects with the bladder neck and prevents the urine from leaking out of the bladder. Both the bladder and the sphincter are supplied by nerves that are under your control. When the bladder is filled (it can normally hold up to sixteen ounces of urine), the brain sends signals to it via those nerves either to contract or to relax the sphincter muscle depending on your wishes. When you're ready to pee, and not a moment sooner, urine flows into the urethra.

You become incontinent when you develop some problem with the muscles of the bladder and/or sphincter or their nerves that causes you to lose control over them.

Incontinence is either acute or chronic. *Acute incontinence* comes on suddenly and is usually due to infection of the bladder, prostate, urethra, or vagina, or occurs when you're severely constipated (stool presses on the bladder and compresses the urethra). Treating the infection or having a bowel movement cures this type of incontinence. You may also become temporarily incontinent if you take a diuretic (water pill), certain tranquilizers, or antihistamines, or drink too many fluids or perform high-impact exercises while your bladder is full, or eat spicy foods and drink too much coffee.

Chronic or persistent incontinence is a more common and important problem. It develops over time, stays with you and is usually due to weakness of the bladder or the muscles in the pelvis that support it; or to neurological problems such as a stroke, multiple sclerosis, Parkinson's disease, diabetes, and others; pelvic surgery; radiation therapy; hormonal deficiency. Here are the most important types of chronic incontinence:

- *Stress incontinence,* the most prevalent type, has nothing to do with emotional stress. It's more common in women (especially after menopause) whose pelvic muscles have been stretched by multiple births, or who've gained a lot of weight, or who have had pelvic surgery. The stretched muscles can no longer support the bladder and allow it to drop. When you cough, sneeze, lift something heavy, dance, jump, laugh, or strain when having a bowel movement, you lose control of your urine because of the sudden increase of abdominal pressure.

- *Urge incontinence* accounts for two-thirds of cases in the elderly. You have a sudden, overwhelming need to urinate and you can't make it to the bathroom in time. This urgency can sometimes be precipitated by the sound of running water or after you drink some liquid. It often occurs in various neurological disorders such as Parkinson's disease, multiple sclerosis, and strokes, and can also be caused by enlargement of the prostate, alcohol, diabetes, and after menopause.

- *Mixed incontinence* is a combination of the stress and urge types, and affects women more than men.

- *Overflow incontinence* is common in men whose enlarged prostate presses on the urethra and prevents the urine from flowing out freely. Urine accumulates in the bladder, which then overflows when it can no longer accommodate all that keeps coming in from the kidneys. The excess just dribbles out—against your will. Prostate surgery usually cures this type of incontinence. Spinal cord injury and neurological disorders such as multiple sclerosis can also result in overflow incontinence.

- *Reflex incontinence* develops when the nerves that control urination are damaged or diseased. Such individuals may not be aware that they're leaking urine.
- *Prostate surgery* leaves some men incontinent. This is usually a temporary complication that occurs more often after an operation for cancer of the prostate than for the relief of benign enlargement.
- *Functional incontinence* is what happens when an otherwise normal individual needs to urinate but just can't make it to the bathroom in time because of severe arthritis or paralysis, or being stuck in a car going sixty miles an hour on the freeway with no rest stop in sight! Unfortunately, we're not camels!

Many who suffer from incontinence are too ashamed to tell anyone about it, including their doctor—and most doctors don't ask. That's a pity because once the cause of incontinence is determined, it can often be helped or even cured—by behavioral therapy, medication, exercises, mechanical devices, and as a last resort, surgery.

A good urologist, gynecologist, or urogynecologist can determine why you're incontinent by means of a thorough physical exam, a detailed history, and a few specific tests. You can help by keeping a log of your voiding pattern during a seventy-two hour period. For example, you may be asked to drink several glasses of water and then empty your bladder. A small catheter is then inserted into your bladder, and the amount of urine remaining in the bladder after you think you've emptied it is measured. This volume of "residual" urine can also be estimated fairly accurately with a sonogram that, in addition, also reveals any abnormalities of the kidneys, bladder, and prostate. If the residual amount of urine is abnormally high, your doctor may perform cystoscopy, in which a thin telescope-like tube is inserted into your bladder to look for evidence of disease in that organ. A urodynamics test may also be necessary: The doctor fills the bladder with fluid and then evaluates how well you void, and whether or not you leak, especially when you cough and strain.

The management of incontinence depends on its cause. Here are some of the more common and important treatments available:

- *Behavior training and exercises.* This is the first route to go. You are taught how to contract and relax the muscles in the pelvis that surround the bladder and sphincter. Your gynecologist, urologist, nurse practitioner, or physiotherapist can teach you how to do these Kegel exercises. A biofeedback monitor can be used to indicate whether you're contracting the right muscles and how effectively you're doing so.
- *Medication.* Some menopausal women may become incontinent because their urogenital tissues have been weakened by estrogen deficiency. Replacing the missing hormone often improves symptoms. There are also several drugs that help control abnormal bladder contractions. These include oxybutynin (marketed as Ditropan; look for the new long-acting Ditropan XL), propantheline (ProBanthine), flavoxate (Urispas), and dicyclomine (Benyl). Detrol, the latest addition to the list, is said to cause less constipation, eye problems, and dry mouth than the others. Your doctor should supervise use of these drugs.
- *Surgery.* This should be your last resort. Don't have any operation unless there's no other way. Since most stress incontinence is caused by the bladder dropping down, the surgeon makes an incision in the vagina or abdomen and restores the bladder to its normal position. Inserting a wide sling can also provide support for the bladder.
- *Electrical simulators* can be implanted in the spine. Electrodes placed in the vagina or rectum stimulate weakened pelvic muscles and make them contract. They generate tiny electric impulses that reduce involuntary

bladder contractions. Electrical stimulation can have the same result as exercise.

- Bulking materials such as collagen can be injected into the tissues around the urethra to tighten the sphincter. They usually take about a month to work, and their benefit is often short-lived. I don't advise this therapy for my patients.

There are several other ingenious surgical procedures that specialists can perform, but make sure that you have exhausted your other options before having *any* operation. If you want more details, ask the American Urological Association for its official surgical guidelines.

When incontinence can't be successfully treated or cured, there is usually some device that can alleviate it. For example, you may need:

- *Catheterization* of your bladder on a regular basis. A tube (catheter) is inserted every few hours into the bladder through the urethra. Many patients learn to do this themselves but be scrupulously careful to avoid chronic infection. When the bladder muscles can't contract, the catheter may be left in permanently. This usually happens after spinal cord or other surgery, or when bladder muscle tone is very bad. A special device is available for men who might otherwise need an indwelling catheter. It's an external-collecting device that fits over the penis like a condom and empties through a tube into a drainage bag strapped to the leg. This avoids the need to leave the catheter in the urethra, and so reduces the risk of infection.
- A *urethral plug,* a cylinder with a balloon at its tip, can be inserted into a woman's urethra and filled with air to prevent it from leaking. When it's time to void, the woman pulls a string that in turn deflates the balloon and the plug is removed.

- A *pessary* is a plastic device that is inserted into the vagina to support a dropped bladder. The problems with pessaries is that you have to keep wearing them and they are a potential source of vaginal and urinary tract infections. They are not predictably effective against incontinence.
- *Absorbent pads* and underwear help keep you dry if none of the other measures do the job.

If you suffer from incontinence, regardless of whatever else you do, here are some additional tips that can improve the quality of your life:

- Consume as little caffeine as possible—in any form. It's diuretic properties are something you certainly don't need.
- Since you want to keep your bladder as close to empty as possible, void even when the urge to do so is not overwhelming. And take your time. Stay on or at the john as long as it takes to empty the bladder.
- If you can predict the time intervals when you lose control of your urine, say, every three or four hours, empty your bladder beforehand. Buy a wrist alarm to remind you.
- Wear clothes and trousers that are easy to open or remove quickly, so that you don't lose time fumbling when you need to void.
- Reduce your intake of alcohol, fruit juices, carbonated beverages, spicy foods, dairy products, sugar, and artificial sweeteners, all of which can irritate the bladder and worsen your symptoms.
- Don't wear tight girdles, corsets, pants, or high heels, all of which can weaken pelvic muscles that control urination.
- Don't smoke. Women who do are twice as likely to become incontinent.
- Cross your legs before you sneeze or cough. Chances are you'll leak less.

WHAT TO INSIST ON IF YOU HAVE URINARY INCONTINENCE

Urinary incontinence can be acute and temporary, usually as a result of some infection in the pelvis. The incidence of chronic incontinence increases with age. It can often be successfully managed. *Insist on access to a urologist or gynecologist who can provide* behavioral training, teach you how to do special pelvic exercises, refer you for biofeedback or electrical simulation, and prescribe medications. Surgery can also help the problem, but it should be a last resort.

CHECKUP OR CHECKOUT

The foregoing chapters deal with the diagnosis and treatment of disease. But an ounce of prevention is worth a pound of cure. You need your doctor to diagnose and treat your illness—but only *you* can prevent it.

The new car I bought the other day came with a 50,000-mile or four-year warranty *provided* that I bring it in for regularly scheduled maintenance exams. After spending all that money, I have no intention of missing a single one of those checkups. Repairs are expensive and I don't want to be stuck in a stalled car somewhere in the middle of no-man's-land. Most people who are very good about their automobile service appointments can't be bothered to have a regular medical exam. That's ironic because the human body is far more complex and vulnerable than any machine—and the consequences of its malfunction potentially much more threatening and expensive. Implicit in the warranty on our bodies—good for much longer than four years—is the same requirement for "service" at regular intervals.

Almost twenty-five years ago I wrote my first book. *The Complete Medical Exam,* in which I explained how important it is to have a regular checkup and what it should consist of.

No one seriously disagreed with the need for a routine physical back in the 1970s, when most of us paid our own medical bills (they were affordable then). Nowadays, however, its cost effectiveness is being questioned by Medicare (for those over sixty-five), and private insurance carriers, and managed care companies, who usually pick up the tab for these workups. Remember that all these third party payers are either on a budget or in business to make money. Most of them will only allow you to see your doctor when you're sick; they will not reimburse you for the cost of a checkup. Of course, that's shortsighted because it costs much less to save a life *now* than it is to treat a chronic illness years later.

There are three main reasons why you should have a checkup even if you're feeling perfectly well.

- *To detect silent disease.* Every year, in the course of routine examinations, millions of "healthy" Americans are found to have previously unsuspected diseases. Among the more important ones are diabetes, vascular problems in the heart (masquerading as "indigestion"), brain, and other organs, cancer (more and more cases are found early enough to be controlled or cured), tuberculosis (by no means wiped out), AIDS, hepatitis, and high blood pressure (the silent killer whose early therapy prolongs and saves life).
- *To establish and maintain an ongoing doctor-patient relationship* so that you can be advised and reminded over the years how to maintain a healthy lifestyle. Even if your checkup does not reveal any disease, it allows your doctor to define your normal health baseline. No two of us are exactly alike in any respect, and no given individual, as he or she grows older, stays the same. Appearance, weight, stamina, energy levels, the electrocardiogram, and the results of various blood tests all change over the years. The objective progression from "health" to early "disease" can be very subtle. For ex-

ample, certain variations in your electrocardiogram may be of no significance if they've been there right along. But their appearance since the last workup may indicate a beginning cardiac problem. Or suppose that your blood pressure has always run around 110/76 and now is suddenly 148/86—still normal but higher—a warning that you must be carefully monitored in the future. And so it is with your weight, heart size, cholesterol level, and many other examination results. Recording these values over the years establishes a *trend* in your health status—permitting intervention before it's too late.

- To gain *reassurance*—the peace of mind that cannot be measured in dollars or cost-effectiveness. If you're anxious about your health because several members of your family died of breast cancer, premature heart disease, Alzheimer's, or stroke, it's comforting to be told every now and then that you're in good health.

Where Should You Get Your Checkup?

Be careful about having a general checkup by a specialist who may focus on one specific area and gloss over the rest of you. You're better off seeing your family doctor or general internist.

Ask what your checkup will consist of and how much it will cost. Most physicians have the training and access to the equipment needed to perform the majority of the tests themselves. If not, they can arrange for the rest to be done by colleagues, or at a nearby clinic. Find out how long it will take. If you're told that you'll be through in less than half an hour, that's not enough. It should take between 45 minutes and an hour, exclusive of any special X rays or ECG stress testing. If your doctor has a busy general practice devoted to treating the sick, sees fifty or sixty patients a day and spends only five or ten minutes with each, he probably does not have the time to give you a thorough checkup. A cursory "nonexamiantion" masquerading as the real thing is worse than no examination at all, because it gives you a false sense of security.

When Should You Have Checkups and at What Intervals?

The National institutes of Health and the Mayo Clinic both suggest two routine checkups between ages eighteen and thirty, three between forty and fifty, five from fifty to sixty and an annual exam after age sixty. Here are my own recommendations:

Childhood

Parents routinely take their children to the pediatrician primarily to be immunized, measured, and weighed, for advice on diet, and to have the doctor fill out school or summer camp forms. These visits are sometimes brief, usually squirming and noisy. In such a setting, subtle disease may not be detected. So I recommend a thorough physical exam during adolescence—looking for malignancies (especially if other children in the family have suffered from cancer); chronic low-grade infections (many youngsters have worms, anemia, and lingering diseases of which the parents may not be aware); heart murmurs (which may have been missed at birth); high blood pressure (5 percent of "normal" children have hypertension); hernias; visual and hearing defects, and other unrecognized handicapping conditions, many of which are corrective. A great number of youngsters who do poorly in school because they are thought to be emotionally disturbed are in reality physically sick or disabled.

Some youngesters should be more frequently examined for specific vulnerabilities. For example, if a parent, grandparent, brother, sister, or even an aunt or uncle has diabetes, analyses of blood and urine for sugar should be done at regular intervals.

Fatal collapse in children and especially in athletes is all too common and may be due to an abnormality in the cardiac electrical system or to certain deformities in the structure of the heart present since birth. Most of these life-threatening conditions can be treated—with medication, pacemakers, or surgery.

Adult Life

If you were a healthy child and adolescent, and have a good family history, a routine examination should ideally be performed every five years between the ages of twenty-one and thirty-five. However, women in this age group should see a gynecologist every year to be tested for cancer of the breast and cervix.

Between the ages of thirty-five and forty-two, I suggest an exam every three years to detect the presence of heart disease, hypertension, and cancer. In nondiabetic women with normal blood pressure, such examinations need not include a special search for arteriosclerosis because that generally becomes apparent in females *after* menopause. All these checkups should include a battery of diagnostic blood tests for cholesterol, sugar, kidney and liver function, and several others that are part of the "package." I also routinely include a blood test for thyroid function, especially in anyone who is chronically tired.

For patients between the ages of forty-two and fifty, I advise a routine physical exam every two years. In men this should always include a rectal exam, and after they reach fifty, a PSA, looking for the evidence of prostate cancer.

Smokers and those with the risk factors for vascular disease should have cardiac stress testts.

Between fifty and sixty years of age, the checkup for both men and women should be done annually. After sixty, a shorter, more targeted evaluation should be performed six months after the yearly one. Its purpose is to detect those diseases that begin to take their toll in this age group—high blood pressure, arteriosclerosis, cancer, emphysema, and chronic bronchitis, arthritis, and behavioral changes, especially depression.

Woven through this schedule are tests such as the colonoscopy (which you should have at age fifty and every five years thereafter, but more frequently if you have gastrointestinal symptoms, a persistent change in bowel habits or blood in the stool, polyps previously removed, and a family history of colon cancer), mammography, bone density tests, PSA levels, and the more frequent monitoring of any abnormalities that may have been previously detected.

Remember this: Be sure to tell your doctor about your vulnerability to any disease, real or feared; and your family history. Describe any symptoms you've had for so long you assumed they were "normal." You can't imagine how many lives have been changed by a diagnosis of lactose deficiency, hypothyroidism, and the lack of various other hormones.

If you can possibly do so, get a health policy that pays for your checkup. Some companies do, and it's worth your finding one. Finally, if you're not insured, or belong to a plan that doesn't reimburse you for routine checkups, tell your doctor about it. There are always ways to get what you need at a price you can afford.

Epilogue

Having read this book, you now know that there is a wide array of diagnostic and therapeutic options when you're sick, some of which are clearly more effective than others. The average patient normally has no way of knowing which procedure or medication is best for him or her in any particular circumstance. In the past, such knowledge didn't matter very much because you could always count on your doctor to prescribe what he or she believed to be in your best interest. That's no longer always true, given the state of today's health-care system.

Whether or not we care to admit it, health care is now rationed for most Americans. Decisions that affect diagnosis and treatment are being made—or at least influenced—by people other than your own physician. They "suggest" to your doctor, who may well be in their employ, how he or she should "best" treat you. Those recommendations more often than not are based on economics, not medical science. Failure of your doctor to comply with these recommendations may result in termination of employment.

I wrote *Power to the Patient* to help you understand all the options that should be made available to you when you're sick. That knowledge can help you regain the sense of security about your medical care that you once had; it should make it possible for you to discuss with your caregiver how to receive that to which you are entitled—the best care. If you know from these pages that this is not the case, there are appeal mechanisms available to you—independent panels with the authority to reverse unfair, arbitrary, and unhealthy (for you) decisions. Don't hesitate to take advantage of them when you are dissatisfied with what your insurance carrier will "allow." Request your doctor to initiate an appeal process for you as soon as possible.

You can never know too much about your own body. I believe this book presents a fair, balanced, comprehensive, and current view of all your options when you're sick—not only *what to insist on,* but also *why* to do so. Read these options carefully and use them wisely. More power to you!

Index